Local Anesthesia
of the Oral Cavity

Local Anesthesia
of the Oral Cavity

J. Theodore Jastak, DDS, PhD

Professor and Chairman
Division of Oral and Maxillofacial Surgery
Faculty of Dentistry
University of British Columbia
Vancouver, British Columbia

John A. Yagiela, DDS, PhD

Professor of Oral Biology and Coordinator of Anesthesia and Pain Control,
 School of Dentistry
Professor of Anesthesiology, School of Medicine
University of California, Los Angeles
Los Angeles, California

David Donaldson, BDS, FDS, RCS, MDS

Professor and Head
Department of Oral Medical and Surgical Sciences
Faculty of Dentistry
University of British Columbia
Vancouver, British Columbia

Chapter 14—Electronic Dental Analgesia contributed by

Frederick C. Quarnstrom, DDS

Clinical Assistant Professor
Department of Dental Public Health Sciences
School of Dentistry
University of Washington
Seattle, Washington

Christine L. Quinn, DDS, MS

Adjunct Assistant Professor of Oral Biology
School of Dentistry
University of California, Los Angeles
Los Angeles, California

W.B. SAUNDERS COMPANY
A Division of Harcourt Brace & Company
Philadelphia London Toronto
Montreal Sydney Tokyo

W.B. SAUNDERS COMPANY

A Division of Harcourt Brace & Company

The Curtis Center
Independence Square West
Philadelphia, PA 19106

Library of Congress Cataloging-in-Publication Data
Jastak, J. Theodore.
Local anesthesia of the oral cavity / J. Theodore Jastak, John
A. Yagiela, David Donaldson.
p. cm.
ISBN 0-7216-2357-3
1. Anesthesia in dentistry. 2. Local anesthesia.   I. Yagiela,
John A.   II. Donaldson, David, MD.   III. Title.
[DNLM: 1. Anesthesia, Dental. 2. Anesthesia, Conduction.   WO 460
J39r 1995]
RK510.J3 1995
617.9′676—dc20
DNLM/DLC   94–8370

LOCAL ANESTHESIA OF THE ORAL CAVITY   ISBN   0–7216–2357–3

Printed in United States of America

Last digit is the print number: 9   8   7   6   5   4   3   2   1

Preface

This text is designed primarily as a basic instructional manual for oral regional anesthesia. As such, it is principally directed at students and practitioners of dentistry and dental hygiene who use oral local anesthesia on a regular basis throughout their careers. This book may also be helpful to physicians, particularly those who specialize in emergency medicine or those who are called upon to treat dental disorders in locations without routine access to dental practitioners. An attempt has been made to be reasonably thorough, although the extent of detailed coverage of subjects varies from chapter to chapter. Extensive discussion has been given to the relevant neurophysiology, basic pharmacology, local anesthetic preparations, injection techniques, and complications. Discussion in other chapters has been limited to specific issues important in providing safe and effective local anesthesia.

This text is based on a prior book co-authored many years ago by two of us (JTJ and JAY). However, it has been extensively rewritten and considerably expanded, with added chapters on choice of anesthetic technique and causes of anesthetic failure, and electronic dental analgesia. Also, advances in understanding of the pharmacology of local anesthesia necessitated an expansion of the relevant material from one to three chapters. The discussion of various local anesthetic techniques has been organized into four separate chapters consisting of basic principles, maxillary anesthesia, mandibular anesthesia, and supplemental injection techniques. In this process, most of the artwork and photography have been redone and improved.

During the preparation of this text, we received considerable help, advice, and critical commentary from many interested persons. However, we would especially like to thank Dr. David Godin for his comments on the pharmacology of local anesthetics and Dr. Alan Hannam for his advice on trigeminal anatomy.

v

We received much help and laborious work on the manuscript from Karen Guthreau, Laurie Holst, and Leslie Soon, as well as expert photographic assistance from Bruce McCaughey and artwork from Irene Petravicius. Finally, we wish to thank the staffs of the W.B. Saunders Company and P.M. Gordon Associates, Inc., for their patience and support during the preparation of this text.

J. Theodore Jastak
John A. Yagiela
David Donaldson

Contents

Anatomy and Physiology of the Peripheral Nervous System

L ocal anesthetics provide pain control by preventing noxious stimuli from reaching the brain. The mechanism of action, pharmacologic profile, and even the clinical application of these agents can be understood only in the context of the anatomic and physiologic characteristics of the peripheral nervous system.

Neuroanatomy

The peripheral nervous system is the primary conduit through which sensory information concerning the internal state and external environment of the body is relayed to the spinal cord and brain. It is also the primary medium for efferent transmissions from the central nervous system (CNS) to the various effector organs and tissues of the body (i.e., muscles and glands). The fundamental unit of the peripheral nervous system is the neuron.

THE NEURON

Figure 1–1 depicts a typical sensory neuron capable of conveying pain sensations from the oral mucosa to the CNS. The neuron is composed of three major parts.[1,2] The most distal segment, the dendritic zone, is an arborization of nerve endings that are responsive to various factors associated with real or potential tissue damage. Detection of an appropriate stimulus (such as bradykinin, a "pain mediator" produced during cellular injury) activates dendritic branches to depolarize and initiate nerve conduction. Information is then relayed from the periphery to the CNS by a thin, cable-like structure called the axon. Terminal branches of the axon distribute incoming signals to the various CNS nuclei responsible for

1

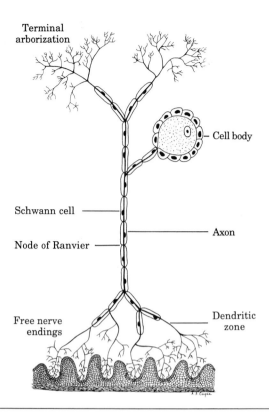

Figure 1–1.   Diagram of a sensory neuron innervating the oral mucosa. In this illustration, the relative length of the axon is foreshortened by a factor of 1,000.

their processing. The third part of the neuron is the cell body, or soma. In neurons subserving general senses, the cell body is not directly involved in nerve transmission, being located well off the conducting pathway of the axon. The soma is responsible, however, for metabolic support of the nerve cell. Cell bodies of sensory neurons supplying the oral tissues are located in the trigeminal ganglion.

Afferent neurons affiliated with proprioception and with exteroceptive sensations other than pain are structurally similar to the "pseudounipolar" neuron described above. The only major differences are in the specialized receptors at the dendritic ends of the nerve cells and in the terminal circuitry within the CNS. Motor neurons, however, are fundamentally dissimilar. In addition to supporting transmission in the opposite (or efferent) direction, motor neurons are arranged so that the cell body separates the dendrites from the axon. The soma of the motor neuron is thus directly involved in nerve transmission.

THE NERVE FIBER

The long, slender axons of peripheral nerves are supported by a variety of connective tissues. Without question, the connective tissue element most intimately associated with individual axons is the Schwann cell (or neurolemma). The union of axon and Schwann cell is so complete that the term "nerve fiber" is often used to denote this functional organization,[3] a practice that will be followed here.

Figure 1–2 illustrates the longitudinal and cross-sectional morphology of a Schwann cell investing a number of small axons. An important feature of this arrangement is that the Schwann cell limits exposure of its associated axons to interstitial fluid. In these small nerve fibers, communication between the invaginated axons and the extracellular compartment is largely reduced to a narrow (10 to 15 nm) cleft separating the enclosing plasma membranes. In isolated areas where a portion of the axon is not covered by Schwann cell processes, there remains a layer of basal lamina separating the axonal membrane from the surrounding environment.

Larger axons are even more thoroughly enveloped (Fig. 1–3). By spirally wrapping its plasma membrane around the single embedded axon, the Schwann cell produces a multilayered covering referred to as myelin.

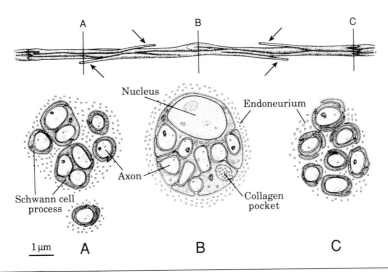

Figure 1–2. Schwann cell investing several small axons (unmyelinated). *Top,* longitudinal view (relative length is foreshortened by a factor of 3). Cytoplasmic processes (arrows) make connection with adjacent Schwann cells (not shown), providing for interchange of axons among anastomosing nerve fibers. Vertical lines indicate the locations of the cross-sectional views depicted below. *Bottom,* cross-sectional view of the Schwann cell and associated axons. **A.** Along much of its length, the Schwann cell is divided into several cytoplasmic processes, each containing one or more axons embedded within. In the bottom case, where the axon leaves to join an adjacent collection of nerve fibers, cytoplasmic tongues of the abutting Schwann cells overlap. Dashed lines surrounding the nerve fibers represent the basal lamina. **B.** At the level of the Schwann cell nucleus, all of the small axons associated with the Schwann cell are enveloped within cytoplasmic troughs. Also entrapped is a "collagen pocket" consisting of invaginated endoneurial fibers. **C.** At the Schwann cell periphery, couplings with other Schwann cells create a complex pattern of axonal investments.

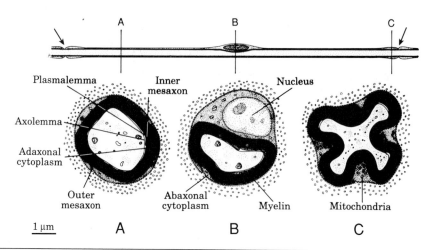

Figure 1–3. Small myelinated nerve fiber. *Top*, longitudinal view (relative length is foreshortened by a factor of 3). The Schwann cell invests a single axon. Arrows highlight the nodes of Ranvier, marking the junctions with adjoining Schwann cells. Vertical lines indicate the locations of the cross-sectional views depicted below. *Bottom*, cross-sectional views. **A.** Internodal region. The periaxonal space, a gap of 15 to 20 nm between the axonal membrane (axolemma) and the plasma membrane of the Schwann cell (plasma-lemma), is separated from the external environment by a tight junction running the length of the inner mesaxon. A small amount of adaxonal Schwann cell cytoplasm exists between the innermost layer of the myelin sheath and the plasmalemma surrounding the axon. Composed of multiple layers of compacted plasmalemma, the myelin sheath serves as a powerful insulator for the axon. (Not shown are the incisures of Schmidt-Lanterman, channels through the myelin that connect the adaxonal cytoplasm with the abaxonal cytoplasm exterior to the myelin sheath.) Dashed line represents the basal lamina. **B.** Internodal region at the level of the Schwann cell nucleus. The myelinated axon is flattened by the presence of the Schwann cell nucleus and its surrounding cytoplasm. **C.** Paranodal region. The myelin sheath is crenated, possibly to accommodate volume changes associated with high rates of neuronal activity. The abaxonal cytoplasm of the Schwann cell contains large numbers of mitochondria.

The myelin sheath almost completely insulates the axon from the outside. Only at the nodes of Ranvier, where the Schwann cells abut one another and the sheath is interrupted, does the myelinated axon have any direct contact with the extracellular space. However, as is illustrated in Figure 1–4, electron micrographs reveal that even at the nodes (which are only 1 to 1.5 μm in length) Schwann cells remain in intimate contact with the axon.[3,4]

Schwann cells play a vital role in support of the peripheral nervous system. When a nerve is damaged and its axons degenerate, complete recovery of innervation can occur, but only if the surrounding Schwann cells remain viable.[5] At the functional level, it is believed that Schwann cells may modulate nerve conduction by altering the external environment of associated axons, by providing direct metabolic support in the form of adenosine triphosphate (ATP) and protein synthesis, and/or by releasing "trophic factors" required for optimal neuronal function.[4,6,7]

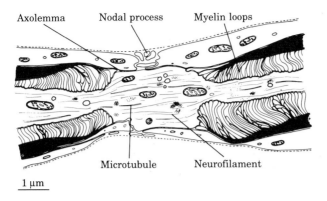

Axolemma   Nodal process   Myelin loops

Microtubule   Neurofilament

1 μm

Figure 1–4.   Longitudinal section through a node of Ranvier. Close apposition of the terminal loops of the myelin lamellae with the axolemma restricts access between the extracellular nodal space and the periaxonal space. Schwann cell processes within the nodal space form a collar that interdigitates with nodal processes from the adjacent Schwann cell and sends fingerlike projections to within approximately 5 nm of the axolemma. The remainder of the nodal space is filled with a mucopolysaccharide "gap substance." Microtubules and neurofilaments running longitudinally along the axon provide a support framework and transport mechanism for the axon. Dashed lines represent the basal lamina.

The influence of myelination on nerve conduction is described in the section on neurophysiology.

CLASSIFICATION OF NERVE FIBERS

The various fibers of peripheral nerves, including those innervating the orofacial region, may be classified into several distinct categories on the basis of electrophysiologic and morphologic differences (Table 1–1).[8] Type A fibers are the largest fibers present in mammalian nerves. With the rate of impulse transmission directly proportional to fiber diameter, this group also comprises the most rapidly conducting axons. Type A fibers are further divided into four groups, α through δ. Although differences in study methods, animal species, and peripheral nerves used by various investigators have led to a confusing array of classification approaches (including a Roman numeral scheme for sensory neurons that separates Aα fibers into two subgroups and lumps the Aβ and Aγ sizes into a single category), the hybrid classification shown in Table 1–1 has functional validity in that the various subdivisions provide dissimilar motor and sensory innervations.

Type B fibers are preganglionic autonomic neurons. Although easily characterized as a group by their relative homogeneity and restricted pattern of distribution, B fibers are almost indistinguishable from Aδ fibers, differing only in certain electrophysiologic properties (not covered in Table 1–1).

Table 1–1.   **CLASSIFICATION OF PERIPHERAL NERVE FIBERS**

Fiber Type*	Fiber Diameter (μm)	Conduction Velocity (m/sec)	Function (Structures)
Aα			
motor	12–20	65–120	Muscle contraction (fast twitch fibers)
Ia sensory	13–22	70–130	Proprioception (muscle spindles)
Ib sensory	12–20	65–120	Proprioception (Golgi tendon organs)
Aβ			
motor	7–14	40–80	Muscle contraction (slow twitch fibers)
II sensory†	5–15	20–80	Proprioception (muscle spindles, joints), discriminatory touch and pressure, vibration
Aγ			
motor	2–10	10–50	Muscle contraction (intrafusal fibers)
II sensory†	5–15	20–80	Proprioception (muscle spindles, joints), discriminatory touch and pressure, vibration
Aδ			
III sensory	1–7	5–40	Fast pain, temperature, crude touch and pressure
B			
preganglionic autonomic	1–5	4–25	Motor control (cardiac, smooth muscle), regulation of secretion (glands)
C			
postganglionic autonomic	0.2–2	0.2–2	Motor control (cardiac, smooth muscle), regulation of secretion (glands)
IV sensory	0.2–2	0.2–2	Slow pain, itch, temperature, crude touch and pressure, visceral sensations

* *Fibers are classified in general according to size and conduction velocity. A separate classification scheme, used exclusively for sensory neurons, is indicated by Roman numerals.*

† *In the sensory classification scheme, group II comprises both Aβ and Aγ fiber sizes and does not distinguish between them.*

The most numerous fibers in the peripheral nervous system are of type C. Unlike types A and B, C fibers are unmyelinated. Type C fibers transmit (at an admittedly leisurely pace) a wealth of sensory information to the CNS. Additional C fibers, the postganglionic autonomic axons, carry effector signals to the smooth muscle and glandular tissues of target organs.

Noxious stimuli are transmitted to the CNS by way of Aδ and C fibers. The lightly myelinated Aδ fibers are responsible for the conduction of sharp, bright pain, whereas the unmyelinated C fibers conduct dull or burning pain. It should be emphasized, however, that these types of fibers also serve other sensations besides pain. Moreover, signals transmitted along larger sensory neurons (Aβ–γ, or type II) serve to modulate nociceptive information within the CNS.[9]

The oral cavity is richly innervated by nociceptive nerve fibers. For example, the human mandibular first premolar contains approximately 500 Aδ and 1800 C fibers.[10] Although pain is usually associated with activation of these neurons, a tingling sensation sometimes referred to as "prepain" may accompany low intensity stimulation.[11]

CONNECTIVE TISSUE INVESTMENTS

Individual axons, with their respective Schwann cell coverings, are organized into a single nerve trunk by three connective tissue investments. The innermost of these, the endoneurium, contains the basal lamina that surrounds each nerve fiber and a loose collection of fine collagen fibrils running parallel with the individual nerve fibers (see Fig. 1–2). Fibroblasts, fixed tissue macrophages, and capillaries are dispersed throughout the endoneurium.

Nerve fibers and interstitial endoneurium are grouped into discrete bundles, or fascicles, by the perineurium (Fig. 1–5). A concentrically laminated sheath (which in large fascicles may contain as many as 15 lamella), the perineurium is composed of sheets of flattened, polygonal cells united by tight junctions and surrounded by basal lamina. Collections of collagen fibrils run concentrically, obliquely, and longitudinally within and around the perineurium, and septa given off by the perineurium may subdivide larger fascicles into several compartments. The perineurium is thought to provide a barrier to the diffusion of hydrophilic chemicals.[12] Electron microscopic studies reveal that perineurial cells are actively engaged in endocytosis, which suggests the cells may transport needed nutrients into the fascicular interior.[13]

Finally, the epineurium is the outermost connective tissue covering of the nerve. It comprises one third to two thirds of the cross-sectional area of a typical peripheral nerve, joins together the various fascicles, and provides structural support for blood and lymphatic vessels serving the nerve proper. Small collections of fat cells are scattered among the fibroblasts and longitudinally oriented collagen fibers of the epineurium.

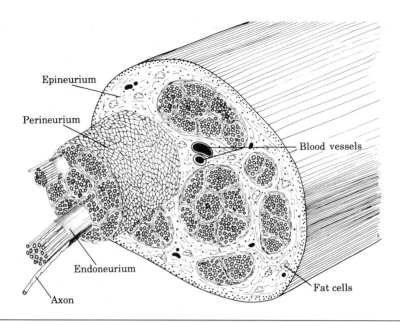

Figure 1–5.   Cross section of a peripheral nerve. Myelinated and unmyelinated fibers are represented by dark and light circles, respectively. Blood vessels and other connective tissue elements are enmeshed within the longitudinally oriented collagen fibers of the epineurium. Extending from the nerve trunk is a single large fascicle of nerve fibers ensheathed by cells of the perineurium. Intrafascicular collagen fibrils of the endoneurium are also illustrated.

Collectively, the connective tissue sheaths of the peripheral nerve provide a physical barrier to drug distribution. The influence of this barrier on regional anesthesia is marked. Indeed, tetrodotoxin and saxitoxin, two of the most potent local anesthetics yet discovered, are clinically unsuited for blocking peripheral nerves because they simply cannot penetrate to reach the axons encased within.

Neurophysiology

Peripheral nerve fibers carry information to or from the CNS in the form of electrical impulses. Known as action potentials, these impulses propagate along the nerve fiber as self-regenerating waves of membrane depolarization. The ability of neurons to initiate and conduct action potentials is based on an asymmetric distribution of ions across the nerve membrane and on variations in permeability of the nerve membrane to these ions.

ION TRANSPORT, PERMEABILITY, AND DISTRIBUTION

The plasma membrane of the neuron is composed of a lipid bilayer that acts as a hydrophobic barrier to the passage of molecules. Being lipid insoluble, most ionized molecules diffuse across the membrane with great difficulty if at all. However, selected ions, such as sodium (Na^+), potassium (K^+), and other small electrolytes, can traverse the membrane with relative ease because embedded in the membrane are "intrinsic" proteins that promote their movement.[14] Many of these proteins serve as channels through which ions such as Na^+ and K^+ may flow in relation to their respective electrochemical gradients. Others involved in ion translocation provide for the active transport of electrolytes. With respect to nerve conduction, the most important active transport system is the Na^+/K^+-activated adenosine triphosphatase pump, more commonly referred to as the Na^+/K^+ pump. The Na^+/K^+ pump is a globular protein made up of two subunits, an α subunit with a molecular weight of about 100,000 daltons and a β subunit with a molecular weight of 45,000.[8] The binding sites for both Na^+ and K^+ and the ATPase activity that enables the ionic exchange are all associated with the α subunit. Because the molecular weight of the smallest active pump particle isolated to date is about 300,000 daltons, it is assumed that the native Na^+/K^+ pump is a tetramer ($\alpha_2\beta_2$).[15] The Na^+/K^+ pump uses energy in the form of ATP to eject Na^+ from the cell while concentrating K^+ within. The stoichiometry for the reaction is usually 3 Na^+ eliminated from the axoplasm for every 2 K^+ taken up and 1 ATP hydrolyzed. When maximally active, a single Na^+/K^+ pump can transport about 300 Na^+ per second. An average neuron may have a million or more individual pumps scattered over its surface.

How the Na^+/K^+ pump establishes and maintains electrochemical gradients across the nerve membrane is illustrated by the hypothetical situation in which the electrolyte concentrations are equal on both sides of the membrane.[16] (It is also assumed that the coupling of Na^+-K^+ exchange is 1:1 under these nonphysiologic conditions). As the Na^+/K^+ pump is activated, Na^+ would begin to accumulate on the outside of the neuron and K^+ on the inside. By virtue of the chemical gradients established, back diffusion of the ions across the membrane would also begin to occur. Although K^+ would be able to migrate out of the cytoplasm with relative ease, the inward flow of Na^+ would be hampered by an ionic permeability only a small fraction of that for K^+. An electrical gradient would then be established by the unbalanced movements of cations across the plasma membrane. Chloride (Cl^-) and other anions capable of penetrating the membrane would then migrate out of the neuron toward the electropositive exterior, and further egress of K^+ would be inhibited. Eventually, a steady state would be reached in which Na^+ and Cl^- are concentrated in the extracellular fluid, K^+ and membrane-impermeable anions are sequestered inside the neuron, and a resting membrane potential of about -70 mV is achieved (Fig. 1–6). The metabolic cost of sustaining such an electrochemical disequilibrium is significant. During periods of high activity, well over half of the neuron's total energy consumption may be devoted to the Na^+/K^+ pump.

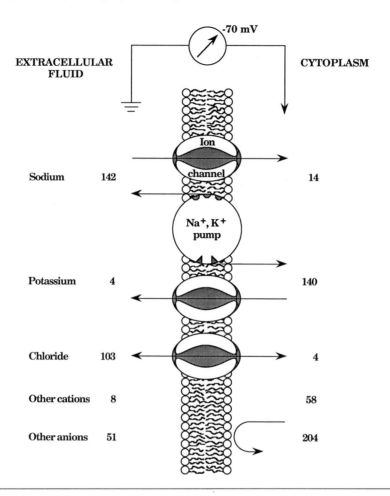

Figure 1–6.   Electrochemical gradients across the neuronal membrane. Active transport by the Na^+/K^+ pump counterbalances the passive influx of Na^+ and efflux of K^+ during the steady state. Chloride ions in peripheral nerve move through the membrane in accordance with the membrane potential, but most organic anions within the nerve cell are prevented from leaving by the hydrophobicity of the plasma membrane. Numbers indicate the milliequivalent concentrations of the various ions in the extracellular fluid (*left*) and cytoplasm (*right*).

   Although the Na^+/K^+ pump may contribute an "electrogenic" component of several millivolts to the resting potential (through the net extrusion of cations from the neuron) and is ultimately responsible for its maintenance, the potential largely is the direct result of the transmembrane concentration gradients and membrane permeabilities of the ions listed in Figure 1–6. The *constant field equation* relates these ionic variables to the membrane potential under steady-state conditions (i.e., when the net ionic flux across the membrane is zero). As originally described by Goldman[17] and by Hodgkin and Katz,[18] who focused on Na^+, K^+, and Cl^- as the primary ions of interest in establishing the membrane potential

(E_m), the constant field equation can be simplified to:

$$E_m = -61 \log \frac{[Na^+]_i P_{Na^+} + [K^+]_i P_{K^+} + [Cl^-]_o P_{Cl^-}}{[Na^+]_o P_{Na^+} + [K^+]_o P_{K^+} + [Cl^-]_i P_{Cl^-}}$$

where P indicates the permeability coefficient of each ion, the subscripts o and i reflect the extracellular and intracellular ionic concentrations, respectively, and the temperature is 37° C. Using the concentrations given in Figure 1–6 and the relative ionic permeabilities of the squid giant axon ($P_{K^+} : P_{Na^+} : P_{Cl^-} = 1 : 0.04 : 0.05$), a resting potential of −71 mV is obtained. Similar calculations and direct potential measurements of other neurons and excitable tissues yield values ranging from −40 to −95 mV. This spectrum of resting potentials is caused by cellular variances in relative membrane permeabilities and (to a lesser degree) in intracellular ionic concentrations.

THE ACTION POTENTIAL

An essential characteristic of the neuron is its excitability. Depending on the fiber, a variety of stimuli—chemical, electrical, mechanical, and thermal—may perturb the nerve membrane and alter the resting potential. Any factor that increases Na^+ permeability will partially depolarize the membrane (i.e., make the cytoplasm less electronegative with respect to the extracellular fluid) as Na^+ ions flow into the cell. The reverse is also true: depolarization augments Na^+ permeability. For a single small stimulus, the depolarization and increase in Na^+ conductance are limited in scope and duration.* If the membrane potential is sufficiently depressed, however, a critical threshold is reached at which the depolarization becomes self-generating (Fig. 1–7). An explosive rise in Na^+ permeability (up to 5,000 times baseline) induces a rapid influx of Na^+ through the Na^+-selective channels spanning the membrane. Within a fraction of a millisecond, the inrushing Na^+ reverses the membrane potential from a negative value to one of approximately +40 mV.[19] The depolarization is likewise brief in duration, however, because two additional changes in membrane permeability occur that serve to repolarize the membrane. First, the increase in Na^+ permeability dissipates. Na^+ channels opened by depolarization close spontaneously, and the Na^+ conductance falls to prestimulus conditions. Second, depolarization increases the permeability of the membrane to K^+. Although the elevation of K^+ conductance develops relatively slowly, the egress of K^+ through activated K^+-selective channels persists until the Na^+ incursion is neutralized and the steady-state membrane potential is restored. As shown in Figure 1–7, a

---

* *Permeability and conductance are measures of the ease with which a substance crosses a membrane in relation to its chemical and electrical gradients, respectively. In this discussion, the two terms are used rather interchangeably because a change in ionic permeability causes a parallel alteration in ionic conductance.*

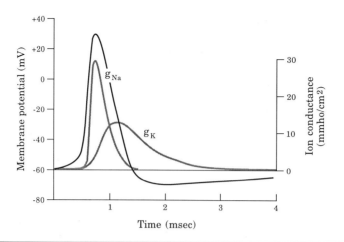

Figure 1–7.   Graphic representation of the action potential of the squid giant axon. Dashed lines indicate the Na$^+$ and K$^+$ conductance changes (g_{Na} and g_K, respectively) responsible for membrane depolarization and recovery. (Adapted from Hodgkin, A.L., and Huxley, A.F.: J. Physiol. (Lond.), *117*:500–544, 1952.)

time lag in closure of the K$^+$ channels once the cell has repolarized produces a period of membrane hyperpolarization known as the "positive afterpotential."

The ionic movements that constitute the action potential do not require energy as such. Neurons exposed to metabolic inhibitors such as cyanide continue to function for some time thereafter. Even axons whose entire cytoplasmic contents have been removed and replaced with a K$^+$ salt solution can conduct normally. Since each action potential exchanges only a minute fraction of the neuron's K$^+$ for Na$^+$, dozens of impulses in small unmyelinated axons and up to 200,000 impulses in large myelinated axons can be propagated in these experimental situations before the Na$^+$ and K$^+$ concentrations become too distorted to support normal conduction. As described previously, the energy actually needed for the system to work is used by the Na$^+$/K$^+$ pump to maintain the electrochemical gradients that provide the foundation for excitation and conduction. Since the intracellular concentration of Na$^+$ is a primary regulator of the Na$^+$/K$^+$ pump, repeated depolarizations of a nerve will produce measurable increases in pump activity, ATP hydrolysis, and oxygen consumption.

ELECTROTONIC CURRENTS

The progression of an action potential along the axon is dependent on the electrotonic spread of membrane depolarization. Local currents created by the inward movement of Na$^+$ circulate passively from the active region of the membrane to adjacent unaffected areas, depolarizing the latter and permitting the action potential to course down the nerve (Fig.

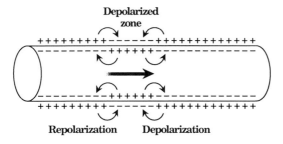

Figure 1–8. Propagation of the action potential in an unmyelinated axon. Large arrow indicates the direction of the action potential. The entry of Na^+ into the axon and reversal of membrane polarity cause the electrotonic spread of current to adjacent areas, initiating further depolarization and progression of the action potential. Once the advancing wave of depolarization has passed, repolarizing currents, including the outward flow of K^+, reestablish the resting membrane potential.

1–8). This process is best understood by viewing the axon as an electrically conducting cable with the following properties: (1) a resistance to current flow through the axon interior (R_i) directly proportional to axonal length and inversely proportional to cross-sectional area; (2) a resistance to transmembrane flow (R_m) inversely proportional to surface area; and (3) a membrane capacitance (C_m) directly proportional to surface area. Electrotonic currents that depolarize the axon do not cross the resting membrane in the form of ions to complete the circuit. Instead, they discharge the membrane, which has a C_m of about 1 μF/cm^2.

The release of membrane capacitance is not instantaneous. The time required for the axonal membrane to lose 63% (or reach $1/e$) of its original charge, known as the time constant, or τ, is equal to $C_m\sqrt{R_mR_i}$. This relationship can be used to predict the influence of fiber diameter on the speed of conduction. Assume, for instance, that the diameter of an unmyelinated axon is doubled. C_m would increase and R_m would decrease by a factor of 2 because the surface area would also double. The R_i would fall to one-fourth its original value because of the increased cross-sectional area. The net effect of these changes would be to reduce τ by a factor of $\sqrt{2}$ and speed conduction by the same amount. Additional variables that govern the rate of membrane depolarization include the density of Na^+ channels in the membrane, their responsiveness to changes in the transmembrane potential (both of which greatly influence R_m), and the presence of myelin (discussed later in this chapter). Measurements reveal that conduction velocity in unmyelinated fibers varies with a power between 0.5 and 0.8 of the axon diameter.[20,21]

A second cable descriptor influencing nerve conduction is the length constant, or λ, which indicates the length down the axon over which a local current loses 63% of its original magnitude. Equal to $\sqrt{R_m/R_i}$, λ varies directly as the square root of the diameter in unmyelinated axons, with typical values ranging from 1 to 3 mm.[20] Obviously, an electrotonic current can affect only a small length of nerve, demonstrating the absolute necessity for a self-sustaining action potential to carry impulses from peripheral tissues to the CNS. As discussed in Chapter 2, λ is an essential governor of the length of nerve that must be exposed to a local anesthetic in order to achieve conduction blockade.

GATING MECHANISMS

The conformational changes that occur in the Na^+ and K^+ channels during an action potential are not fully understood. Nevertheless, a graphic representation of the major events can be drawn, as in Figure 1–9.[22,23] In the unstimulated nerve, most of the Na^+ channels are in a closed, resting state. Na^+ ions are prevented from passing through the channel by a barrier termed the activation, or m, gate. This gate, shown in Figure 1–9 as a constriction in the channel's diameter, is strongly voltage dependent. Under appropriate conditions a depolarization of as little as 9 mV can open enough channels to increase Na^+ permeability tenfold.[22] Near the peak of the action potential, when most activation gates are in the open position, Na^+ conductance may be several hundred to several thousand times normal. The subsequent reduction in Na^+ permeability is due to erection of a second voltage-dependent barrier, the inactivation, or h, gate. Here, depolarization closes the gate. As a population, Na^+ channels once inactivated cannot be induced to open by a

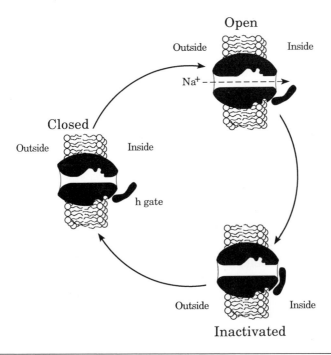

Figure 1–9.   Conformational changes of the Na^+ channel during an action potential.

depolarizing current until repolarization of the nerve membrane has permitted conversion from the inactivated to the closed configuration.

Regulation of voltage-sensitive K^+ channels in peripheral nerves is more straightforward. As with Na^+ channels, these K^+ channels exist largely in the resting state until their activation gates are opened by depolarization. K^+ channels open rather sluggishly, however, permitting the abrupt Na^+ influx to reverse the membrane potential. Because these K^+ channels have no counterpart to the Na^+ inactivation gate, they remain open until the K^+ efflux successfully repolarizes the membrane. Thereafter, the majority of the K^+ channels revert back to the resting conformation.

The concept of channel gating is a useful one. For instance, the rapid inactivation of Na^+ channels, coupled with the prolonged increase in K^+ permeability, offers a molecular explanation for the phenomenon of post-stimulation refractoriness. The *absolute refractory period*, the time after the initiation of an action potential when the nerve fiber cannot be stimulated to propagate another impulse, extends from the opening of the Na^+ channels, through the inactivation phase, to the point of membrane repolarization at which a sufficient fraction of Na^+ channels have returned to the closed state to support a second action potential. Beyond this point, and for the duration of the positive afterpotential, the axon can be activated, but only if a supranormal stimulus is applied. An initial deficit of responsive Na^+ channels and the protracted delay in K^+ channel closure provide the basis for this *relative refractory period*. As discussed in Chapter 2, the gating mechanism also yields important insights into the pharmacology of local anesthetics.

THE Na^+ CHANNEL

Because of the central role of the Na^+ channel in nerve conduction, considerable research efforts have been made to understand its properties at the molecular level. Since 1980, advances in molecular biology and neurophysiology have contributed pivotal discoveries regarding the structure and function of the Na^+ channel.

Using various neurotoxins that bind selectively and avidly to specific sites on the Na^+ channel as molecular markers and as ligands in affinity chromatography, investigators have successfully isolated Na^+ channels from several excitable tissues, including mammalian brain and skeletal muscle. The Na^+ channel in rat brain consists of a major α subunit with a molecular weight of 260,000 daltons, and two minor components, labeled β_1 and β_2, with respective molecular weights of 36,000 and 33,000.[24] All three subunits are heavily glycosylated and are therefore thought to be exposed in vivo to the extracellular space. Reconstitution studies in which the channel glycopeptides are incorporated into phospholipid bilayers reveal that the α constituent contains the channel passageway and that the β_1 subunit confers functional stability to the channel.[25] Although

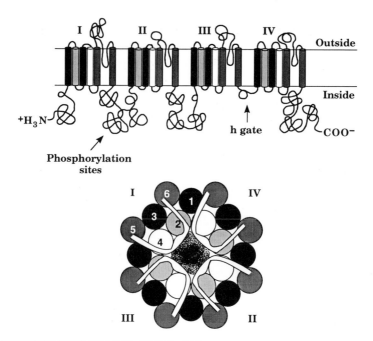

Figure 1–10.   Structural model of the Na$^+$ channel (α subunit). *Top*, the channel is composed of four homologous units (I, II, III, and IV), each of which contains six helical segments (designated S1 through S6) spanning the membrane. A portion of the S5-S6 linkage lines the pore itself and confers ion selectivity to the channel. Parts of the channel extending beyond the membrane constitute three fourths of the polypeptide by weight and are shown in approximate relative size. *Bottom*, proposed spatial orientation of transmembrane subunits as viewed perpendicular to the membrane from the external surface. Positive charges from arginine and lysine residues in S4 are balanced electrostatically by negative charges in S1, S3, and S2 (the last of which also contains positively charged groups and is electrically neutral). Segments S5 and S6 are uniformly hydrophobic. The horseshoe-like figures represent the S5-S6 segments lining the pore. (Adapted with permission from Noda, M., Ikeda, T., et al.: Nature, *320*:826–828, 1986, and from Sato, C., and Matsumoto, G. Biochem: Biophys. Res. Commun., *186*:1158–1167, 1992.)

the β_2 polypeptide is covalently linked to the α subunit through a disulfide bond, its removal causes no discernible change in channel activity.

Recombinant DNA techniques have permitted the complete amino acid sequencing of the α subunit. In rat brain, multiple isoforms of the α subunit have been identified. The first two of these to be sequenced are composed of 2,009 and 2,005 amino acid residues, respectively. The α polypeptides are 87% homologous in structure and are also closely related to other α subunits isolated from brain tissue, cardiac and skeletal muscle, and even the electric organ of *Electrophorus electricus*.[26,27] As illustrated in Figure 1–10, the α polypeptide is composed of four homologous domains, each containing six peptide helices that are believed to cross the membrane. Although the exact arrangement of these segments within the membrane is unclear, the configuration depicted is consistent with what is known about the channel, including its 0.3 × 0.5 nm effective internal diameter predicted from permeability studies of organic cations of different molecular size.[25,28] Studies of the K^+ channel encoded by the *Drosophila Shaker* gene[29] and more recent work with Na^+ channels from various sources[27,30] indicate that the actual Na^+-channel pore is lined by a portion of the peptide chain connecting each S5 and S6 pair.

The Na^+ channel depicted in Figure 1–10 provides a useful foundation for linking molecular structure with physiologic function. Gating currents and Na^+ channel activation can be accounted for by a "helical screw" model in which ionic charges are carried across the membrane by an outward twisting of the positively charged S4 segment.[25] Originally hypothesized by Hodgkin and Huxley in 1952[19] and then detected experimentally in the early 1970s,[31] gating currents immediately precede channel opening and arise from conformational changes in the Na^+ channel induced by electrotonic depolarization of the membrane. Reciprocal currents occur when channels return to the resting state. The currents are feeble in magnitude—the equivalent of four to six charges per Na^+ channel—but they are fundamental to the activation process. In the helical screw model, the S4 segments are proposed to be in a metastable state, with their positively charged amino acid residues neutralized by pairings with negatively charged groups on adjacent segments (S1 through S3).[25] With depolarization and the loss of stabilization afforded by an electronegative inner surface of the membrane, each S4 helix undergoes independently an outward rotation of at least 60 degrees and 0.5 nm, which exposes one or two charges per segment to the exterior. Concomitant with these changes is an opening of the channel pore such that Na^+ can traverse the channel when all S4 segments have become extruded.*

Channel inactivation has been ascribed to a peptide segment connecting domains III and IV (h gate, Fig. 1–10). Intracellular injection of the proteolytic enzyme pronase and removal of the h gate results in Na^+ channels that open normally in response to membrane depolarization but which remain open until the membrane is repolarized artificially. Inactivation is also modified by administration of antibodies specific for this peptide segment. Although inactivation was originally considered to be a voltage-sensitive process independent of channel activation, the reverse now seems to be the case.[25,31] One possible explanation for the *inter*dependence of activation and inactivation is that the outward displacement of S4 segments enhances association of the h-gate peptide with the channel opening. Thus, whenever channels are activated (open), inactivation soon follows. Return to the resting state hinges on the inward return of the S4 segments once the membrane has fully repolarized.

The technique of patch clamping, in which a small area (i.e., patch) of membrane is made to adhere by suction to the polished tip of a micropi-

---

* An alternative proposal suggests that the electronegative S5-S6 linkers lining the channel pore serve as the voltage sensors, with their inward slide along each S4 helix causing the activation gating current.[28]

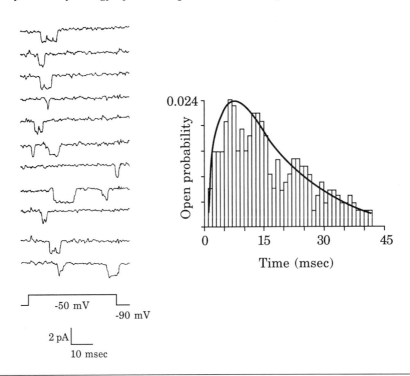

Figure 1–11. Patch-clamp recording of ionic currents from single Na⁺ channels (NIE-115 neuroblastoma cells, 10° C). *Left*, 11 individual recordings in response to a depolarizing voltage to -50 mV from a holding potential of -90 mV. A mean inward current (downward deflection in the graph) of 1.12 pA per open channel was obtained from 128 consecutive recordings. *Right*, histogram of the mean probability of a single Na⁺ channel being open as a function of time from the beginning of the depolarizing pulse. (Adapted from Quandt, F.N., and Narahashi, T.: Proc. Natl. Acad. Sci. U.S.A., 79:6732–6736, 1982.)

pet electrode, has recently permitted the measurement of Na⁺ currents through single Na⁺ channels.[32,33] Individual recordings, as represented in Figure 1–11, indicate that the Na⁺ channel is either completely closed or fully open to the passage of Na⁺. A current of 1.12 pA per open channel is equivalent to 7 million Na⁺ traversing the channel per second. The opening of any given channel is a stochastic event, with an overall occurrence rate that exhibits a Poisson distribution strongly dependent on transmembrane voltage and time. As the number of channels measured increases, the mean probability of the Na⁺ channel existing in the open state gradually assumes a smooth function equivalent to the changes in Na⁺ conductance that take place during an action potential as determined by conventional voltage clamp methodology.

Given recent advances in understanding of the Na⁺ channel, it is appropriate to expand on the chain of events outlined in Figure 1–9 by including a series of closed channel configurations synonymous, for example, with the number of S4 segments in the externally rotated state, and arrows indicating the reversible nature of the transformations at the molecular level:

$$Closed_0 \rightleftharpoons Closed_1 \rightleftharpoons Closed_2 \rightleftharpoons Closed_3 \rightleftharpoons Open$$
$$Inactivated$$

Future studies will undoubtedly refine this scheme as more is learned about the structure and function of the Na^+ channel.

MYELINATION AND SALTATORY CONDUCTION

No discussion of the physiology of the peripheral nervous system would be complete without some consideration of the effects of myelination on nerve conduction. As described in preceding sections, the action potential in unmyelinated neurons is propagated as a continuous wave, with local currents depolarizing adjacent segments of the membrane. Action potentials in myelinated fibers, however, can be supported only at the nodes of Ranvier. Elsewhere, the heavy internodal insulation (representing as many as 300 layers of lipoid membrane tightly wrapped around the axon) precludes ionic flow across the axolemma. Local depolarizing currents are thus constrained to flow between adjacent nodes, and the impulse is propagated in a saltatory fashion (saltatory is derived from *saltare*, the Latin verb meaning to leap), skipping from one node to the next down the axon (Fig. 1–12).

Several important advantages are realized by myelination. For instance, the velocity of conduction is greatly enhanced. Illustrative of this fact is the influence of a myelin sheath on the cable properties of an axon. Should a Schwann cell wrap around an axon 50 times, it will produce a myelin layer 100 times as thick as the axolemma. A proportional increase in R_m occurs because local currents must cross 100 additional membranes (resistors arranged in series) to complete their circuits. This change would tend to slow conduction according to the previously mentioned

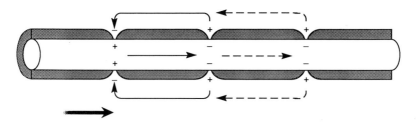

Figure 1–12. Saltatory nerve conduction in a myelinated axon. The large arrow indicates the direction of the action potential. Depolarizing electrotonic currents generated by the action potential (solid and dashed arrows) are constrained to adjacent nodes of Ranvier by the myelin insulation.

formula $\tau = C_m\sqrt{R_m R_i}$ (τ being inversely proportional to conduction velocity). However, C_m is reduced at the same time to 1% of its former value, because membrane capacitors in series add according to the formula:

$$\frac{1}{C_m} = \frac{1}{C_1} + \frac{1}{C_2} + \cdots + \frac{1}{C_n}.$$

Assuming no change in R_i, τ is reduced and conduction velocity is enhanced tenfold. The diameter of the fiber would admittedly be increased 40% by myelination; nevertheless, the gain in conduction velocity is much greater than the 18% increase that would occur from simply enlarging the unmyelinated axon a comparable amount. The 40% increase in fiber thickness assumes an axon/myelinated fiber diameter ratio of 0.7. This ratio provides the optimal balance between axonal diameter and myelin thickness for nerve conduction theoretically, and it is the one that occurs naturally. Because the ratio is maintained over a wide range of fiber sizes, larger myelinated fibers must have thicker myelin coverings. Consideration of cable properties indicates that both the conduction velocity and the length constant in myelinated axons vary directly with fiber diameter (and not the square root of the diameter, as is the case theoretically with unmyelinated axons). Since the length constant is a limiting factor influencing internodal distance, it is not surprising that internodal length maintains a fixed ratio of 100 to 200 times the fiber diameter. Combining this relationship with diameter and conduction velocity values provided in Table 1–1 allows one to conclude that the action potential leaps from node to node as rapidly as every 20 μsec.[34] Even so, it should be recognized that, in a large axon with an action potential spike duration of only 0.4 msec, a minimum of 20 nodes are involved in some phase of the same action potential at any given moment.

Restriction of transmembrane currents to the nodal region has been accompanied by specialization of the nodal axolemma. Whereas Na^+ channels are scattered evenly across the surface of the unmyelinated axon, with a mean density of about 110 channels/μm^2, myelinated axons contain 1,200 to 1,500 Na^+ channels/μm^2 at the nodes and few if any Na^+ channels elsewhere along the axon.[34,35] An opposite distribution of voltage-sensitive K^+ channels is also in evidence. The heavy concentration of Na^+ channels at each node increases the depolarization rate of the membrane and provides sufficient local currents to activate the next node. With the absence of nodal K^+ channels, membrane repolarization is totally dependent on Na^+ inactivation. Inactivation is quite rapid in mammalian nodes, however, and freedom from stabilizing K^+ currents after an action potential permits large myelinated axons to conduct at frequencies up to 2,500 Hz.[8] It is theorized that internodal K^+ channels contribute to nerve conduction indirectly by maintaining the internodal resting potential and preventing spontaneous firing of the node from persisting depolarization of the paranodal region.[35] Because relatively few

Na^+ and K^+ ions are exchanged per action potential in myelinated nerves, correspondingly less Na^+/K^+ pump activity is required to restore the ionic balance. The savings in energy utilization are considerable, equaling 90% to 99% of what would otherwise be required to drive Na^+ transport.

In summary, myelination enables nerve fibers to be small enough to exist in numbers large enough for fine sensory discrimination and motor control and yet be fast enough to transmit impulses at conduction velocities and frequencies sufficient for all needs, from maintaining balance while the animal is standing to withdrawing quickly from a potentially injurious stimulus.

References

1. Fawcett, D.W.: A Textbook of Histology, 11th ed. Philadelphia, W.B. Saunders Co., 1986.
2. Cormack, D.H.: Ham's Histology, 9th ed. Philadelphia, J.B. Lippincott Co., 1987.
3. Thomas, P.K., and Ochoa, J.: Microscopic anatomy of peripheral nerve fibers. *In* Dyck, P.J., Thomas, P.K., Lambert, E.H., and Bunge, R., eds.: Peripheral Neuropathy, 2nd ed. Philadelphia, W.B. Saunders Co., 1984.
4. Landon, D.N.: Structure and function of nerve fibres. *In* Swash, M., and Kennard, C., eds.: Scientific Basis of Clinical Neurology. Edinburgh, Churchill Livingstone, 1985.
5. Mathers, L.H., Jr.: The Peripheral Nervous System: Structure, Function, and Clinical Correlations. Menlo Park, Calif., Addison-Wesley Publishing Co., 1985.
6. Orkand, R.K.: Glial cells. *In* Kandel, E.R., ed.: Handbook of Physiology. Section 1. The Nervous System. Vol. 1. Cellular Biology of Neurons, part 2. Bethesda, Md., American Physiology Society, 1977.
7. Gray, P.T.A., Bevan, S., Chiu, S.Y., Shrager, P., and Ritchie, J.M.: Ionic conductances in mammalian Schwann cells. *In* Ritchie, J.M., Keynes, R.D., and Bolis, L., eds.: Ion Channels in Neural Membranes. New York, Alan R. Liss, Inc., 1986.
8. Guyton, A.C.: Basic Neuroscience: Anatomy and Physiology. Philadelphia, W.B. Saunders Co., 1987.
9. Wall, P.D.: The gate control theory of pain mechanisms: A re-examination and restatement. Brain, *101*:1–18, 1978.
10. Johnsen, D.C., Harshbarger, J., and Rymer, H.D.: Quantitative assessment of neural development in human premolars. Anat. Rec., *205*:421–429, 1983.
11. Mumford, J.M.: Pain perception threshold and adaptation of normal human teeth. Arch. Oral Biol., *10*:957–965, 1965.
12. Noback, C.R., and Demarest, R.J.: The Human Nervous System: Basic Principles of Neurobiology, 3rd ed. New York, McGraw-Hill Book Co., 1981.
13. Thomas, P.K., and Olsson, Y.: Microscopic anatomy and function of the connective tissue components of peripheral nerve. *In* Dyck, P.J., Thomas, P.K., Lambert, E.H., and Bunge, R., eds.: Peripheral Neuropathy, 2nd ed. Philadelphia, W.B. Saunders Co., 1984.
14. Stevens, C.F.: The neuron. Sci. Am., *241*(3):54–65, 1979.
15. Hille, B.: Transport across cell membranes: Carrier mechanisms. *In* Patton, H.D., Fuchs, A.F., Hille, B., Scher, A.M., and Steiner, R., eds.: Textbook of Physiology, 21st ed. Vol. 1. Excitable Cells and Neurophysiology. Philadelphia, W.B. Saunders Co., 1989.

16. Woodbury, J.W.: The cell membrane: Ionic and potential gradients and active transport. *In* Ruch, T.C., and Patton, H.D., eds.: Physiology and Biophysics, 20th ed. Philadelphia, W.B. Saunders Co., 1974.

17. Goldman, D.E.: Potential, impedance, and rectification in membranes. J. Gen. Physiol., *27*:37–60, 1943.

18. Hodgkin, A.L., and Katz, B.: The effect of sodium ions on the electrical activity of the giant axon of the squid. J. Physiol. (Lond.), *108*:189–236, 1949.

19. Hodgkin, A.L., and Huxley, A.F.: A quantitative description of membrane current and its application to conduction and excitation in nerve. J. Physiol. (Lond.), *117*:500–544, 1952.

20. Kutchai, H.C.: Generation and conduction of action potentials. *In* Berne, R.M., and Levy, M.N., eds.: Physiology, 3rd ed. St. Louis, Mosby–Year Book, Inc., 1993.

21. Hille, B.: Membrane excitability: Action potential propagation in axons. *In* Patton, H.D., Fuchs, A.F., Hille, B., Scher, A.M., and Steiner, R., eds.: Textbook of Physiology, 21st ed. Vol. 1. Excitable Cells and Neurophysiology. Philadelphia, W.B. Saunders Co., 1989.

22. Hille, B.: Gating in sodium channels of nerve. Annu. Rev. Physiol., *38*:139–152, 1976.

23. Keynes, R.D.: Ion channels in the nerve-cell membrane. Sci. Am., *240*(3):126–135, 1979.

24. Catterall, W.A.: The molecular basis of neuronal excitability. Science, *223*:653–661, 1984.

25. Catterall, W.A.: Structure and function of voltage-sensitive ion channels. Science, *242*:50–61, 1988.

26. Villegas, R., Villegas, G.M., Rodriguez-Grille, J.M., and Sorais-Landaez, F.: The sodium channel of excitable and non-excitable cells. Q. Rev. Biophys., *21*:99–128, 1988.

27. Satin, J., Kyle, J.W., Chen, M., Bell, P., Cribbs, L.L., Fozzard, H.A., and Rogart, R.B.: A mutant of TTX-resistant cardiac sodium channels with TTX-sensitive properties. Science, *256*:1202–1205, 1992.

28. Sato, C., and Matsumoto, G.: Proposed tertiary structure of the sodium channel. Biochem. Biophys. Res. Commun., *186*:1158–1167, 1992.

29. Yellen, G., Jurman, M.E., Abramson, T., and MacKinnon, R.: Mutations affecting internal TEA blockade identify the probable pore-forming region of a K^+ channel. Science, *251*:939–942, 1991.

30. Backx, P.H., Yue, D.T., Lawrence, J.H., Marban, E., and Tomaselli, G.F.: Molecular localization of an ion-binding site within the pore of mammalian sodium channels. Science, *257*:248–251, 1992.

31. Hille, B.: Voltage-gated channels and electrical excitability. *In* Patton, H.D., Fuchs, A.F., Hille, B., Scher, A.M., and Steiner, R., eds.: Textbook of Physiology, 21st ed. Vol. 1. Excitable Cells and Neurophysiology. Philadelphia, W.B. Saunders Co., 1989.

32. Patlak, J., and Horn, R.: Effect of *N*-bromoacetamide on single sodium channel currents in excised membrane patches. J. Gen. Physiol., *79*:333–351, 1982.

33. Quandt, F.N., and Narahashi, T.: Modification of single Na^+ channels by batrachotoxin. Proc. Natl. Acad. Sci. U.S.A., *79*:6732–6736, 1982.

34. Rasminsky, M.: Conduction in normal and pathological nerve fibers. *In* Swash, M., and Kennard, C., eds.: Scientific Basis of Clinical Neurology. Edinburgh, Churchill Livingstone, 1985.

35. Ritchie, J.M.: The distribution of sodium and potassium channels in mammalian myelinated nerve. *In* Ritchie, J.M., Keynes, R.D., and Bolis, L., eds.: Ion Channels in Neural Membranes. New York, Alan R. Liss, Inc., 1986.

Pharmacology of Local Anesthetics

L ocal anesthetics are drugs that reversibly block nerve conduction when applied to a circumscribed area of the body. Although numerous substances display local anesthetic activity on injection, only a few are sufficiently reliable and selective enough to be used for regional anesthesia. Most local anesthetics of proven clinical worth are identified by the suffix *caine*.

Historical Development

Cocaine, the first local anesthetic, has an intriguing history.[1,2] Centuries before the first European description of the coca plant was published by Pedro Cieza de Leon in 1532, Peruvian Indians had discovered that chewing "khoka" leaves mixed with lime produced exhilaration and relief from fatigue and hunger. In 1855, Gaedcke isolated an alkaloid from leaves of the coca plant, now given the botanical designation of *Erythroxylon coca,* and named the substance erythroxyline. Albert Niemann improved the extraction process and obtained the alkaloid in pure form in 1859. He also renamed the drug cocaine, to indicate its source (coca) and the fact that it is an alkaloid (ine). Initially, cocaine was pronounced kō'-ka-ēn', but the pronunciation gradually changed to the modern kō'-kān, with the *caine* suffix assuming the etymological significance of a drug having local anesthetic activity. Niemann recognized the anesthetic effect of cocaine when he wrote that "it benumbs the nerves of the tongue, depriving it of feeling and taste."[1] Several subsequent investigators, notably Moreno Y Maize (1868) and Von Anrep (1880), went so far as to suggest its use as a local anesthetic but stopped short of demonstrating its value clinically.[2]

In the early 1880s, cocaine was described as possessing the ability to relieve addiction to morphine and alcohol.[3] Sigmund Freud, then a young physician at the University of Vienna, administered cocaine in an effort to free a colleague of morphine dependence. Freud achieved mixed success—his patient was able to overcome morphine craving, only to become dependent on cocaine. Freud also performed a number of experiments with the drug and published a review of its properties in July 1884. Carl Koller, a junior resident in the Ophthalmological Clinic, helped Freud in some of these experiments.

Aspiring to a faculty appointment, Koller was interested in making a strong contribution to research in his chosen field. In the summer of 1884, after Freud had left for an extended visit with his fiancee, Koller decided to test cocaine for topical anesthetic activity. He was successful in rendering the corneas of various animals and himself insensible to pain. On September 11, 1884, Koller performed the world's first operation using local anesthesia on a patient with glaucoma.[4] News of Koller's achievement spread rapidly. A summary of his preclinical studies was read on September 15 at the Congress of Ophthalmology in Heidelberg. Attendees at the Congress transmitted the discovery of local anesthesia throughout the world. Within 30 days, even before Koller had had the opportunity to describe his clinical success at the October 17 meeting of the Vienna Medical Society, ophthalmologists in New York had successfully used cocaine in their clinical practices.[3] (Koller followed his discovery to the United States several years later, his appointment the victim of personal enmity.)

William Halsted, a noted American surgeon, was the first person to inject cocaine for conduction anesthesia. In November 1884, he performed infraorbital and inferior alveolar nerve blocks for dental operations, and subsequently he developed numerous other regional nerve blocks.[4] Halsted became addicted to cocaine (self-administration being commonly practiced in medical research) but was able to "recover" through the abuse of morphine. Two of his assistants and many other early workers were even less fortunate.

Two major drawbacks of cocaine were its toxicity and the fact that anesthesia was of short duration, necessitating injection of large amounts of drug with potentially severe side effects. One technique used to increase the duration of anesthesia, and hence limit the dose of cocaine required, was to apply a tourniquet near the operating site. This approach was only partially successful and added to the danger of local tissue damage. It was also impractical for certain regions, such as the oral cavity. In 1903, Heinrich Braun reported that epinephrine could be used as a "chemical tourniquet."[5] When added to a solution of cocaine, this drug would decrease the rate of absorption and thus prolong anesthesia and lower the dosage of cocaine required.

As the problems of cocaine toxicity and addiction became apparent, chemists turned their attention to analyzing the cocaine molecule to identify that portion responsible for the anesthetic effect in hopes of producing a synthetic substitute without cocaine's undesirable properties. Alfred Einhorn and his associates in Munich synthesized several anesthetics, including orthoform, neoorthoform, and nirvanin, which were good topical anesthetics but too toxic for parenteral administration.[6] Finally, in 1904, they discovered procaine (which was subsequently marketed under the trade name Novocain). The discovery was reported by Einhorn in 1905; the drug was immediately accepted as a substitute for cocaine. Procaine is still considered a safe, effective local anesthetic, and some writers contend that its discovery marked the beginning of the modern era of regional anesthesia.[6] Nevertheless, in 1943 the Swedish chemist Nils Löfgren synthesized lidocaine (Xylocaine), the first amide anesthetic derived from xylidine.[7] More potent and less allergenic than procaine, it displaced procaine and other esters as the drug of choice for most purposes and remains one of the most popular local anesthetics in clinical practice.

Table 2–1 summarizes salient events in the historical development of local anesthesia. Anesthetic agents and the methods and devices for administering them have all undergone remarkable improvement in the past century. Judging from ongoing research efforts, it is clear that progress is continuing toward the ultimate aim of achieving technologies that provide effective local anesthesia limited to the area of the operation and to the duration of the procedure while being completely free of undesirable side effects, including the discomfort of needle penetration. Until

Table 2–1. **LANDMARK DEVELOPMENTS IN LOCAL ANESTHESIA FOR DENTISTRY**

Year	Person/Company	Contribution
1859	Niemann	Isolation of cocaine in pure form; recognition of its topical anesthetic property
1884	Koller	Clinical introduction of cocaine topical anesthesia
1884	Halsted	Clinical introduction of cocaine regional anesthesia
1885	Corning	Application of a tourniquet to retard cocaine absorption
1903	Braun	Report on use of epinephrine as a ''chemical tourniquet''
1904	Einhorn	Synthesis of procaine
1905	Braun	Clinical introduction of procaine
1920	Cook Laboratories	Marketing of the anesthetic cartridge and syringe
1943	Löfgren	Synthesis of lidocaine
1948	Astra	Marketing of lidocaine for dentistry
1947	Novocol Co.	Marketing of the dental aspirating syringe
1957	Ekenstam	Synthesis of bupivacaine
1959	Cook-Waite, Roehr Co.	Marketing of the disposable sterile needle
1983	Cook-Waite	Marketing of bupivacaine for dentistry

then, the effective and safe use of local anesthetics will depend on a clear understanding of the pharmacology of these agents.

Classification and Structure–Activity Relationships

The typical local anesthetic molecule is composed of three parts: an aromatic group, an intermediate chain, and a secondary or tertiary amino terminus (Fig. 2–1). Each component is an important determinant of anesthetic potency. The aromatic residue confers lipophilic (or, more accurately, hydrophobic) properties on the molecule, and the amino

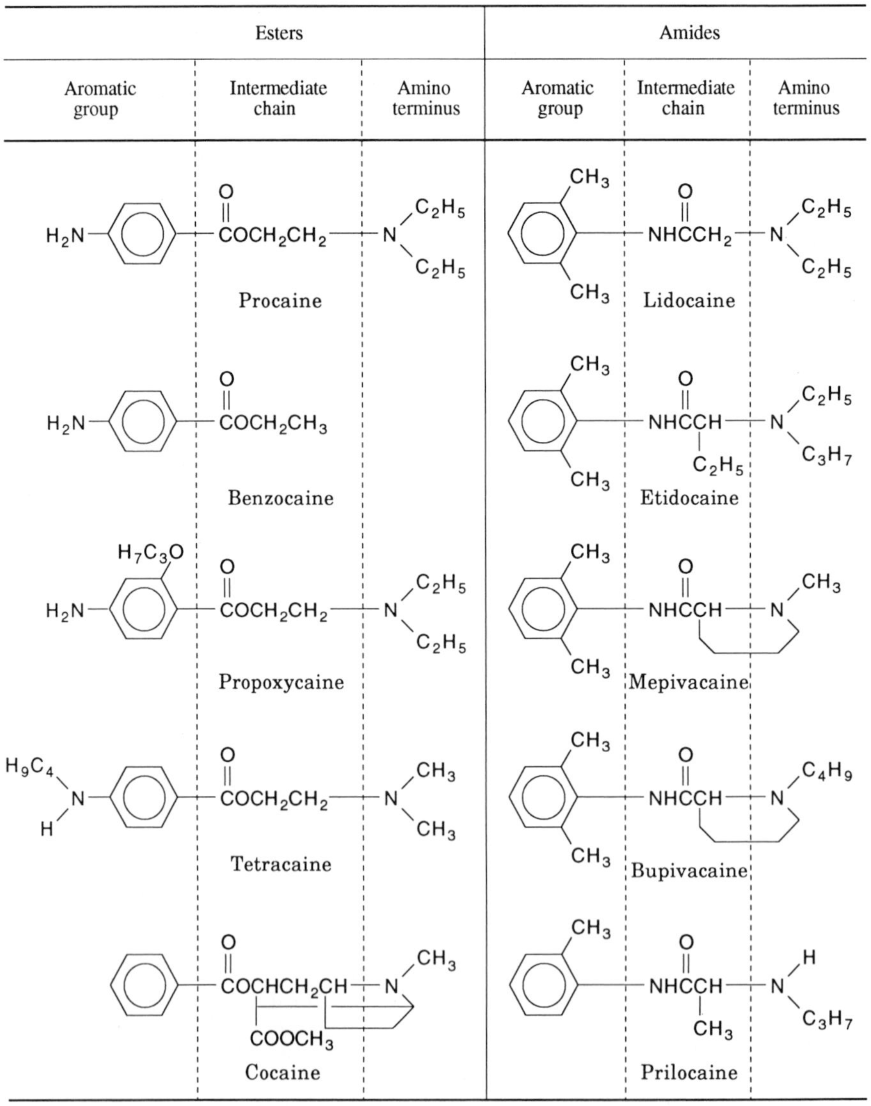

Esters			Amides		
Aromatic group	Intermediate chain	Amino terminus	Aromatic group	Intermediate chain	Amino terminus
Procaine			Lidocaine		
Benzocaine			Etidocaine		
Propoxycaine			Mepivacaine		
Tetracaine			Bupivacaine		
Cocaine			Prilocaine		

Figure 2–1.   Structural formulas of local anesthetics used in dentistry.

group furnishes water solubility. Both features are necessary for the full expression of local anesthetic activity. Lipid solubility is essential for penetration of the various anatomic barriers existing between an administered drug and its site of action. Water solubility ensures that, once injected in an effective concentration, the drug will not precipitate on exposure to interstitial fluid. The intermediate portion of the molecule is significant in two respects. First, it provides the necessary spatial separation between the hydrophobic and hydrophilic ends of the local anesthetic. Second, the chemical link between the central hydrocarbon moiety and the aromatic group serves as a suitable basis for classifying conventional local anesthetics into two groups, the esters (—COO—) and the amides (—NHCO—). This distinction is useful, since there are marked differences in allergenicity and metabolism between the two drug categories. A few compounds fall outside this taxonomy, but these agents currently either have little or no clinical application (e.g., tetrodotoxin, a highly potent and dangerous anesthetic) or are restricted to topical use (e.g., dyclonine, a ketone). Local anesthetics may also be categorized on the basis of certain pharmacologic properties.[8-10] Table 2–2 lists several such discriminators and their physicochemical correlates. Anesthetic agents, for example, may be grouped according to potency or duration of action, attributes proportional to the organic:aqueous distribution coefficient (Q). Alternatively, the rate of onset of anesthesia, a characteristic dependent on the dissociation constant (as reflected in the

Table 2–2.   **PHYSICOCHEMICAL AND CLINICAL PROPERTIES OF LOCAL ANESTHETICS**

Drug	pK$_a$*	Rate of Onset	Q*	Relative Potency†	Duration of Anesthesia	MW	Phasic Block‡
Amides							
Lidocaine	7.8	Fast	110	2	Moderate	234	Low
Mepivacaine	7.7	Fast	42	2	Moderate	246	Medium
Prilocaine	7.8	Fast	55	2	Moderate	220	Low
Bupivacaine	8.1	Medium	560	8	Long	288	High
Etidocaine	7.9	Fast	1853	6	Long	276	Medium
Articaine§	7.8	Fast	~40	2	Moderate	284	Medium
Esters							
Procaine	8.9	Medium	3	1	Short	236	Low
Propoxycaine§	8.9	Medium	?	6	Moderate	294	High
Tetracaine	8.4	Medium	541	8	Long	264	Medium

* *Data from Strichartz, et al.[8] pK$_a$ (dissociation constant) and Q (octanol:buffer distribution coefficient) were measured at 36° C in buffered (pH 7.4) isotonic saline solution. Values for prilocaine are extrapolated from measurements taken at 25° C.*

† *Data from Covino.[9] Tonic block; peripheral nerve in vitro.*

‡ *Data from Courtney.[10] Potency was determined in peripheral nerve in vitro.*

§ *Estimated values (except molecular weight).*

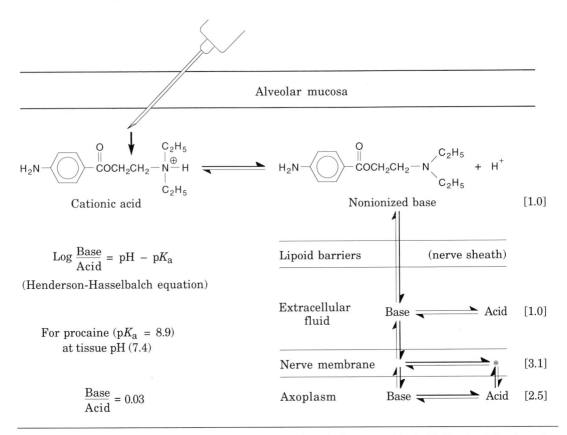

$$\log \frac{\text{Base}}{\text{Acid}} = \text{pH} - \text{p}K_a$$

(Henderson-Hasselbalch equation)

For procaine ($\text{p}K_a = 8.9$)
at tissue pH (7.4)

$$\frac{\text{Base}}{\text{Acid}} = 0.03$$

Figure 2–2.   Distribution of a local anesthetic (procaine) during nerve block. Following injection of the local anesthetic, a portion of the cationic acid is converted to the free base. Estimated using the Henderson-Hasselbach equation is the base/acid ratio for procaine in the extracellular fluid at equilibrium (0.03). Thick arrows depict the major pathway followed by a local anesthetic in reaching its site of action within the nerve membrane. Values in brackets on the right indicate the relative concentrations of total drug (acid + base) in the extracellular fluid, nerve membrane, and axoplasm, assuming an intracellular pH of 7.0, a membrane/extracellular fluid distribution coefficient (Q) of 3.1, and no protein binding in any tissue compartment (less than 10% of procaine is normally bound to nerve homogenates).

$\text{p}K_a$, the negative log of the dissociation constant of the acidic form of the drug), may be employed.

By virtue of the substituted amino group, most local anesthetics are weak bases, with $\text{p}K_a$ values ranging from 7.5 to 9.0. However, a local anesthetic intended for injection is usually converted to the acidic salt by adding hydrochloric acid. This practice improves water solubility, which facilitates the manufacture and sterilization of the anesthetic formulation and increases the stability of the drug in aqueous media. Once injected, the acidic local anesthetic solution is neutralized by tissue fluid buffers, and a fraction of the cationic form is converted back to the nonionized base. As represented by the Henderson-Hasselbalch equation (Fig. 2–2), the percentage of drug converted depends primarily on the local anesthetic pK_a and the tissue pH. Because only the base form can diffuse rapidly into the nerve, drugs with high pK_a values tend to have a slower onset of action than similar agents with more favorable dissociation constants. Tissue acidity, as may occur with certain diseases, can impede the development of local anesthesia. Acidic products of inflammation can lower the pH of the affected tissue and limit formation of the free base. Ionic entrapment of the local anesthetic in the extracellular space not only delays the onset of local anesthesia but may preclude effective nerve blockade. Clinically, failure to obtain satisfactory pain relief in inflamed tissue is well documented.[11] (Other potential reasons for local anesthetic failure associated with tissue inflammation are discussed in Chapter 12.)

Because local anesthetics exist in both cationic and uncharged forms at tissue pH, the question arises as to which drug species is actually responsible for nerve blockade. Experiments involving intact nerve trunks have shown that anesthesia is enhanced in vitro by increasing the pH of the bathing medium.[12] Although this finding seemingly supports the notion that the nonionized base is the active form (alkalization favoring dissociation to the free base), additional studies utilizing desheathed nerve fibers have conclusively demonstrated that both forms are active and that most of the anesthetic effect is produced by the cationic species.[13] Alkalization merely improves the ability of the drug to reach its site of action within the axonal membrane.

Mechanism of Anesthesia

Local anesthetics block the sensation of pain by interfering with the propagation of peripheral nerve impulses. Both the generation and the conduction of action potentials are inhibited. Electrophysiologic data indicate that local anesthetics do not significantly alter the normal resting potential of the nerve membrane; instead, they impair certain dynamic responses to nerve stimulation.[14]

EFFECTS ON IONIC PERMEABILITY

The inactive nerve membrane is relatively impermeable to sodium (Na^+) ions. Excitation of the axolemma by an appropriate stimulus, however, will temporarily increase Na^+ conductance and cause the nerve cell to become less electronegative with respect to the outside. If the transmembrane potential is sufficiently depressed, a critical threshold is reached at which the depolarization becomes self-generating. A marked increase in Na^+ permeability induces a rapid influx of Na^+ through Na^+-selective channels traversing the nerve membrane. The inward Na^+ current creates an action potential of approximately $+40$ mV, which is then propagated down the nerve. The action potential is quite transient at any given segment of membrane; inactivation of Na^+ permeability (closure of the

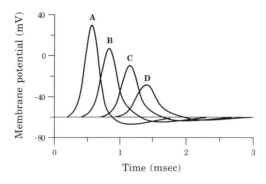

Figure 2–3.   Onset of local anesthetic block in a single axon. **A**, control action potential. **B**, beginning of local anesthetic block. Enough sodium channels are blocked to cause a fall in the amplitude of the action potential and a slowing in the rate of conduction in the area of local anesthetic exposure. **C**, progressive decline in the rate of depolarization and the height of the action potential. **D**, cessation of axonal conduction. Enough channels are blocked that electrotonic depolarization of the adjacent, drug-free membrane is insufficient to generate a self-replicating action potential.

Na$^+$ channels) and, in unmyelinated nerve, an outward flow of potassium (K$^+$) quickly repolarize the membrane. (See Chapter 1 for a more comprehensive review of nerve transmission.)

Local anesthetics interfere with nerve conduction by blocking the influence of stimulation on Na$^+$ permeability. A developing local anesthetic block is characterized by a progressive reduction in the rate and extent of depolarization and a slowing of conduction (Fig. 2–3). Since the onset and rate of repolarization are not greatly affected by local anesthetics, the safety factor for transmission decreases. When depolarization is retarded such that repolarization processes develop before the threshold potential can be reached, nerve conduction fails.

THEORIES OF NERVE BLOCKADE

Several theories have been advanced to account for the selective effects of local anesthetics on Na$^+$ permeability. These theories are not mutually exclusive, and it may be that a combination of drug actions contributes to regional anesthesia.

Specific Receptor Binding

Perhaps the most plausible and compelling theory of regional anesthesia asserts that local anesthetics abolish nerve conduction by binding to specific receptor sites on or within Na$^+$ channels. Considerable support for the specific receptor hypothesis has been obtained using structural analogues of conventional local anesthetics. For example, the specificity of receptor binding has been demonstrated by structure–activity testing in which components of the local anesthetic molecule are systematically

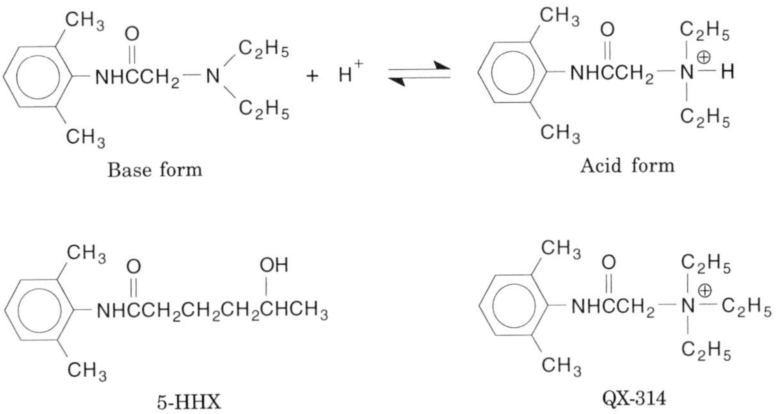

Figure 2–4. Structural formulas of lidocaine in its base and acid forms and of the corresponding neutral and charged analogues 5-HHX and QX-314.

altered.[15,16] Although results indicate that considerable modifications of molecular structure can be accommodated without loss of anesthetic activity, sufficient specificity does exist to suggest that discrete binding sites are involved in regional anesthesia. Certain local anesthetics, such as mepivacaine and bupivacaine, have chiral carbon constituents and are marketed as racemic mixtures.[16,17] Up to tenfold differences in anesthetic potency between paired stereoisomers suggest a specific receptor locus for these drugs.

Analogues of local anesthetic cations have been particularly useful in identifying where the receptors may be situated. The experimental drug QX-314 is a quaternary ammonium derivative of lidocaine that always carries a positive charge (Fig. 2–4). External application of QX-314 to a nerve fiber has no effect on Na^+ conductance.[18] Upon internal infusion, however, the drug stabilizes the membrane as efficiently as does lidocaine. An interesting feature of the block produced by QX-314 is that repetitive stimulation of the nerve fiber dramatically enhances the development of anesthesia. These observations of a *use-* or *frequency-dependent block*, also known as a *phasic block,* suggest that the site of action of local anesthetics is accessible to hydrophilic cations only from the axoplasmic side of the membrane and then only when Na^+ channels are in the open state.*[19] Benzocaine, a procaine derivative without an amino terminus (Fig. 2–1), 5-HHX, a nonelectrolyte derivative of lidocaine, and conventional local anesthetics in the free base form may bind to the same receptor, but they do not exhibit the same marked dependence on nerve

* *Follow-up studies have shown that charged molecules can also reach the receptor when the channel is partially activated, as represented by the closed$_1$, closed$_2$, and closed$_3$ states (described in Chapter 1).[18] Thus, partial depolarizations of the membrane insufficient to open Na^+ channels completely nevertheless increase local anesthetic blockade.*

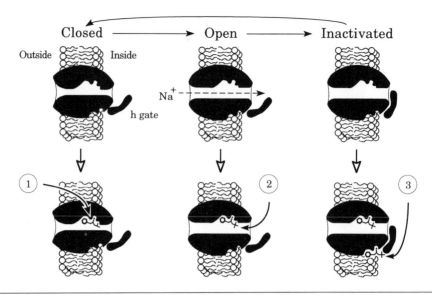

Figure 2–5.   Specific receptor theory of anesthesia. The top row illustrates the major transformations of the sodium channel during an action potential; the bottom row depicts the binding of local anesthetics to specific channel receptors. *1*, uncharged anesthetic molecules can reach the active site within the channel through a hydrophobic route and may therefore bind to open or closed channels. *2*, local anesthetic cations are restricted to a hydrophilic pathway and therefore depend on channel activation for exposing the receptor to the drug. *3*, inactivation traps charged local anesthetics within the channel. Also shown is the possibility that the binding site may be exterior to the pore itself.

stimulation. Being lipid soluble, these nonionized drugs can reach the receptor through hydrophobic pathways. They are not constrained to migrate only into the activated Na^+ channel. Figure 2–5 represents the blockade of a Na^+ channel by a local anesthetic.

What are the consequences of local anesthetic binding to or within the channel? One possibility is a physical obstruction of the channel itself. Local anesthetics, approximately 15 Å in length, are seemingly large enough to block the pore of the open Na^+ channel, which at its most constricted point is probably only 3 by 5 Å in cross section.[20] However, measurements of Na^+ channel gating currents (see Chapter 1) indicate that local anesthetics prevent the Na^+ channel from opening in response to a depolarizing current. Figure 2–6 depicts the Na^+ flow and the gating currents before and after the administration of benzocaine.[21] Inhibition of the conformational changes that underlie the activation gating current (e.g., outward extrusion of the positively charged S4 segments of the channel) parallels the reduction in Na^+ entry. (A corresponding reduction in the gating current–associated return of Na^+ channels to the resting state is also evident.) Therefore, physical obstruction of the pore is probably irrelevant to the blocking action of benzocaine. With procaine and other local anesthetic agents, Na^+ conductance is reduced more than the gating currents,[18] and physical occlusion may play a secondary role in

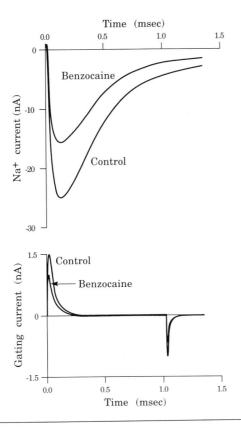

Figure 2–6.   Parallel inhibition of sodium influx (Na^+ current) and the channel gating current by 1 mM benzocaine in myelinated frog axons. *Top*, Na^+ current measured in a single node of Ranvier voltage-clamped at −32 mV and then depolarized to +100 mV. Benzocaine reduced the Na^+ influx to 64% of control. *Bottom*, gating currents recorded from a single node of a different axon (same stimulus parameters, 1 msec depolarization). Charge displacement across the membrane was reduced to 66% of control for the ''on'' current (outward movement of fixed membrane charges during channel activation, as described in Chapter 1) and to 67% for the ''off'' current (inward movement of charges at 1 msec, associated with return of channels to the resting state). The smaller off current, irrespective of benzocaine, indicates that many channels remain inactivated after return of the membrane potential to −32 mV. (Adapted from Neumcke, B., Schwarz, W., and Stämpfli, R.: Pflugers Arch., *390*:230–236, 1981.)

blocking nerve conduction. Alternatively, procaine-like drugs may prevent only a specific portion of the activation process, thus leaving some of the gating currents intact. They may also restrict Na^+ influx independently of effects on channel activation by distorting the local electrical field and/or by causing a conformational change in the pore.

It is not known where local anesthetics bind to produce channel blockade. Most[18,22] but not all[23] data are consistent with a single site per channel for conventional local anesthetic molecules. This site provides hydrophobic interactions with the aromatic moiety and with alkyl groups on the amino terminus and in the intermediate chain.[16] An ionic component to binding for charged anesthetic molecules is evident from the ability of externally applied Na^+ to inhibit receptor binding.[22,24]

Membrane Interaction

The membrane interaction theory holds that local anesthetics associate nonspecifically with hydrophobic constituents of the axolemma to prevent the conformational transformations of the Na^+ channel that subserve nerve transmission. As illustrated in Figure 2–7, one variant of this hypothesis focuses on the ability of anesthetic molecules to disorder or "fluidize" membrane lipids.[25] The resultant loss of lateral compressibility effectively prohibits activation of Na^+ channels.

A considerable body of evidence supports the notion that local anesthetics, both the neutral and charged forms, interact with phospholipid constituents of the nerve membrane.[18,26] Charged local anesthetics tend to concentrate on or near the outermost layer of the membrane, where the quaternary amino group can interact with fixed negative charges on the membrane surface, and the ester or amide linkage with the high-

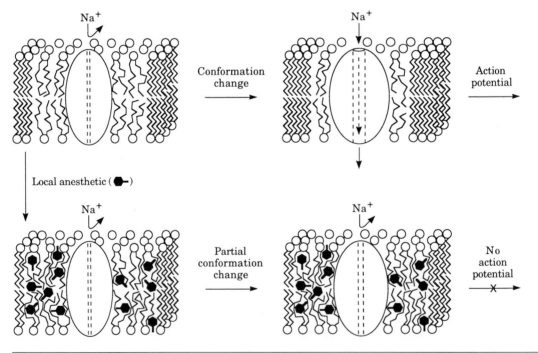

Figure 2–7.   Membrane fluidization theory of anesthesia. **A.** Sodium channel in the closed position. **B.** Sodium channel in the open position, allowing the influx of ions. **C.** Absorption of local anesthetic by the membrane, causing fluidization of the membrane lipids or disorganization of the channel–membrane interface. **D.** Inability of the sodium channel to open in response to membrane depolarization because of a reduction in the lateral compressibility of the membrane. (Adapted from Trudell, J.R.: Anesthesiology, *46*:5–10, 1977.)

dipole region of the membrane. Local anesthetic molecules without a formal charge are able to penetrate into the nonpolar interior of the membrane.

Local anesthetics such as procaine and lidocaine have been shown to disorder the nerve membrane.[27,28] In clinically achievable concentrations, local anesthetics are also known to influence the action of membrane proteins other than Na^+ channels: K^+ channels, calcium (Ca^{2+}) channels, nicotinic and muscarinic receptors, adenylate and guanylate cyclase enzymes, adenosine triphosphatases, calmodulin-dependent proteins, and phospholipases A_2 and C.[18,28-31] The breadth of these activities is best explained by a single fundamental action on the membrane, such as fluidization.* On the other hand, the stereospecific block of some local anesthetics (especially as seen in Na^+ channels activated by batrachotoxin, a potent toxin produced by the Colombian frog *Phyllobates aurotaenia*[22]) cannot be readily explained by nonspecific membrane interactions, nor can major aspects of use-dependent block, such as its strong dependence on molecular weight and specific structural features of the local anesthetic.[10,32] Because the specific receptor and membrane interaction hypotheses are not mutually exclusive, it is quite possible that both activities may contribute to the overall pharmacology of local anesthetics.

Lastly, it should be mentioned that a highly unusual feature of the Na^+ channel is its acylation with up to 50 molecules of mostly saturated fatty acids.[33] Inasmuch as the orientation of these acyl residues is dependent on the tertiary structure of the Na^+ channel, the possibility of stereospecific interactions between these fatty acids and local anesthetics is enhanced. In addition to stabilizing the channel within the nerve membrane, they may help regulate gating functions of the channel. Thus, local anesthetics diffusing into this region could produce nonreceptor-mediated channel-blocking effects independently of their actions on the bulk membrane.

TONIC AND USE-DEPENDENT BLOCK

Inhibition of Na^+ channels by local anesthetics has two components: a tonic element independent of neuronal activity and a use-dependent or phasic block correlated with the frequency of depolarization (Fig. 2–8).[32] With infrequent stimulation of a nerve exposed to a local anesthetic, a stable inhibition of Na^+ flux is observed relative to the anesthetic concen-

---

* The membrane interaction theory can also be applied to numerous unrelated inhibitors of nerve conduction. It is especially attractive regarding general depressants of the central nervous system (inhalation anesthetics, alcohols, etc.) and topical anodynes present in some dental salves (e.g., chlorobutanol), agents whose similarity of pharmacological effect belies marked dissimilarities in molecular structure. The emphasis that this hypothesis places on nonspecific hydrophobic interactions embodies the fact that the anesthetic potency of these various drugs is largely controlled by the membrane:buffer partition coefficient.

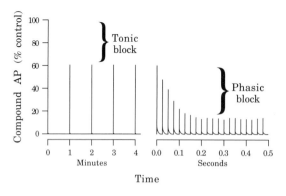

Figure 2–8.   Influence of stimulation frequency on nerve block by 1 mM lidocaine. *Left,* at very low rates of stimulation (e.g., 0.016 Hz), a basal, or tonic, inhibition of the compound action potential is observed. *Right,* with stimulation at relatively high rates (e.g., 40 Hz), an additional frequency-dependent, or phasic, block occurs. Return to low-frequency stimulation releases the nerve from phasic block (not shown). (Adapted from Bokesch, P.M., Post, C., and Strichartz, G.: J. Pharmacol. Exp. Ther., *237*:773–781, 1986. © William & Wilkins, 1986.)

tration. This tonic block arises from the local anesthetic interacting with resting Na^+ channels through a hydrophobic pathway. During repeated stimulation, an additional, transient depression of Na^+ flux occurs. Minimal with benzocaine irrespective of pH and with lidocaine-like anesthetics exposed to an alkaline external pH, this phasic increment predominates with positively charged drugs such as QX-314 and with lidocaine-like drugs in an acidic external environment. As was discussed earlier, charged drugs require channel activation to reach their site of action. However, phasic block is more complicated than a simple issue of receptor access. It also involves increased binding to channel configurations other than the resting state.[14,18] Increased binding may arise because local anesthetics have greater affinity for one or more of these configurations or because the drugs become physically trapped and unable to diffuse away from the site of action. In either case, the result is an increased proportion of Na^+ channels blocked by the local anesthetic. Cessation of repeated stimulation allows the membrane channels to return to the resting state, resulting in decreased local anesthetic binding and recovery from phasic block.

    Several factors besides the degree of protonation influence phasic block. In contrast to tonic inhibition, extremes of hydrophobicity (both high and low) increase potency of phasic block.[10,32] Phasic block is also greatly influenced by molecular size and shape. Large, bulky anesthetics such as bupivacaine (see Fig. 2–1) exert significant use-dependent inhibition at low frequencies of stimulation (e.g., 0.5 Hz), whereas smaller, more flexible drugs, such as lidocaine, require higher frequencies (more than 2 Hz) for phasic block to develop. These associations suggest that the binding site for local anesthetics is a narrow pocket surrounded by a

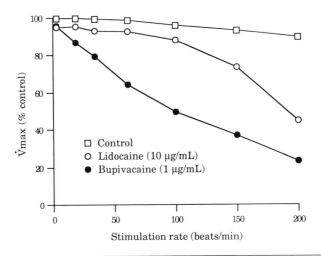

Figure 2–9.   Influence of local anesthetics and heart rate on the maximum upstroke velocity ($\dot{V}$max) in guinea pig papillary muscle. A small tonic block at 3 beats/min is observed for both lidocaine and bupivacaine. All values are normalized against the control $\dot{V}$max measured at 3 beats/min. (Adapted from Clarkson, C.W., and Hondeghem, L.M.: Anesthesiology, *62*:396–405, 1985.)

hydrophobic environment. Charged molecules exit this pocket through a passageway whose effective diameter is only about 7.2 Å. Table 2–2 lists the relative tendency of injectable local anesthetics to cause phasic nerve block.[10]

Use-dependent block has several important clinical implications. As noted below, a differential blockade of fibers carrying high frequencies of impulses can occur. Thus, sensations encoded in rapid bursts of nervous activity may be blocked preferentially to sensations causing lesser frequencies of stimulation. Of toxicologic significance is the tendency of bupivacaine and several other local anesthetics to block cardiac Na^+ channels at normal heart rates. Figure 2–9 illustrates the progressive phasic block that occurs as the stimulation of a heart papillary muscle exposed to bupivacaine is increased in frequency.[34] The maximum upstroke velocity of the action potential ($\dot{V}$max) is a measure of peak Na^+ conductance. The clinical sequellae of its depression are bradycardia and an increased risk of dysrhythmia. Lidocaine also causes a use-depressant block, but only at heart rates above normal. Therefore, lidocaine has clinical value as an antiarrhythmic agent for ventricular tachydysrhythmias.

DIFFERENTIAL NERVE BLOCK

Peripheral neurons vary according to fiber size and type in their susceptibility to local anesthetics.[35,36] Autonomic functions subserved by preganglionic B and postganglionic C fibers are more easily disrupted by local anesthetics than is motor function, which depends on large Aα and Aγ fibers. Sensory neurons are quite heterogeneous in size and therefore exhibit a wide range of sensitivity. Modalities listed in increasing order of resistance to conduction block include the sensations of dull pain, warmth, cold, sharp pain, touch, pressure, and proprioception. In general, the more susceptible a fiber is to a local anesthetic agent, the faster it is blocked and the longer it takes to recover.

These observations, most readily seen clinically after spinal and epidural anesthesia, should not be construed as proof that large myelinated axons are inherently more resistant to local anesthetics than are smaller fibers. Indeed, careful study of individual axons reveals that for both myelinated and unmyelinated nerves the minimum blocking concentration of a local anesthetic is independent of fiber diameter.[37,38] A ''differential block,'' in which small C and Aδ fibers are affected but larger fibers are not, can be obtained, but only when the length of compound nerve exposed to the drug is restricted and the local anesthetic concentration is within a set range. Differential sensitivities of fibers of unequal diameter result from variations in the ''critical length'' that must be exposed to a given concentration of local anesthetic for conduction to fail.[37]

In myelinated nerves, action potentials are propagated from one node of Ranvier to the next in saltatory fashion, with a safety factor such that three consecutive nodes must be completely blocked in order for impulse transmission to be interrupted. Because internodal distance is directly related to fiber diameter, it is understandable that small neurons appear to be more sensitive clinically than large fibers to conduction block. As a local anesthetic diffuses into the nerve trunk, it reaches an effective concentration over a length required to inhibit small axons before it spreads sufficiently to block large fibers. Anatomic barriers to diffusion, nonuniform distribution of drug, or the use of a minimal amount of local anesthetic may preclude some large axons from ever being affected. As local anesthesia fades, small neurons are the last to recover because circumscribed areas of drug concentrations adequate for their inhibition remain along the nerve after the more substantial areas required for large axons have broken up.

When the local anesthetic concentration is insufficient to completely block all Na$^+$ channels in three successive nodes, conduction may still fail if a longer chain of nodes is partially blocked.[39,40] A partially blocked node yields an action potential that is delayed in onset and reduced in size. The resulting electrotonic currents produce a weaker stimulus for the depolarization of adjacent nodes. If more than 70% of the Na$^+$ channels are blocked in successive nodes, the action potential will continue to degrade until it is no longer self-sustaining.[40] As shown in Figure 2–10, a differential block can then occur even if the length of nerve exposed to drug is 2 cm or more.

The critical length concept may also be applied to unmyelinated axons as a group. Here, the length constant of the neuron (λ), which is propor-

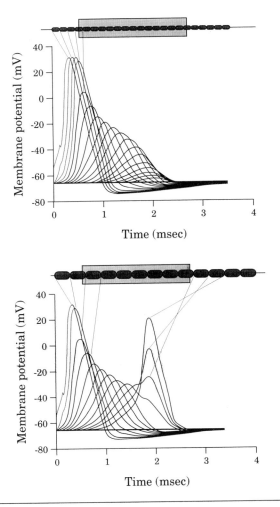

Figure 2–10. Decremental conduction and differential nerve block. *Top,* impulses arising from successive nodes of a small myelinated axon are plotted versus time. Exposure of 14 nodes to a specific concentration of local anesthetic causes conduction to fail. *Bottom,* identical exposure of an adjacent axon twice in size results in seven nodes being affected, an insufficient number to prevent conduction at this local anesthetic concentration.
(Adapted from Raymond, S.A., Thalhammer, J.G., and Strichartz, G.R. *In* Dimitrievic, M.R., ed.: Restorative Neurology: Altered Sensation and Pain. Basel, S. Karger, 1989.)

tional to the square root of the diameter of unmyelinated axons (reviewed in Chapter 1), determines the amount of nerve that must be exposed to a given concentration of local anesthetic in order to prevent electrotonic depolarizing currents from traversing the blocked region to excite the adjacent drug-free portion of the fiber.

In addition to critical length, fiber type and the pattern of impulse traffic normally carried in situ by these different axons may contribute to differential nerve block. When critical length is removed as a controlling influence, unmyelinated axons appear to be somewhat more resistant to local anesthetics than myelinated fibers.[38] A possible explanation for this difference is the role played by K^+ channels during the recovery phase of the action potential in C fibers. Partial inhibition of K^+ channels by the local anesthetic would inhibit repolarization and help sustain depolarizing electrotonic currents in unmyelinated axons. Because myelinated fibers do not rely on K^+ efflux for repolarization, they would be more readily blocked.

As previously discussed, local anesthetics inhibit high-frequency trains of impulses more readily than they do single action potentials. Noxious stimuli and sympathetic nervous system transmission, both of which are encoded in rapid bursts of impulses, are particularly susceptible to local anesthetics. Motor function, however, usually involves low-frequency discharges and is relatively resistant to drug interference.

Systemic Effects

Although primarily used to depress peripheral nerve conduction, local anesthetics can prevent the propagation of action potentials in any excitable tissue. Most prominent of the systemic effects of local anesthetics are those associated with the cardiovascular and central nervous systems, but virtually any organ dependent on nervous or muscular activity may be affected. Local anesthetics may also influence a variety of tissues through actions unrelated to disturbances in Na^+ conductance. (Systemic effects that are associated with specific drugs and not common to other local anesthetics are described in Chapter 4.)

CENTRAL NERVOUS SYSTEM

Local anesthetics easily pass from the peripheral circulation into the brain. Because central nervous system (CNS) activity is particularly sensitive to local anesthetics, blood concentrations incapable of altering axonal conduction peripherally may profoundly influence CNS function (Table 2–3). In general, the concentrations of local anesthetics required to elicit CNS effects are inversely proportional to their anesthetic potencies.

Local anesthetics are especially adept at interfering with nervous transmission across synapses. In addition to blocking Na^+ channels, local anesthetics may inhibit the ability of postsynaptic membrane receptors to respond effectively to their neurotransmitters. Inhibition of Ca^{2+} channels and calmodulin-dependent events can decrease the ability of presynaptic depolarization to cause neurotransmitter release. At synapses with low safety factors for transmission, even modest inhibition of one or more of these several processes may lead to effective blockade.[18,31]

Table 2–3. **EFFECTS OF LIDOCAINE ON THE CENTRAL NERVOUS SYSTEM (CNS) AND CARDIOVASCULAR SYSTEM (CVS)**

Concentration (μg/mL)	CNS Effect*	CVS Effect*
<5	Anticonvulsant activity Mild sedation Analgesia	Antiarrhythmic activity Mild increases in mean blood pressure and peripheral vascular resistance and decrease in stroke volume Mild increase in heart rate
5–10	Light-headedness, slurred speech, drowsiness, euphoria Nausea, dysphoria, sensory disturbances, diplopia, muscle twitching	
10–15	Disorientation Uncontrollable tremors Respiratory depression Unconsciousness Tonic-clonic seizures	Cardiovascular instability
15–20	Coma Respiratory arrest	
>20		Profound myocardial depression, vasodilation Cardiovascular collapse

* CNS and CVS effects are listed in approximate order of occurrence with increasing blood concentration.

Psychomotor testing indicates that CNS effects occur with plasma concentrations that are easily achieved during oral surgery. For lidocaine, a concentration of approximately 1.0 μg/mL improved mean performance on the digit symbol substitution test* even as subjects reported feeling mildly drowsy.[41] Increasing the concentration to about 1.8 μg/mL led to a sharper, transient decrease in psychomotor performance and heightened reports of somnolence. For comparison, a mean venous serum concentration of 1.15 μg/kg was measured 7 minutes after completion of injections for the surgical removal of third molars (mean dose of 3.16 mg/kg; lidocaine administered as a 2% solution with 1:100,000 epinephrine).[42] Other effects observed with subtoxic concentrations of local anesthetics include anticonvulsant activity and analgesia.[43]

Initial signs and symptoms of a CNS toxic effect are usually excitatory in nature and include light-headedness and dizziness, followed by visual

* While improved performance may seem paradoxical in this setting, antianxiety drugs at doses producing mild sedation yield similar outcomes.

and auditory disturbances, apprehension, disorientation, and localized involuntary muscular activity. Depressant responses such as slurred speech, drowsiness, and unconsciousness may also occur and are especially prominent with certain drugs (e.g., lidocaine). As higher blood concentrations of drug are attained, muscle fasciculations and tremors intensify and develop into generalized tonic-clonic convulsions. On termination, seizure activity is often succeeded by a state of CNS depression identical to general anesthesia. With excessively large doses, respiratory impairment becomes manifest; if untreated, death may ensue.

The CNS excitation sometimes observed after local anesthesia is intriguing, since the sole action ascribed to these agents is depression. Indeed, studies involving topical application of local anesthetics to exposed cortical or spinal cord neurons document that the only direct effect of procaine and related drugs is to inhibit electrical activity.[44] The apparent stimulation observed clinically is best explained on the basis that inhibitory cortical neuron synapses are highly susceptible to transmission block. Initial marked disruption of these pathways disinhibits excitatory neurons, which presents clinically as stimulation.

Local anesthetic seizures appear to arise from disinhibition of the amygdala, a core component of the limbic system that is associated with olfactory input to the brain and with autonomic and behavioral arousal.[45] Electrical activity recorded from the amygdala as lidocaine is slowly infused intravenously in the cat mirrors the sequential sensory and behavioral patterns described above: sedation, excitation, depression, and seizure activity.[46] The sedative phase, which in cats manifests as a cessation of movement, correlates with high-voltage spindles in the amygdala synchronized with respiratory efforts. Concurrent cortical and reticular formation activity is depressed. Excitation, characterized in cats by vocalization, pupillary dilation, and incontinence, is linked to low-voltage spindles in the amygdala. A loss of spindling heralds the late depressive phase, in which cats do not respond to external stimuli and are generally quiescent but swing the head in a stereotypic fashion. The sudden appearance of high-voltage spike trains in the amygdala and throughout the brain marks the onset of tonic-clonic convulsions. With increased infusion rates, preseizure CNS depression becomes less evident. IV bolus injections may lead almost immediately to seizures.

CARDIOVASCULAR SYSTEM

Local anesthetics can exert a variety of effects on the cardiovascular system. Some influences are beneficial therapeutically and serve as a basis for the use of selected agents to treat cardiac arrhythmias; others are not and merely serve to accentuate systemic toxicity.

At nontoxic concentrations, local anesthetics differ somewhat in their electrophysiologic influences on the heart. Whereas lidocaine shortens the action potential duration and the effective refractory period in ventricular tissues, procaine prolongs them. Both drugs, however, increase the effective refractory period relative to the action potential duration, slow conduction velocity, and decrease cardiac automaticity, especially in ectopic pacemakers. These effects are caused by inhibition of myocardial Na^+ conductance.

Hemodynamically, lidocaine in low concentrations causes a modest increase in peripheral vascular resistance and an even smaller increase in mean blood pressure.[47,48] Concurrent with these changes is a decline in the stroke volume (Fig. 2–11). Presumably through their disruption of normal Ca^{2+} metabolism, local anesthetics produce a dose-dependent decrease in myocardial contractility.[49] In response to the negative inotropism (mild at these concentrations) and/or to a local anesthetic-induced depression of baroreceptor input into the CNS, sympathetic nervous system reflexes are activated to support the circulation. Epinephrine and norepinephrine secretion is stimulated,[48] which helps to maintain the cardiac output and, in the case of norepinephrine secreted by sympathetic neurons, to increase peripheral vascular resistance. Lidocaine may also induce vasoconstriction through a direct myogenic effect on vascular smooth muscle.[50] Finally, a centrally mediated disinhibition of sympathetic nervous activity is still another source for the increase in peripheral vascular resistance.[51] Modest cardiovascular effects have also been reported for subconvulsive doses of mepivacaine and bupivacaine. Mepivacaine apparently elicits a different mix of responses, however, since it is more likely to increase both heart rate and cardiac output and to lower peripheral vascular resistance.[52]

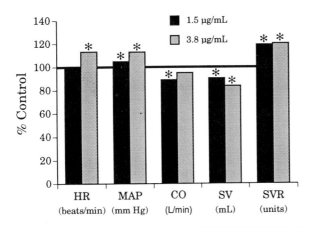

Figure 2–11. Effect of intravenous lidocaine (1.5 and 3.8 μg/mL) on cardiovascular parameters. Asterisks (*) indicate significant differences from preinjection control values. The fall in cardiac output with 1.5 μg/mL was not significantly different from the 4% decrease measured in control patients not receiving lidocaine. (Data from Klein, S.W., Sutherland, R.I.L., and Morch, J.E.: Can. Med. Assoc. J., *99*:472–475, 1968; and Duranteau, J., Pussard, E., et al.: Cardiovasc. Pharmacol., *18*:60–67, 1991.)

Local anesthetic concentrations causing CNS excitation result in tachycardia, hypertension, and increased cardiac output, all of which reflect central sympathetic nervous system arousal. With still higher concentrations and pronounced CNS depression, the direct depressant effects of the local anesthetic are exposed. Peripheral resistance falls as contraction of vascular smooth muscle is impaired directly and as sympathetic nervous system function is interrupted. Membrane excitability and conduction velocity are reduced throughout the heart. Sinus bradycardia and impairment of myocardial contractility contribute to a significant reduction in cardiac output. These effects are magnified by hypoxia, hypercarbia, and hyperkalemia—all possible outcomes of uncontrolled seizures. Even if respiration is supported artificially, circulatory collapse will eventually ensue after excessively large doses.

Strongly hydrophobic local anesthetics exert disproportionate effects on the heart. The clinical significance of this issue was raised by Albright, who noted a pattern of sudden cardiovascular collapse, presumably after accidental intravascular injection of standard doses of bupivacaine or etidocaine.[53] Subsequent research has verified this enhanced cardiotoxicity and suggested several mechanisms by which it occurs.

Table 2–4 lists the relative doses and blood concentrations of local anesthetics infused intravenously that cause convulsions and cardiovascular system collapse in sheep.[54,55] Because the CNS toxicities of the drugs are proportional to their anesthetic potencies, the lower cardiovascular system/CNS ratios for bupivacaine and etidocaine indicate disproportionate cardiotoxicity. Most evidence suggests that cardiac contractility is not unusually depressed by these two drugs.[56] They do appear, however, to trigger ventricular tachycardia and ventricular fibrillation under conditions in which lidocaine and mepivacaine do not. As discussed previously, the propensity of bupivacaine to cause use-dependent block and pronounced disruption of cardiac electrophysiology may play a pivotal role permitting life-threatening dysrhythmias to arise.[34] It has also been suggested that inhibition of myocardial metabolism[57] and disruption of CNS regulation of cardiac function[58,59] may be involved. A factor

Table 2–4. **COMPARATIVE TOXICITIES OF AMIDE LOCAL ANESTHETICS IN SHEEP***

Drug	*CVS/CNS Dose Ratio*	*CVS/CNS Conc. Ratio*
Lidocaine	7.1 ± 1.1	3.6 ± 0.3
Bupivacaine	3.7 ± 0.5	1.6 ± 0.1
Etidocaine	4.4 ± 0.9	1.7 ± 0.2

* The CVS/CNS dose ratio is the dose causing cardiovascular collapse/dose causing seizures. The CVS/CNS concentration ratio is the blood concentration of local anesthetic at the time of cardiovascular collapse/blood concentration at the time of seizure onset. Values represent means ± standard error.
Data from Morishima, et al.[54,55]

contributing to cardiovascular collapse coincident with seizures is the exaggerated effect hypoxia, hypercarbia, and acidosis have on bupivacaine toxicity. The chances for ventricular fibrillation are greatly increased, as both heart rate and myocardial contractility are profoundly depressed.[60,61] Because of bupivacaine's tendency to become sequestered in tissues and produce prolonged effects, resuscitative efforts are rendered more complicated and the results less predictable.

A final consideration of the cardiovascular influences of local anesthetics is their influence on the local circulation. The effects of local anesthetics on discrete vascular beds are varied and complex.[62] In the area of injection, vasodilation predominates. The high concentration of drug directly inhibits myogenic tone in vascular smooth muscle and blocks sympathetic nervous system activity in the area. Local anesthetics listed in approximate order of vasodilatory potential (highest to lowest) include etidocaine, bupivacaine, procaine, lidocaine, prilocaine, mepivacaine, and cocaine.[62,63] Adjacent tissues may show either vasodilation or vasoconstriction, depending on the local anesthetic and the vasomotor tone. For example, thermograms of the face after 1-mL injections over the maxillary canine show evidence of vasoconstriction in the overlying skin when 3% mepivacaine is used, no change in the local circulation with 4% prilocaine, and increasing vasodilation with 2% lidocaine and 2% procaine.[63] Even local anesthetics that produce vasoconstriction in vascular beds at rest cause vasodilation when the blood vessels are under tonic vasoconstrictive influences.

Injection of local anesthetics directly into a blood vessel, as may occur by accident clinically, is more likely to cause vasoconstriction than is injection into the surrounding tissues. Veins are more likely to contract than are arteries. Because of striking differences in sensitivity to various local anesthetics, no other generalizations can be made regarding the local effects of intravascular injection. For example, in the maxillofacial circulation of the rat, lidocaine causes substantial vasoconstriction.[64] No discernible effect occurs in humans after intraarterial injection in the forearm,[65] however, and umbilical arteries yield a dose-dependent relaxation.[66] Because both prilocaine and bupivacaine evoke contractile responses in the umbilical artery, paracervical block with these drugs during childbirth may carry an extra hazard to the fetus.

MISCELLANEOUS EFFECTS

Aside from their influences on cardiovascular and CNS function, local anesthetics in concentrations compatible with life exert few systemic effects. Transmission at the neuromuscular junction and at autonomic ganglia may be affected, but intraarterial administration is usually required for these effects to be observed clinically. A variety of nonvascular smooth muscle actions have also been reported, the clinical significance of which remains obscure, at least for dentistry.

In tissue culture, local anesthetics are capable of disrupting numerous cellular functions: locomotion, endocytosis, exocytosis, axonal transport, cell fusion, and maintenance of normal morphology. These effects have been ascribed to a disconnection of the cytoskeleton (microtubule and microfilament assemblies) from the cell membrane.[67,68] While their therapeutic and toxicologic implications have not been fully explored, several intriguing possibilities for clinical use are emerging. For instance, inhibition of platelet aggregation may help explain why epidural anesthesia is associated with a lower than normal incidence of thromboembolism after major hip surgery.[69]

The ability of local anesthetics in concentrations achievable locally to block locomotion and exocytosis may contribute to enhanced wound healing. Depression of leukocyte function, including decreased migration, superoxide generation, and lysosomal degranulation, has been documented in animals.[70] Additional antiinflammatory effects include inhibition of the synthesis and/or release of interleukins, leukotrienes, prostaglandins, thromboxane, and substance P. One of the first intentional uses of the antiinflammatory property of local anesthetics in humans was the intravenous administration of lidocaine in the treatment of postoperative paralytic ileus. Continuous infusion during the first day after abdominal surgery reduced the duration of bowel paralysis and the need for opioid analgesics.[71]

Although inhibition of inflammation can predispose damaged tissue to infection, the microbicidal action of local anesthetics may negate this concern. Topical application of a commercially available 5% lidocaine liquid is rapidly cidal to bacterial species found in the oral cavity.[72]

A final pharmacologic effect deserving review is the ability of local anesthetics to inhibit peripheral nerve function after systemic administration. Circumoral numbness associated with large but subconvulsive concentrations of local anesthetics may reflect direct inhibition of sensitive sensory neurons.

As early as the 1940s, local anesthetics were administered intravenously for the relief of pain from various chronic conditions. Although the availability of safer, more effective drugs and approaches for this purpose has largely led to abandonment of the technique, interest has resurfaced regarding the infusion of lidocaine for the treatment of neuropathic pain. Damage to peripheral nerve fibers can lead to spontaneous depolarizations of nociceptive nerve endings.[73] Local anesthetics causing use-dependent block of high-frequency discharges successfully relieved pain in patients after nonsteroidal antiinflammatory drugs, opioid analgesics, and tricyclic antidepressants had failed.[74] Local anesthetics have also been used to terminate persistent coughing caused by bronchoscopy and resultant irritation of the respiratory tract.[75] Finally, local anesthetics have been infused for postoperative analgesia and as adjunctive agents for general anesthesia. Especially in these latter uses, CNS activity plays an increasingly significant role.

Absorption, Fate, and Excretion

Pharmacokinetic considerations regarding local anesthetics are vital, since the balance between a local anesthetic's uptake into the systemic circulation and its removal through redistribution, metabolism, and excretion determines in large measure the drug's toxic potential. These processes are graphically represented in Figure 2–12.

LOCAL DISTRIBUTION

Immediately after a local anesthetic is injected, it begins to spread through the local tissues. Early on, hydrostatic pressure governs this distribution. The solution simply courses down the paths of least resistance. Various hard and soft tissue barriers cause a nonuniform spread; if present, the nerve sheath prevents the anesthetic from gaining quick access to the axons encased within. With specific injection techniques, the normal physical barriers to distribution may be circumvented by bulk flow of the anesthetic into the local circulation. In dentistry, the nearly instantaneous onset of pulpal anesthesia after periodontal ligament injection may be a good example of this[76]; in medicine, the Bier block produces anesthesia by the intentional injection of anesthetic into the venous system of a limb isolated from the central circulation by a tourniquet.

Gravity and therefore body position may potentially influence the dispersion of a local anesthetic if the solution has a density different from the surrounding aqueous environment. This factor strongly governs spinal anesthesia and is of some clinical importance with epidural anesthesia. However, there is no objective evidence that manipulating patient

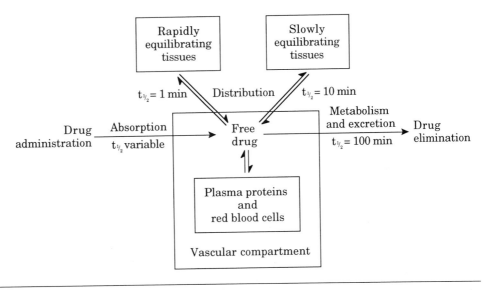

Figure 2–12.   Absorption, distribution, and fate of local anesthetics. Distribution and elimination half-times ($t_{1/2}$) are given in minutes for lidocaine.

position directly influences the success of peripheral nerve blocks, including those used in dentistry.

Once the anesthetic agent has reached the nerve target, diffusion takes over as the driving force for distribution. The perineurium constitutes the greatest barrier to diffusion, but all injectable local anesthetics are able to cross it within several minutes. Terminal nerve networks and free nerve endings, unencumbered by a nerve sheath, are affected within seconds of exposure. Diffusion into nonneural structures, including uptake by adipose tissue and binding to tissue proteins, reduces the concentration gradient for continued diffusion. Uptake by the microvasculature eventually reverses the direction of diffusion and removes the drug from the local tissues.

SYSTEMIC ABSORPTION AND DISTRIBUTION

The rate of absorption into the systemic circulation depends on numerous factors, including the dosage and pharmacologic profile of the drug employed, the presence of a vasoconstrictor agent, and the nature of the administration site. Obviously, the more drug that is injected, the higher its resultant blood concentration will be. Less obvious are the qualitative influences of the anesthetic solution and how these interact with the site of administration. Drugs with potent vasodilating properties, such as procaine and lidocaine, may significantly enhance their own uptake, particularly when injected into a highly vascular space. Inclusion of epineph-

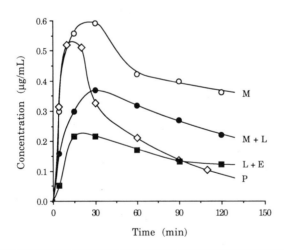

Figure 2–13.   Venous serum (plasma for prilocaine) concentrations of local anesthetics after intraoral injection. M = 1.8 mL 3% mepivacaine HCl (54 mg); M + L = 1.8 mL 2% mepivacaine HCl (36 mg) with 1:20,000 levonordefrin; L + E = 1.8 mL 2% lidocaine HCl (36 mg) with 1:100,000 epinephrine; P = 2 mL 4% prilocaine HCl (80 mg). (Data from Goebel, W., Allen, G., and Randall, F.: Anesth. Prog., 25:52–56, 1978; Goebel, W., Allen, G., and Randall, F.: Anesth. Prog., 26:93–97, 1979; and Cannell, H., and Whelpton, R.: Br. Dent. J., 160:47–49, 1986.)

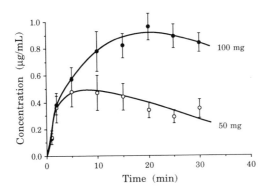

Figure 2–14.   Venous plasma concentrations of lidocaine after aerosol spray of the trachea and lar-
ynx. *Solid circles* represent a dose of 100 mg, *open circles* 50 mg. Bars indicate standard errors. (Data from Scott, D.B., Littlewood, D.G., et al.: Br. J. Anaesth., *48*:899–
902, 1976.)

rine or another vasoconstrictor is especially important in these instances
(as discussed in Chapter 3). Drugs that are not strong vasodilators, such
as mepivacaine and prilocaine, do not markedly accentuate their own
absorption and do not require as much vasoconstrictor to retard uptake.
Etidocaine and other extremely lipid-soluble agents may limit absorption
by being strongly sequestered within the injected tissues.

Figure 2–13 depicts the venous concentrations of standard local anesthetic formulations used in dentistry as a function of time after intraoral
injection.[77-79] In each case, the injection of a single cartridge resulted in
concentrations below those that cause systemic effects.

Absorption after topical application varies widely. Although intact skin
and oral epithelium are relatively impermeable to local anesthetics, these
drugs are readily absorbed from most mucosal surfaces. Instillation of
tetracaine into the piriform fossa, for instance, results in a peak plasma
concentration one-third to one-half that obtained after rapid intravenous
infusion.[80] By comparison, absorption of lidocaine from the tracheobron-
chial tree is much slower, roughly comparable to that associated with
intraoral injection (Fig. 2–14).[81] Regardless of the site of application,
sympathomimetic agents are ineffective topically in delaying absorption.
Uptake may be minimized, however, by using local anesthetics prepared
in the form of an ointment or gel instead of an aqueous spray.

On entering the circulation, a local anesthetic is partially bound by
plasma proteins and red blood cells. Figure 2–15 portrays the plasma
protein binding of several amide anesthetics.[82,83] In general, the more
lipophilic agents are more heavily bound. This relationship indicates a
hydrophobic component to the acceptor sites. In addition, bupivacaine
and mepivacaine, each with a cyclic amino terminus, are more strongly
bound than noncyclic tertiary amines of similar lipophilicity. Prilocaine,
a secondary amine with an octanol:buffer distribution coefficient slightly

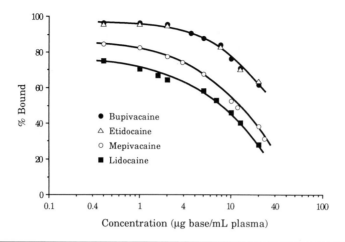

Figure 2–15.   Plasma protein binding of amide local anesthetics as a function of total plasma concentration of drug. (Redrawn with permission from Tucker, G.T., and Mather, L.E.: Br. J. Anesth., *47*:213–224, 1975.)

greater than that of mepivacaine, has the lowest binding (55% in normal plasma concentrations).[84]

Also represented in Figure 2–15 is the fact that the percentage of binding falls as the drug concentration increases, gradually at first and more quickly at high concentrations. Inasmuch as the free drug in the

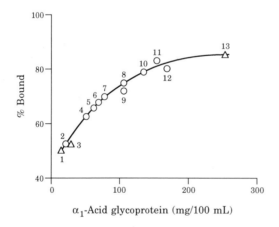

Figure 2–16.   Plasma protein binding of lidocaine as a function of α_1-acid glycoprotein concentration. *Circles* are mean data from various groups; *triangles* are data for individual patients. *1,* patient with nephrotic syndrome; *2,* neonates; *3,* patient with carcinoma of the prostate receiving high-dose estrogen therapy; *4,* females on oral contraceptives; *5,* women under 40 years; *6,* men under 40 years; *7,* adults over 70 years; *8,* epileptic subjects; *9,* renal transplant patients; *10,* chronic renal failure patients; *11,* cancer patients; *12,* myocardial infarction patients; *13,* patient with myocardial infarction. (Redrawn with permission from Tucker, G.T., and Mather, L.E., *in* Cousins, M.J., and Bridenbaugh, P.O., eds.: Neural Blockade in Clinical Anesthesia and Management of Pain, 2nd ed. Philadelphia, J.B. Lippincott Co., 1988.)

plasma governs distribution into the brain, decremental binding results in a disproportionate entry of drug into the brain with increasing doses of highly bound drugs. For bupivacaine, a decrease in binding from 95% to 90% is synonymous with a doubling of the free concentration. With lidocaine, a similar drop (i.e., from 70% to 65%) results in a much smaller increase (12%) in unbound drug.

A globulin specifically identified as α_1-acid glycoprotein (AAG) is the primary plasma protein involved in local anesthetic binding. Albumin also binds local anesthetics, but it has less affinity for the drugs and normally accounts for a small fraction of the total binding. AAG is an acute-phase protein, which means its concentration increases significantly during periods of stress. Medical conditions that stimulate concentrations of AAG include heart attack, cancer, trauma, surgery, uremia, and chronic pain. (Fig. 2–16).[85] Conversely, neonates, pregnant women, women taking oral contraceptives, and patients receiving estrogen tend to exhibit lower AAG binding capacity.

Binding of local anesthetics to AAG is influenced by hypercarbia and acidosis.[86,87] For example (Fig. 2–17), a reduction in pH from 7.4 to 7.0 reduces the binding of 5 μg/mL lidocaine by one-third (from 51% to 35%). It is also possible that competition by other drugs for acceptor sites may interfere with local anesthetic binding[88]; however, no clinically important interactions of this kind have emerged.

Distribution between erythrocytes and plasma varies inversely with the octanol:buffer distribution coefficient. Blood/plasma ratios for amide anesthetics are as follows: prilocaine, 1.00; mepivacaine, 0.92; lidocaine, 0.84; bupivacaine, 0.73; and etidocaine, 0.58.[84]

After distribution throughout the intravascular space, the unbound drug is free to diffuse into the various organs of the body. Because redistribution is a major mechanism responsible for removing slowly metabolized drugs from the bloodstream, an anesthetic agent (e.g., prilo-

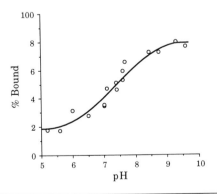

Figure 2–17.   Influence of pH on lidocaine binding to plasma proteins. Total plasma concentration = 5 μg/mL. (Data from Burney, R.G., DiFazio, C.A., and Foster, J.A.: Anesth. Analg., 57:478–480, 1978.)

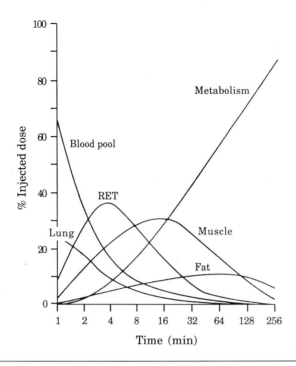

Figure 2–18.   Perfusion model simulation of the distribution of lidocaine in various tissues and its elimination from man following an intravenous infusion for 1 minute. Rapidly equilibrating tissues (RET) = brain, heart, liver, and kidneys. (Redrawn with permission from Benowitz, N., Forsyth, R.P., et al.: Clin. Pharmacol. Ther., *16*:87–98, 1974.)

caine) that leaves the circulation quickly to enter muscle and other tissues will enjoy a reduced toxicity. So-called barriers to diffusion are relatively ineffective against the local anesthetics. In addition to entering the CNS, these drugs readily cross the placenta and may occasionally induce severe cardiac depression in the fetus.

The lungs play an important role in buffering transient large concentrations that follow rapid intravascular injection. The most highly perfused organs of the body, the lungs can temporarily accept as much as 90% of a bolus injection of lidocaine.[89] The local anesthetic leaves the lungs via the pulmonary drainage over the next half minute, but peak concentrations in the coronary and carotid arteries are still reduced by as much as 70%.

By virtue of their own rich blood supplies, the brain, heart, liver, and kidneys are the next organs to reach steady state with the free plasma concentration of the local anesthetic. Subsequently, redistribution of anesthetic to the less well-perfused muscle and fat completes the distribution phase of drug disposition (Fig. 2–18).[90]

METABOLISM AND EXCRETION

The metabolic fate of a particular agent largely depends on the chemical linkage between the aromatic residue and the rest of the molecule. Ester drugs are inactivated by hydrolysis (Fig. 2–19). Derivatives of *p*-amino-

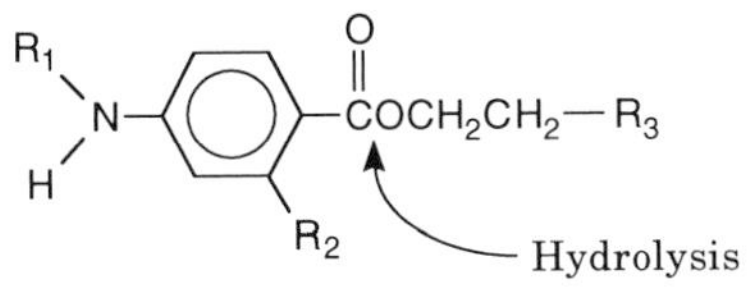

Figure 2–19. Metabolism of typical ester local anesthetics. Various constituent groups are indicated by $R_{(1-3)}$.

benzoic acid (e.g., procaine and tetracaine) are preferentially metabolized in the plasma by pseudocholinesterase; the ratio between plasma and liver hydrolysis with other esters is somewhat variable. Procaine is not a substrate for acetylcholinesterase, and very little drug is broken down in peripheral tissues. Products of hydrolytic cleavage may undergo further biotransformation in the liver before being ultimately eliminated in the urine. Less then 2% of an administered dose of procaine is excreted unchanged by the kidneys.

The rapid hydrolysis of the esters has complicated pharmacokinetic studies. The reported half-life for metabolism of procaine in the plasma is as low as 43 seconds,[84] although intravenous infusion of large doses yields a value of 7.7 minutes.[91]

Metabolism of amide drugs occurs primarily in the liver. The initial reaction is usually N-dealkylation of the tertiary amino terminus (Fig. 2–20). The resultant secondary amine of most amides is susceptible to hydrolysis by hepatic amidase activity, but conjugation, hydroxylation, or further dealkylation may also occur. Inactivation of prilocaine, a secondary amine, is relatively rapid because dealkylation is not required before hydrolysis can take place. Some metabolites retain significant pharmacologic activity and may contribute to drug toxicity. Much of the sedative effect of lidocaine, for example, has been attributed to its deethylated metabolites monoethylglycinexylidide and glycinexylidide.[92] As with ester compounds, small amounts (1% to 20%) of administered amides appear unmetabolized in the urine.

Table 2–5 lists pharmacokinetic parameters for amide anesthetics in humans.[83,93,94] The clearance rate of prilocaine, almost twice the liver blood flow of 1.5 L/min, indicates that extrahepatic metabolism (probably

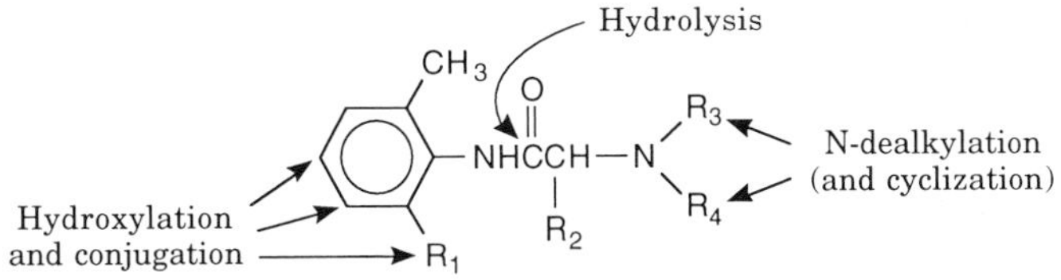

Figure 2–20. Metabolism of typical amide local anesthetics. Various constituent groups are indicated by $R_{(1-4)}$. The relative importance of the metabolic processes listed differs widely with these drugs.

Table 2-5. **PHARMACOKINETIC PARAMETERS OF AMIDE LOCAL ANESTHETICS IN HUMANS***

Drug	$t_{1/2}$ (min)	V_{Dss} (L)	Cl (L/min)
Lidocaine	96	91	0.95
Mepivacaine	114	84	0.78
Prilocaine	93	261	2.84
Bupivacaine	162	73	0.58
Etidocaine	162	133	1.11

* *Abbreviations:* $t_{1/2}$, *elimination half-time;* V_{Dss}, *volume of distribution at steady state; Cl, clearance rate. Data from Tucker and Mather[83,93] and Arthur et al.[94]*

pulmonary and/or renal) accounts for a significant fraction of the breakdown of that drug. Etidocaine and lidocaine, drugs that are metabolized only in the liver, are mostly cleared from the portal circulation in a single pass (hepatic extraction rates of 74% and 72%, respectively.)[84] Hepatic blood flow then becomes an important variable in the metabolism of these amides. Conditions such as congestive heart failure, hypotension, and cirrhosis of the liver have the potential for decreasing hepatic blood flow and retarding amide anesthetic metabolism.[95,96] On the other hand, eating a meal high in protein increases liver blood flow and lidocaine clearance by 20%.[97]

Details on the elimination of specific local anesthetics are provided in Chapter 4. Specific drugs and medical disorders that can significantly influence the disposition of local anesthetics are discussed in Chapter 5.

References

1. Robinson, V.: Victory over Pain. New York, Henry Schuman, 1946.
2. Liljestrand, G.: The historical development of local anesthesia. *In* Lechat, P., ed.: International Encyclopedia of Pharmacology and Therapeutics. Sect. 8. Local Anesthetics. Vol. 1. New York, Pergamon Press, 1971.
3. Fink, B.R.: Leaves and needles: The introduction of surgical local anesthesia. Anesthesiology, *63*:77–83, 1985.
4. Fink, B.R.: History of neural blockade. *In* Cousins, M.J., and Bridenbaugh, P.O., eds.: Neural Blockade in Clinical Anesthesia and Management of Pain, 2nd ed. Philadelphia, J.B. Lippincott Co., 1988.
5. Braun, H.: Ueber den Einfluss der Vitalität der Gewebe auf die ortlichen und allgemeinen Giftwerkungen Localanästhesirender Mittel und über die Bedeutung des Adrenalins für die Localanästhesie. Arch. Klin. Chirurg., *69*:541–587, 1903.
6. Hadda, S.E.: Procaine: Alfred Einhorn's ideal substitute for cocaine. J. Am. Dent. Assoc., *64*:841–845, 1962.
7. Dobbs, E.C.: A chronological history of local anesthesia in dentistry. J. Oral Ther. Pharmacol., *1*:546–549, 1965.

8. Strichartz, G.R., Sanchez, V., Arthur, G.R., Chafetz, R., and Martin, D.: Fundamental properties of local anesthetics: II. Measured octanol:buffer partition coefficients and pK_a values of clinically used drugs. Anesth. Analg., *71*:158–170, 1990.

9. Covino, B.G.: Toxicity and systemic effects of local anesthetic agents. *In* Strichartz, G.R., ed.: Local Anesthetics. Handbook of Experimental Pharmacology. Vol. 81. Berlin, Springer-Verlag, 1987.

10. Courtney, K.R.: Structure–activity relations for frequency-dependent sodium channel block in nerve by local anesthetics. J. Pharmacol. Exp. Ther. *213*:114–119, 1980.

11. de Jong, R.H.: Local Anesthetics, 2nd ed. Springfield, Ill., Charles C Thomas, 1977.

12. Hille, B.: The pH-dependent rate of action of local anesthetics on the node of Ranvier. J. Gen. Physiol., *69*:475–496, 1977.

13. Narahashi, T., Moore, J.W., and Poston, R.N.: Anesthetic blocking of nerve membrane conductances by internal and external applications. J. Neurobiol., *1*:3–22, 1969.

14. Strichartz, G.R., and Ritchie, J.M.: The action of local anesthetics on ion channels of excitable tissues. *In* Strichartz, G.R., ed.: Local Anesthetics. Handbook of Experimental Pharmacology. Vol. 81. Berlin, Springer-Verlag, 1987.

15. Courtney, K.R., and Strichartz, G.R.: Structural elements which determine local anesthetic activity. *In* Strichartz, G.R., ed.: Local Anesthetics. Handbook of Experimental Pharmacology. Vol. 81. Berlin, Springer-Verlag, 1987.

16. Wang, G.K.: Binding affinity and stereoselectivity of local anesthetics in single batrachotoxin-activated Na^+ channels. J. Gen. Physiol., *96*:1105–1127, 1990.

17. Luduena, F.P., Bogado, E.F., and Tullar, B.F.: Optical isomers of mepivacaine and bupivacaine. Arch. Int. Pharmacodyn., *200*:359–369, 1972.

18. Butterworth, J.F., IV, and Strichartz, G.R.: Molecular mechanisms of local anesthesia: A review. Anesthesiology, *72*:711–734, 1990.

19. Hille, B.: Local anesthetics: Hydrophilic and hydrophobic pathways for the drug-receptor reaction. J. Gen. Physiol., *69*:497–515, 1977.

20. Catterall, W.A.: Structure and function of voltage-sensitive ion channels. Science, *242*:50–61, 1988.

21. Neumcke, B., Schwarz, W., Stämpfli, R.: Block of Na channels in the membrane of myelinated nerve by benzocaine. Pflugers Arch., *390*:230–236, 1981.

22. Wang, G.K.: Cocaine-induced closures of single batrachotoxin-activated Na^+ channels in planar lipid bilayers. J. Gen. Physiol., *92*:747–765, 1988.

23. Huang, L.-Y.M., and Ehrenstein, G.: Local anesthetics QX 572 and benzocaine act at separate sites on the batrachotoxin-activated sodium channel. J. Gen. Physiol., *77*:137–153, 1981.

24. Cahalan, M.D., and Almers, W.: Interactions between quaternary lidocaine, the sodium channel gates, and tetrodotoxin. Biophys. J., *27*:39–56, 1979.

25. Trudell, J.R.: A unitary theory of anesthesia based on lateral phase separations in nerve membranes. Anesthesiology, *46*:5–10, 1977.

26. Boulanger, Y., Schreier S., Leitch, L.C., and Smith, I.C.P.: Multiple binding sites for local anesthetics in membranes: Characterization of the sites and their equilibria by deuterium NMR of specifically deuterated procaine and tetracaine. Can. J. Biochem., *58*:986–995, 1980.

27. Simpkins, H., Panko, E., and Tay, S.: The interaction of procaine with the nonmyelinated nerve axon. Can. J. Biochem., *50*:174–176, 1972.

28. Illiano, G., Chiosi, E., Draetta, G.F., and Laurenza, A.: Relationship between the fluidity of the membrane lipids and the activity of the membrane-bound proteins: The effects of lidocaine on the adenylate cyclase activity of rat myocardium. Gen. Pharmacol. *14*:669–672, 1983.

29. Aguilar, J.S., Criado, M., and De Robertis, E.: Inhibition by local anesthetics, phentolamine and propranolol of [³H]quinuclydinyl benzylate binding to central muscarinic receptors. Eur. J. Pharmacol., *68*:317–326, 1980.

30. Houslay, M.D., Dipple, I., Rawal, S., Sauerheber, R.D., Esgate, J.A., and Gordon, L.M.: Glucagon-stimulated adenylate cyclase detects a selective perturbation of the inner half of the liver plasma-membrane bilayer achieved by the local anesthetic prilocaine. Biochem. J., *190*:131–137, 1980.
31. Volpi, M., Sha'afi, R.I., Epstein, P.M., Andrenyak, D.M., and Feinstein, M.B.: Local anesthetics, mepacrine, and propranolol are antagonists of calmodulin. Proc. Natl. Acad. Sci. U.S.A., *78*:795–799, 1981.
32. Bokesch, P.M., Post, C., and Strichartz, G.: Structure–activity relationship of lidocaine homologs producing tonic and frequency-dependent impulse blockade in nerve. J. Pharmacol. Exp. Ther., *237*:773–781, 1986.
33. Levinson, S.R., Thornhill, W.B., Duch, D.S., Recio-Pinto, E., and Urban, B.W.: The role of nonprotein domains in the function and synthesis of voltage-gated sodium channels. *In* Narahashi, T., ed.: Ion Channels. Vol. 2. New York, Plenum Press, 1990.
34. Clarkson, C.W., and Hondeghem, L.M.: Mechanism for bupivacaine depression of cardiac conduction: Fast block of sodium channels during the action potential with slow recovery from block during diastole. Anesthesiology, *62*:396–405, 1985.
35. Gasser, H.S., and Erlanger, J.: The role of fiber size in the establishment of a nerve block by pressure or cocaine. Am. J. Physiol., *88*:581–591, 1929.
36. Ford, D.J., Raj, P.P., Singh, P., Regan, K.M., and Ohlweiler, D.: Differential peripheral nerve block by local anesthetics in the cat. Anesthesiology, *60*:28–33, 1984.
37. Franz, D.N., and Perry, R.S.: Mechanisms for differential block among single myelinated and nonmyelinated axons by procaine. J. Physiol. (Lond.), *236*:193–210, 1974.
38. Fink, B.R., and Cairns, A.M.: Differential peripheral axon block with lidocaine: Unit studies in the cervical vagus nerve. Anesthesiology, *59*:182–186, 1983.
39. Fink, B.R.: Mechanisms of differential axial blockade in epidural and subarachnoid anesthesia. Anesthesiology, *70*:851–858, 1989.
40. Raymond, S.A., Steffensen, S.C., Gugino, L.D., and Strichartz, G.R.: The role of length of nerve exposed to local anesthetics in impulse blocking action. Anesth. Analg., *68*:563–570, 1989.
41. Armstrong, P.J., Morrison, L.M., Noble, D., Sinclair, W.A., Tiplady, B., and Wildsmith, J.A.W.: Effects of I.V. lignocaine on psychological performance and subjective state in healthy volunteers. Br. J. Anaesth., *67*:532–538, 1992.
42. Scaramella, J., Allen, G.D., Gobel, W.M., and Donaldson, D.: Lidocaine as a supplement to general anesthesia for extraction of third molars: Serum levels. Anesth. Prog., *26*:118–119, 1979.
43. Brose, W.G., and Cousins, M.J.: Subcutaneous lidocaine for treatment of neuropathic cancer pain. Pain, *45*:145–148, 1991.
44. Covino, B.G.: Local anesthesia (first of two parts). N. Engl. J. Med., *286*:975–983, 1972.
45. Garfield, J.M., and Gugino, L.: Central effects of local anesthetic agents. *In* Strichartz, G.R., ed.: Local Anesthetics. Handbook of Experimental Pharmacology. Vol. 81. Berlin, Springer-Verlag, 1987.
46. Seo, N., Oshima, E., Stevens, J., and Mori, K.: The tetraphasic action of lidocaine on CNS electrical activity and behavior in cats. Anesthesiology, *57*:451–457, 1982.
47. Klein, S.W., Sutherland, R.I.L., and Morch, J.E.: Hemodynamic effects of intravenous lidocaine in man. Can. Med. Assoc. J., *99*:472–475, 1968.
48. Duranteau, J., Pussard, E., Edouard, A., and Berdeaux, A.: Lidocaine and cardiovascular reflex responses to simulated orthostatic stress in normal volunteers. J. Cardiovasc. Pharmacol., *18*:60–67, 1991.
49. Perlmutter, N., Wilson, R., Joyce, M., Angello, D., and Gee, D.: Effect of lignocaine on coronary blood flow, systolic myocardial function and myocardial high energy phosphate stores in swine. Clin. Exp. Pharmacol. Physiol., *17*:697–706, 1990.

50. Johns, R.A., DiFazio, C.A., and Longnecker, D.E.: Lidocaine constricts or dilates rat arterioles in a dose-dependent manner. Anesthesiology, *62*:141–144, 1985.

51. Löfström, J.B.: Physiological effects of local anaesthetics on circulation and respiration. *In* Löfström, J.B., and Sjöstrand, U., eds.: Local Anaesthesia and Regional Blockade. Monographs in Anaesthesiology. Vol. 15. Amsterdam, Elsevier Science Publishers, 1988.

52. Jorfeldt, L., Löfström, B., Pernow, B., Persson, B., Wahren, J., and Widman, B.: The effect of local anaesthetics on the central circulation and respiration in man and dog. Acta Anaesthesiol. Scand., *12*:153–169, 1986.

53. Albright, G.A.: Cardiac arrest following regional anesthesia with etidocaine or bupivacaine. Anesthesiology, *51*:285–287, 1979.

54. Morishima, H.O., Pederson, H., Finster, M., et al.: Bupivacaine toxicity in pregnant and nonpregnant ewes. Anesthesiology, *63*:134–139, 1985.

55. Morishima, H.O., Pederson, H., Finster, M., Feldman, H.S., and Covino, B.G.: Etidocaine toxicity in the adult, newborn, and fetal sheep. Anesthesiology, *58*:342–346, 1983.

56. Covino, B.G.: Clinical pharmacology of local anesthetic agents. *In* Cousins, M.J., and Bridenbaugh, P.O., eds.: Neural Blockade in Clinical Anesthesia and Management of Pain, 2nd ed. Philadelphia, J.B. Lippincott Co., 1988.

57. Eledjam, J.J., de La Coussaye, J.E., Brugada, J., et al.: In vitro study on mechanisms of bupivacaine-induced depression of myocardial contractility. Anesth. Analg., *69*:732–735, 1989.

58. Thomas, R.D., Behbehani, M.M., Coyle, D.E., and Denson, D.D.: Cardiovascular toxicity of local anesthetics: An alternative hypothesis. Anesth. Analg., *65*:444–450, 1986.

59. Heavner, J.E.: Cardiac dysrhythmias induced by infusion of local anesthetics into the lateral cerebral ventricle of cats. Anesth. Analg., *65*:133–138, 1986.

60. Rosen, M.A., Thigpen, J.W., Shnider, S.M., Foutz, S.E., Levinson, G., and Koike, M.: Bupivacaine-induced cardiotoxicity in hypoxic and acidotic sheep. Anesth. Analg., *64*:1089–1096, 1985.

61. Sage, D.J., Feldman, H.S., Arthur, G.R., et al.: Influence of lidocaine and bupivacaine on isolated guinea pig atria in the presence of acidosis and hypoxia. Anesth. Analg., *63*:1–7, 1984.

62. Blair, M.R.: Cardiovascular pharmacology of local anaesthetics. Br. J. Anaesth., *47*:247–252, 1975.

63. Lindorf, H.H.: Investigation of the vascular effect of newer local anesthetics and vasoconstrictors. Oral Surg. Oral Med. Oral Pathol., *48*:292–297, 1979.

64. Pateromichelakis, S.: Circulatory and respiratory effects of lidocaine administered into the rat maxillofacial circulation. J. Oral Maxillofac. Surg., *50*:724–727, 1992.

65. Jorfeldt, L, Löfström, B., Pernow, B., and Wahren, J.: The effect of mepivacaine and lidocaine on forearm resistance and capacitance vessels in man. Acta Anaesthesiol. Scand., *14*:183–201, 1970.

66. Tuvemo, T., and Willdeck-Lund, G.: Smooth muscle effects of lidocaine, prilocaine, bupivacaine and etidocaine on the human umbilical artery. Acta Anaesthesiol. Scand., *26*:104–107, 1982.

67. Nicolson, G.L.: Cell shape changes and transmembrane receptor uncoupling induced by tertiary amine local anesthetics. J. Supramol. Struct. 5:65–72, 1976.

68. Eichhorn, J.H., and Peterkofsky, B.: Local anesthetic-induced inhibition of collagen secretion in cultured cells under conditions where microtubules are not depolymerized by these agents. J. Cell Biol. *81*:26–42, 1979.

69. Borg, T., and Modig, J.: Potential anti-thrombotic effects of local anaesthetics due to their inhibition of platelet aggregation. Acta Anaesthesiol. Scand., *29*:739–742, 1985.

70. Eriksson, A.S., Sinclair, R., Cassuto, J., and Thomsen, P.: Influence of lidocaine on leukocyte function in the surgical wound. Anesthesiology, *77*:74–78, 1992.

71. Rimbäck, G., Cassuto, J., and Tollesson, P.-O.: Treatment of postoperative paralytic ileus by intravenous lidocaine infusion. Anesth. Analg. *70*:414–419, 1990.

72. Morrow, M.E., and Berry, C.W.: Antimicrobial properties of topical anesthetic liquids containing lidocaine or benzocaine. Anesth. Prog., *35*:9–13, 1988.

73. Tanelian, D.L., and Brose, W.G.: Neuropathic pain can be relieved by drugs that are use-dependent sodium channel blockers: Lidocaine, carbamazepine, and mexiletine. Anesthesiology, *74*:949–951, 1991.

74. Tanelian, D.L., and MacIver, M.B.: Analgesic concentrations of lidocaine suppress tonic A-delta and C fiber discharges produced by acute injury. Anesthesiology, *74*:934–936, 1991.

75. Christensen, V., Ladegaard-Pedersen, H.J., and Skovsted, P.: Intravenous lidocaine as a suppressant of persistent cough caused by bronchoscopy. Acta Anaesthesiol. Scand. Suppl., *67*:84–86, 1978.

76. Smith, G.N., and Walton, R.E.: Periodontal ligament injection: Distribution of injected solutions. Oral Surg. Oral Med. Oral Pathol., *55*:232–238, 1983.

77. Goebel, W., Allen, G., and Randall, F.: Circulating serum levels of mepivacaine after dental injection. Anesth. Prog., *25*:52–56, 1978.

78. Goebel, W.M., Allen, G., and Randall, F.: Comparative circulating serum levels of mepivacaine with levo-nordefrin and lidocaine with epinephrine. Anesth. Prog., *26*:93–97, 1979.

79. Cannell, H., and Whelpton, R.: Systemic uptake of prilocaine after injection of various formulations of the drug. Br. Dent. J., *160*:47–49, 1986.

80. Adriani, J., and Campbell, B.: Fatalities following topical application of local anesthetics to mucous membranes. J.A.M.A., *162*:1527–1530, 1956.

81. Scott, D.B., Littlewood, D.G., Covino, B.G., and Drummond, G.B.: Plasma lignocaine concentrations following endotracheal spraying with an aerosol. Br. J. Anaesth., *48*:899–902, 1976.

82. Tucker, G.T., Boyes, R.N., Bridenbaugh, P.O., and Moore, D.C.: Binding of anilide-type local anesthetics in human plasma: I. Relationships between binding, physicochemical properties, and anesthetic activity. Anesthesiology, *33*:287–303, 1970.

83. Tucker, G.T., and Mather, L.E.: Pharmacokinetics of local anaesthetic agents. Br. J. Anaesth., *47*:213–224, 1975.

84. Arthur, G.R.: Pharmacokinetics of local anesthetics. *In* Strichartz, G.R., ed.: Local Anesthetics. Handbook of Experimental Pharmacology. Vol. 81. Berlin, Springer-Verlag, 1987.

85. Tucker, G.T., and Mather, L.E.: Properties, absorption, and disposition of local anesthetic agents. *In* Cousins, M.J., and Bridenbaugh, P.O., eds.: Neural Blockade in Clinical Anesthesia and Management of Pain, 2nd ed. Philadelphia, J.B. Lippincott Co., 1988.

86. Burney, R.G., DiFazio, C.A., and Foster, J.A.: Effects of pH on protein binding of lidocaine. Anesth. Analg., *57*:478–480, 1978.

87. Apfelbaum, J.L., Shaw, L.M., Gross, J.B., Caldwell, C.B., and Spaulding, B.C.: Modification of lidocaine protein binding with CO_2. Can. Anaesth. Soc. J., *32*:468–471, 1985.

88. McNamara, P.J., Slaughter, R.L., Pieper, J.A., Wyman, M.G., and Lalka, D.: Factors influencing serum protein binding of lidocaine in humans. Anesth. Analg., *60*:395–400, 1981.

89. Jorfeldt, L., Lewis, D.H., Löfström, J.B., and Post, C.: Lung uptake of lidocaine in healthy volunteers. Acta Anaesthesiol. Scand., *23*:567–574, 1979.

90. Benowitz, N., Forsyth, R.P., Melmon, K.L., and Rowland, M.: Lidocaine disposition kinetics in monkey and man: I. Prediction by a perfusion model. Clin. Pharmacol. Ther., *16*:87–98, 1974.

91. Seifen, A.B., Ferrari, A.A., Seifen, E.E., Thompson, D.S., and Chapman, J.: Phar-

macokinetics of intravenous procaine infusion in humans. Anesth. Analg., *58*:382–386, 1979.

92. Strong, J.M., Parker, M., and Atkinson, A.J., Jr.: Identification of glycinexylidide in patients treated with intravenous lidocaine. Clin. Pharmacol. Ther., *14*:67–72, 1973.

93. Tucker, G.T., and Mather, L.E.: Clinical pharmacokinetics of local anaesthetics. Clin. Pharmacokinet., *4*:241–278, 1979.

94. Arthur, G.R., Scott, D.H.T., Boyes, R.N., and Scott, D.B.: Pharmacokinetic and clinical pharmacological studies with mepivacaine and prilocaine. Br. J. Anaesth., *51*:481–485, 1979.

95. Nation, R.L., and Triggs, E.J.: Lignocaine kinetics in cardiac patients and aged subjects. Br. J. Clin. Pharmacol., *4*:439–448, 1977.

96. Feely, J., Wade, D., McAllister, C.B., Wilkinson, G.R., and Robertson, D.: Effect of hypotension on liver blood flow and lidocaine disposition. N. Engl. J. Med., *307*:866–869, 1982.

97. Elvin, A.T., Cole, A.F.D., Pieper, J.A., Rolbin, S.H., and Lalka, D.: Effect of food on lidocaine kinetics: Mechanism of food-related alteration in high intrinsic clearance drug elimination. Clin. Pharmacol. Ther., *30*:455–460, 1981.

Pharmacology of Vasoconstrictors

Local anesthetic solutions often contain a vasoconstrictor agent in order to reduce blood flow in the area of injection and thus impede systemic absorption of the anesthetic. The adrenergic (or sympathomimetic) amines most commonly used for this purpose—epinephrine, norepinephrine, and levonordefrin—are described in this chapter. Following consideration of these adrenergic drugs, some special features of felypressin, a polypeptide vasoconstrictor available outside the United States and Canada, will also be addressed.

Rationale for Use

Several major benefits may be obtained by incorporating vasoconstrictors into local anesthetic solutions. First, the duration of anesthesia may be considerably prolonged. As shown in Table 3–1, the duration of pulpal anesthesia afforded in the maxilla by 2% lidocaine is increased nine times and that in soft tissue is increased four times when 1 : 100,000 epinephrine is added to the anesthetic solution.[1,2] This dramatic effect on the duration of anesthesia arises because the maxillary arch is richly supplied with blood and because lidocaine causes vasodilation. Without epinephrine, lidocaine is rapidly absorbed from the administration site. Although some anesthesia of the oral mucosa is obtained, insufficient amounts of lidocaine gain access to nerve fibers innervating the pulp to produce more than a transient blockade of conduction. Epinephrine allows the anesthetic to remain in the tissues long enough for profound anesthesia to develop and to last an extended period.

A second advantage of vasoconstrictor inclusion is that the depth of anesthesia may be enhanced. Figure 3–1 illustrates this point. Although

Table 3–1.   **INFLUENCE OF EPINEPHRINE ON THE DURATION OF LIDOCAINE ANESTHESIA IN THE ANTERIOR MAXILLA***

Preparation	Pulpal Anesthesia (min)†	Soft Tissue Anesthesia (min)‡
2% Lidocaine plain	5	42
2% Lidocaine with 1 : 200,000 epinephrine	34	166
2% Lidocaine with 1 : 100,000 epinephrine	45	168

*Data from Berling.[1]

†Determined by electric pulp testing.

‡Determined by return of normal lip sensations.

1% lidocaine is incapable of providing pulpal anesthesia after supraperiosteal injection in the oral cavity, the same concentration becomes highly effective if administered with a small amount of epinephrine.[3] However, this example is admittedly extreme, as other local anesthetic formulations often exhibit less potentiation by epinephrine.

A final major consequence of vasoconstrictor addition is that the peak concentration of anesthetic in the blood may be significantly reduced. Figure 3–2 presents data from an investigation of the systemic absorption of lidocaine following intraoral injection.[4] Although considerable differences existed among individuals within each treatment group in this study, epinephrine did retard overall the absorption of lidocaine from

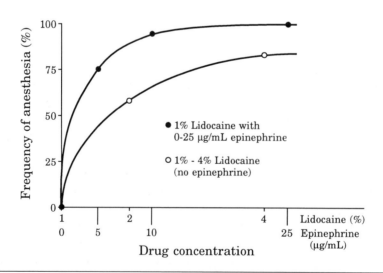

Figure 3–1.   Influence of local anesthetic and vasoconstrictor concentrations on anesthetic efficacy after supraperiosteal injection of the maxillary lateral incisor. (Data from Björn, H., and Huldt, S.: Sven. Tandlak. Tidskr., *40*:831–851, 1947.)

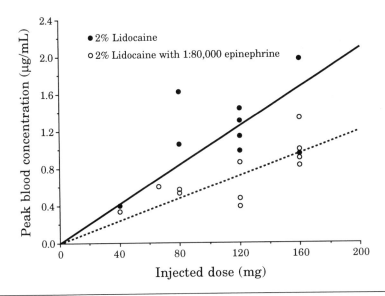

Figure 3–2.   Influence of epinephrine on the maximum venous blood concentration of lidocaine after intraoral injection. Plasma concentrations were converted to blood values using a blood/plasma distribution ratio of 0.85. (Data from Cannell, H., Walters, H., et al.: Br. Dent. J., *138*:87–93, 1975.)

perioral tissues. This finding implies that a given dose of lidocaine with vasoconstrictor should be less toxic than the same dose without vasoconstrictor, provided that the adrenergic agent causes no adverse effects of its own or exacerbates those of the local anesthetic. In view of the widespread acceptance that vasoconstrictors reduce local anesthetic toxicity,[5,6] it is interesting that neither of these postulates has been proved.[7] Indeed, adrenergic vasoconstrictors are known to cause a variety of side effects[8,9] and rare instances of serious systemic toxicity.[10–12] Probably the major contribution of vasoconstriction to local anesthetic safety is indirect. By enhancing the efficiency of nerve blockade, the vasoconstrictor may render the operative procedure less stressful to the patient, and less volume of drug may have to be administered. Moreover, because lower concentrations of local anesthetics are often effective when epinephrine is employed, the total dose necessary for regional anesthesia may be reduced.

Although the benefits of vasoconstrictor inclusion in local anesthetic solutions apply generally, the actual gains realized vary with the local anesthetic, its concentration, and the site of administration. Mepivacaine and prilocaine, for instance, are not strong vasodilators and may even cause moderate vasoconstriction in some vascular beds. These agents, particularly prilocaine, are less dependent than lidocaine on epinephrine-like drugs, especially when deposited in tissues not as well perfused as the maxillary periodontium. Thus, when 4% prilocaine is injected into the pterygomandibular space to block the inferior alveolar nerve, epinephrine has little effect on the duration of anesthesia.[13] Similarly, the consensus of several clinical trials is that epinephrine increases the incidence of successful anesthesia with prilocaine by only 3% to 5%.[13-15] Local blood flow, at least as it is influenced by epinephrine, is apparently not always the rate-limiting factor in the removal of prilocaine from its site of action.

Structure–Activity Relationships

Vasoconstrictors employed in regional anesthesia are structurally related to, if not identical with, the natural mediators of the sympathetic nervous system—epinephrine and norepinephrine (Fig. 3–3). Because these drugs produce effects similar to those caused by stimulation of adrenergic nerves, they are collectively referred to as *sympathomimetic* or *adrenergic* drugs. The term *catecholamine* (after catechol, *o*-dihydroxybenzene) is also appropriate for these agents. Highly unstable and sparingly soluble in water, they are usually manufactured for injection in the form of hydrophilic salts (e.g., epinephrine bitartrate).

The basic structure of the adrenergic amines is reminiscent of the local anesthetics: a substituted aromatic ring separated from a nitrogen moiety by a small aliphatic connector. Unlike the situation with local anesthetics, however, even minor changes in the molecular structure of an adrenergic amine almost invariably yield dramatic alterations in drug effect. For example, removal of the *m*-hydroxyl group of epinephrine yields phenylephrine, a vasoconstrictor 20 times less potent than epinephrine and virtually devoid of cardiostimulatory activity. Obviously, the receptors that combine with these drugs to elicit pharmacologic responses are much more selective than those postulated for local anesthetics. Because the ligand binding sites of adrenergic receptors are open to the exterior surface of the plasma membrane of effector cells, access to the receptors is not governed by lipid solubility, and lipid:buffer partition coefficients

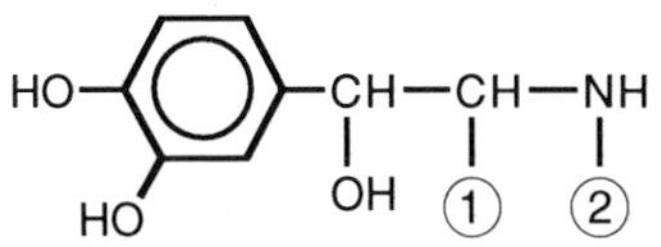

	①	②
Epinephrine	H	CH$_3$
Levonordefrin	CH$_3$	H
Norepinephrine	H	H

Figure 3–3.   Structural formulas of sympathomimetic amines commonly used as vasoconstrictors in local anesthesia for dentistry.

of the catecholamine vasoconstrictors are much less than those of conventional local anesthetics.

Mechanism of Action

Epinephrine, norepinephrine, and levonordefrin cause vasoconstriction by activating adrenergic receptors located on the myocytes of blood vessels. Although all blood vessels containing smooth muscle may be affected by these drugs, the constriction of resistance arterioles and precapillary sphincters is primarily responsible for limiting local blood flow in the injected tissue. Once the drug is absorbed into the systemic circulation, side effects may occur from stimulation of adrenergic receptors at distant sites.

ADRENERGIC RECEPTORS

Careful study of the structure–activity relationships of adrenergic amines has revealed that several different classes of adrenergic receptors (also referred to as adrenoceptors) exist. In 1948, Ahlquist[16] recognized the existence of two types of receptors, α and β, based on the excitatory (usually α) and inhibitory (usually β) actions of catecholamines on smooth muscle. Noting the differing effects of epinephrine and norepinephrine on lipolysis and cardiac function versus bronchial and vascular smooth muscle relaxation, Lands et al.[17] subdivided β receptors into β_1 (adipocytes, cardiac muscle) and β_2 (most other sites) subtypes. A similar categorization of α receptors was subsequently predicated[18] on differences in α-receptor location and function (α_1, postsynaptic–excitatory; α_2, presynaptic–inhibitory). In recent years, the synthesis of highly selective ligands for adrenoceptors and the cloning of adrenoceptor genes have demonstrated additional heterogeneity. A third β receptor (β_3) has been identified,[9] and multiple subtypes of α_1 and α_2 receptors are under investigation.[19] Studies have also indicated that the distribution and function of the various adrenoceptors are more complex than previously thought. Thus, α and β receptors exhibit both excitatory and inhibitory actions in a variety of tissues; β_2 receptors exist in the heart, and β_1 receptors in the viscera; and α_2 receptors exert excitatory effects at postsynaptic sites.

All adrenergic receptors belong to the same family of plasma membrane–bound proteins. Their basic structure is represented in Figure 3–4.[19,20] Composed of a single peptide chain approximately 450 to 500 amino acids in length, each adrenoceptor comprises seven hydrophobic α helices spanning the membrane. Serine residues on segment V form hydrogen bonds with the catechol hydroxyl groups of epinephrine, a phenylalanine on segment VI interacts with the phenyl ring, and an aspartate on segment III provides an ionic association with the amino terminus.

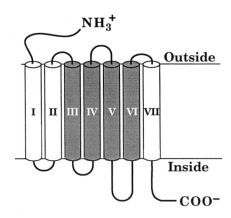

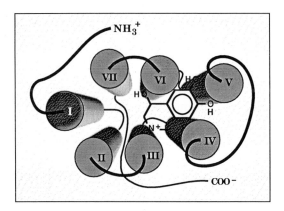

Figure 3–4. Structural model of the adrenergic receptor. *Top,* the receptor contains seven α-helical segments that span the membrane. The shaded segments (III through VI) contribute to the ligand binding site. The connector between segments V and VI interacts with the G protein to elicit the pharmacologic response. *Bottom,* possible spatial orientation of the transmembrane subunits as viewed perpendicular to the membrane from the external surface. An epinephrine molecule occupies the ligand binding site. (Adapted from Ostrowski, J., Kjelsberg, M.A., et al.: Annu. Rev. Pharmacol. Toxicol., *32*:167–183, 1992. Reproduced, with permission, from the Annual Review of Pharmacology and Toxicology, Volume 32, © 1992, by Annual Reviews Inc.)

CONSEQUENCES OF RECEPTOR BINDING

Adrenergic receptors are incapable by themselves of generating cellular responses to drug binding. Instead, they regulate the activity of effector proteins (enzymes, ion channels, etc.) indirectly through their actions on a second family of membrane constituents known as guanine nucleotide–binding proteins or, more simply, G proteins. G proteins are linked to adrenoceptors on the inner surface of the cell membrane. Binding of an agonist to the adrenoceptor causes an allosteric effect on the coupled G protein. The G protein, in turn, binds a guanosine triphosphate (GTP) molecule, which enables it to activate, or in some cases inhibit, the effector protein to which it is linked. Within several seconds, the GTP is hydrolyzed to guanosine diphosphate (GDP) and the signal is turned off. The cycle will then repeat itself so long as agonist continues to stimulate the receptor.

The primary steps involved in adrenergic amine–induced vasoconstriction are outlined in Figure 3–5.[9,19] The adrenoceptors mediating the effect in mucosal tissues are α_1 and α_2 receptors. The α_1 receptor is found in the smooth muscle of blood vessels throughout the body, generally in close association with sympathetic nerve terminals. Its activation by endogenously released norepinephrine or by exogenously administered drug causes, through stimulation of a specific G protein, a temporary opening of the calcium (Ca^{2+}) ion channel. Ca^{2+} flows into the cell down its electrochemical gradient. The resulting activation of calmodulin-dependent myosin light chain kinase causes contraction. Through stimulation of a separate G protein linked to phospholipase C, α_1 receptors effect the hydrolysis of the membrane lipid phosphatidylinositol-4,5-biphosphate. The second messenger products of this reaction—inositol-1,4,5-triphosphate (IP_3) and diacylglycerol—promote contraction, respectively, by facilitating the release of Ca^{2+} from intracellular storage sites and by fostering Ca^{2+} activation of protein kinase C, which recruits metabolic support for contraction.

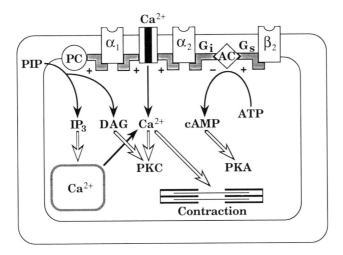

Figure 3–5.   Intracellular responses to receptor binding. Adrenergic receptors directly influencing vascular tone are coupled via guanine nucleotide–binding proteins (G_s, G_i, and unlabeled shaded connectors) to effector proteins: adenylate cyclase (AC), phospholipase C (PC), and calcium (Ca^{2+}) channels. Signal transduction by effector proteins (shown in black arrows) results in altered concentrations of second messengers: cyclic adenosine monophosphate (cAMP), Ca^{2+}, inositol-1,4,5-triphosphate (IP_3), and diacylglycerol (DAG). The second messengers in turn activate (white arrows) various enzymes such as protein kinase A (PKA) and protein kinase C (PKC), and cause ionic fluxes (such as release of Ca^{2+} from intracellular storage sites). Increased Ca^{2+} activates muscle contraction and vasoconstriction.

Vasoconstrictor stimulation of α_2 receptors also causes a G protein–dependent opening of plasma membrane Ca^{2+} ion channels. A second effect of α_2-receptor activation is inhibition (mediated by an inhibitory G protein, G_i) of the enzyme adenylate cyclase. Exactly how this latter outcome supports smooth muscle contraction is unknown; however, it is clear that stimulation of adenylate cyclase by β_2-receptor activation results in vasodilation. Postsynaptic α_2 receptors are not closely associated with sympathetic synapses and therefore may be more responsive to circulating catecholamines than to neuronally released norepinephrine.

Sparsely distributed in mucous membranes and skin, β_2 receptors are prevalent in some tissues, such as the vasculature of the heart, lungs, skeletal muscle, and some abdominal viscera. Agonist binding by this receptor and activation of its stimulatory G protein (G_s) and associated adenylate cyclase promotes synthesis of the second messenger adenosine $3'$, $5'$-monophosphate (cyclic AMP, or cAMP). In turn, cAMP modulates the activity of intracellular enzymes such as protein kinase A. One possible outcome is increased Ca^{2+} sequestration within the subcellular organelles, which would reduce the concentration of free Ca^{2+} available for muscle contraction.

Like the β_2 receptor, the β_1 receptor is coupled via the G_s protein to adenylate cyclase. Although the β_1 receptor is not directly involved in the regulation of vascular tone (except at a few specific sites), it is the primary adrenoceptor in the heart and an important contributor to various systemic effects of the adrenergic amines.

DIFFERENTIAL BINDING OF VASOCONSTRICTORS

Vasoconstrictors vary greatly in their relative affinities for different adrenoceptors. As shown in Table 3–2, epinephrine is the most potent α agonist.[19,21] On the other hand, with its powerful β_2 stimulant properties,[17] epinephrine is the least selective of these drugs and can generate opposing vascular actions. Two factors dictate whether epinephrine will increase or decrease blood flow through a particular tissue: the local concentration of epinephrine and the relative proportion of α and β_2 receptors in the tissue. Because β_2 receptors are more sensitive to epinephrine than are α receptors, low concentrations of the drug will cause

Table 3–2. **RELATIVE RECEPTOR POTENCIES OF ADRENERGIC VASOCONSTRICTORS***

Drug	α_1	α_2	β_1	β_2
Epinephrine	+++	+++	+++	+++
Norepinephrine	++	++	++	+
Levonordefrin	+	++	++	+

Symbols indicate the relative potency: +++ = high, ++ = intermediate, + = low.

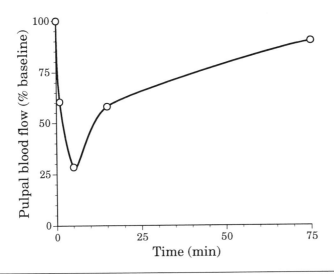

Figure 3–6.   Reduction in maxillary canine blood flow after supraperiosteal injection of 2% lido-caine with 1 : 100,000 epinephrine in dogs. (Data from Kim, S., Edwall, L., et al., J. Dent. Res., *63*:650–652, 1984.)

vasodilation in vascular beds well endowed with β_2 receptors (e.g., skeletal muscle, liver), and β_2-mediated vasodilation may persist after α-mediated vasoconstriction wanes with the decreasing epinephrine concentration. The α response predominates at higher doses, though, and concentrations employed clinically invariably diminished circulation in the area of injection (Fig. 3–6).[22,23] Furthermore, in tissues where β_2 receptors are scarce or nonexistent, such as the gingiva and alveolar mucosa, even minimally effective concentrations of epinephrine produce vasoconstriction. Norepinephrine, by virtue of its feeble β_2 effects, only constricts blood vessels. Levonordefrin, a rather selective α_2 agonist, usually produces vasoconstriction in low systemic concentrations and invariably does so at larger concentrations. As discussed below, the relative receptor affinities of the adrenergic amines can also lead to some marked differences in systemic effects.

Systemic Effects

Depending on the dose and route of administration, sympathomimetic amines can evoke a variety of systemic reactions. Consideration of the distribution of adrenergic receptors in effector tissues and the relative receptor affinities of the individual vasoconstrictors is necessary to understand the pharmacology of these drugs. As listed in Table 3–3,[21,24] the major systemic effects of injected sympathomimetic agents involve the cardiovascular system, pulmonary tree, abdominal viscera, skeletal muscle, and intermediary metabolism. These drugs can also elicit a number of central nervous system reactions.

Table 3–3. **SYSTEMIC EFFECTS OF ADRENERGIC AMINES**

Effector Organ or Function	Receptor*	Response
Cardiovascular system		
Heart rate	β_1, β_2	Increased†
Contractile force	β_1, β_2	Increased
Coronary arterioles	$\alpha_1, \alpha_2/\beta_2$	Constriction/dilation‡
Automaticity	β_1, β_2	Increased
Conduction velocity	β_1, β_2	Increased†
Peripheral resistance	$\alpha_1, \alpha_2/\beta_2$	Increased/decreased
Capacitance veins	α_1/β_2	Constriction/dilation
Respiratory system		
Bronchial smooth muscle	β_2	Relaxation
Bronchial glands	α_1/β_2	Decreased/increased secretion
Pulmonary arterioles	α_1/β_2	Constriction/dilation‡
Gastrointestinal tract		
Motility and tone	$\alpha_1, \alpha_2, \beta_1, \beta_2$	Decreased
Sphincters	α_1	Contraction
Visceral arterioles	α_1/β_2	Constriction/dilation
Liver		
Glucose metabolism	α, β_2	Glycogenolysis, gluconeogenesis
Arterioles	α_1/β_2	Constriction/dilation
Fat		
Lipolysis	$\alpha, \beta_1 (\beta_3)$	Lipolysis
Arterioles	α_1/β_2	Constriction/dilation
Pancreas		
Insulin secretion	α_2/β_2	Decreased/increased
Genitourinary system		
Urinary bladder sphincter	α_1	Contraction
Detrusor muscle	β_2	Relaxation
Trigone muscle	α_1	Contraction
Uterine tone	α_1/β_2	Contraction/relaxation§
Renal arterioles	$\alpha_1, \alpha_2/\beta_1, \beta_2$	Constriction/dilation
Skeletal muscle		
Neuromuscular transmission	α, β_2	Increased
Arterioles	α/β_2	Constriction/dilation
Salivary glands		
Secretion	β	Mucous secretion
Arterioles	α_1, α_2	Constriction
Skin and mucosa		
Arterioles	α_1, α_2	Constriction

*Primary receptors mediating pharmacologic response. Receptors separated by commas yield complementary actions; receptors separated by a slash have differing or opposing actions. Data from Lefkowitz et al.[21] and Brodde.[24]

†Direct effects on the heart may be blocked or reversed by compensatory vagal reflex activity.

‡Local regulatory processes largely govern blood flow.

§Effect depends on stage of menstrual cycle, sexual hormone concentrations, and other factors.

CARDIOVASCULAR SYSTEM

Some misunderstandings exist concerning the cardiovascular effects of adrenergic amines used as vasoconstrictors in regional anesthesia. Until the 1950s, excessive fears were often expressed in the dental literature concerning the dangers these drugs posed, particularly for patients with angina pectoris, hypertension, or a history of myocardial infarction. Subsequently a series of investigations found that patients with cardiovascular disease could tolerate moderate doses of epinephrine-like drugs without mishap.[25,26] Citing studies documenting a lack of effect of epinephrine on arterial blood pressure and values of up to 14 μg/min for the basal release of epinephrine from the resting adrenal medulla (an amount roughly equivalent to the epinephrine content in a 1.8-mL cartridge of 1:100,000 solution), several authors implied that, barring intravascular injection, conventional doses of vasoconstrictors are too small to have any significant effect on the cardiovascular system.[5,27] Such is not the case.

Using improved methods for measuring catecholamines, a number of investigators have shown that epinephrine injected during local anesthesia markedly elevates the resting plasma concentration of the hormone.[28,29] A meta-analysis (Fig. 3–7)[30] of several studies[31–36] using similar designs revealed that the mean resting venous plasma concentration of epinephrine, 39 pg/mL,* is approximately doubled by the intraoral injection of a single cartridge of 2% lidocaine with 1:100,000 epinephrine (18 μg epinephrine). The elevation of epinephrine is linearly dose-dependent and lasts from several minutes to half an hour. Use of radiolabeled epinephrine demonstrated that the injected drug is the source of the increased epinephrine (Fig. 3–8).[38] Figure 3–9[39] compares the concentrations of epinephrine associated with various activities and medical emergencies[40] with those achieved by intraoral injection.[30] The cardiovascular effects of epinephrine administered with lidocaine for brachial plexus block are illustrated in Figure 3–10[41]; similar responses to lidocaine with and without epinephrine injected for inferior alveolar nerve anesthesia are represented in Figure 3–11.[33] A powerful β_1 agonist, epinephrine even at low doses increases the rate (modestly) and the force of contraction. Because the large capacitance veins of the leg and abdomen are constricted by epinephrine, the venous return to the heart and the cardiac stroke volume are increased. Cardiac output, the product of the stroke volume and heart rate, is likewise enhanced. Since moderate doses of epinephrine lower total peripheral resistance (largely by dilating resistance blood vessels in skeletal muscle), the mean arterial pressure may remain unchanged or become slightly reduced. With an elevated

---

* *Under resting conditions, the adrenal medulla secretes 0.009 μg/kg–min.[37] The release of epinephrine into the circulation is intermittent, with brief releases interspersed with periods of no release.*

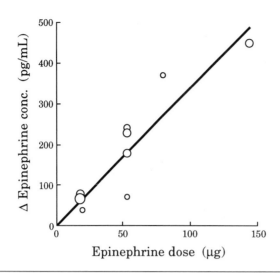

Figure 3–7.   Changes in venous plasma epinephrine concentrations after intraoral injection of 2% lidocaine with 1 : 100,000 epinephrine (1 : 25,000 for the 80-μg dose). Each circle indicates the mean value of a group of subjects; the relative size of the circle is proportional to the number of subjects in the study group (n = 6 to 14). (Data from various sources.[31-36] Redrawn with permission from Yagiela, J.A.: Local anesthetics. *In* Dionne, R.A., and Phero, J.C., eds.: Management of Pain and Anxiety in Dental Practice. New York, Elsevier Science Publishing Co., 1991.)

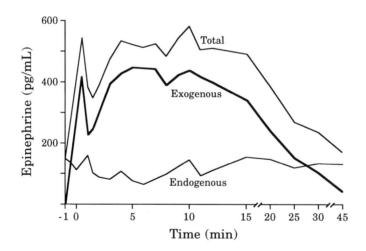

Figure 3–8.   Endogenous and exogenous contributions to venous plasma epinephrine after the injection of 2 mL of 4% articaine with 1 : 100,000 ^{3}H-epinephrine. The early spike at 30 seconds reflects abrupt, massive increases of exogenous epinephrine in four of the 20 subjects; the smaller peak at 10 minutes marks the beginning of dental treatment (deep scaling). (Data from Lipp, M.D.W., Dick, W.F., et al.: Anesthesiology, *69*:A371, 1988.)

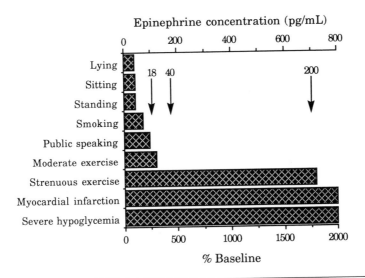

Figure 3–9. Influence of various activities and conditions on venous plasma epinephrine concentrations. (Data from Kopin, I.J., Epinephrine and the compromised heart. *In* Trendelenburg, U., and Weiner, N., eds: Catecholamines. Handbook of Experimental Pharmacology. Vol. 90/II. Berlin, Springer-Verlag, 1989. Redrawn from Yagiela, J.A.: Orofac. Pain Manage., *1*(5):1–8, 1991.)

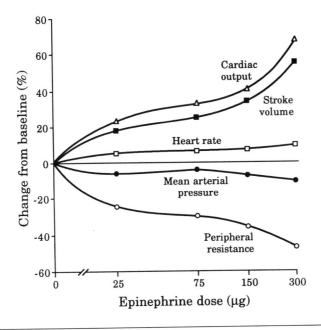

Figure 3–10. Cardiovascular effects of epinephrine when used in regional anesthesia. (Data from Kennedy, W.F., Jr., Bonica, J.J., et al.: Acta Anaesthesiol. Scand., *10*:320–333, 1966.)

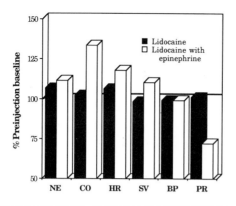

Figure 3–11. Changes in cardiovascular function after intraoral injection of 5.4 mL of 2% lidocaine with or without 1:100,000 epinephrine. Solid line indicates baseline values; NE = venous norepinephrine; CO = cardiac output; HR = heart rate; SV = stroke volume; BP = mean arterial blood pressure; PR = peripheral resistance. (Data from Dionne, R.A., Goldstein, D.S., and Wirdzek, P.R.: Anesth. Analg., *63*:640–646, 1984.)

systolic and lowered diastolic blood pressure, the pulse pressure is increased. Coronary blood flow increases, partly because of β-receptor stimulation, but mostly from local factors (e.g., accumulation of metabolites, release of adenosine). Even so, cardiac efficiency is reduced, and oxygen consumption increases more rapidly than oxygen delivery.

Electrocardiographic changes that mirror the increased rate and force of contraction include accelerated depolarization of the sinoatrial node, an increased amplitude of the QRS complex, and a decrease in the size of the T wave. Conduction of electrical impulses throughout the heart is improved. Automaticity, or the tendency for potential pacemakers in the atrioventricular node and Purkinje system to spontaneously depolarize, is also increased. In patients prone to dysrhythmias, premature ventricular contractions may occur.

The cardiovascular effects of norepinephrine differ from those of epinephrine. Because norepinephrine lacks significant β_2 activity, its vasoconstricting action is unopposed, and the mean arterial pressure is elevated. Although injected norepinephrine is as effective as epinephrine in directly stimulating β_1 receptors, inability to activate cardiac β_2 receptors may attenuate the overall effect on the heart, at least at low doses. Furthermore, compensatory vagal reflex activity initiated by baroreceptors in the aortic arch and carotid sinuses usually surmounts the direct effect, and the heart rate is actually depressed. Inasmuch as the stroke volume remains elevated, the cardiac output is unchanged or falls only slightly below preanesthetic values. Levonordefrin resembles norepinephrine in cardiovascular activity.[42]

In most individuals, even those with heart disease, the cardiovascular effects of conventional doses of adrenergic vasoconstrictors are of little practical concern. Accidental intravascular injection, unusual patient sensitivity, unanticipated drug interactions, or excessive doses, however, can result in potentially serious outcomes.

Intravenous administration of the contents of a local anesthetic cartridge containing epinephrine can lead to transient but dramatic increases in heart rate. Figure 3–12 illustrates the effect of intravenous injection of epinephrine as may occur in clinical practice. On average, 15 μg of epinephrine administered with lidocaine increases the heart rate by 25 beats/min, but some individuals experience increases of more than 70 beats/min.[43,44] The peak effect is generally reached within the first 30 to 60 seconds and then subsides over the next few minutes. The systolic blood pressure is also increased by about 20 mm Hg, with occasional exaggerated responses of more than 70 mm Hg. Premature ventricular contractions may be superimposed on the tachycardia, and the patient may be disturbed by unpleasant palpitation or forceful contractions of the heart. Intravenous administration of levonordefrin or norepinephrine can lead to precipitous (>40 mm Hg) increases in blood pressure and marked bradycardia, effects that patients also find distressing.

Patients with coronary artery disease receiving intravenous infusion of epinephrine exhibit smaller changes in heart rate and myocardial contractility than do normal patients.[45] However, they are more likely to experience ventricular dysrhythmias, chest pain, and ischemic electrocardiographic changes (ST-segment depression). Myocardial oxygen consumption begins to exceed supply in these patients at an epinephrine infusion rate of 0.06 μg/kg-min[46]; clinically evident myocardial ischemia has been shown to occur at plasma epinephrine concentrations ranging from 650 pg/mL to 3,360 pg/mL.[45] Patients with increased susceptibility to the adverse cardiovascular side effects of adrenergic vasoconstrictors

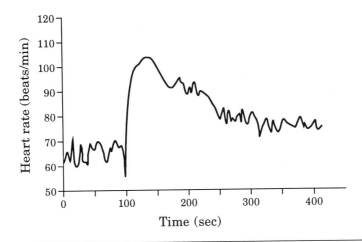

Figure 3–12.   Effect of intravenous epinephrine on heart rate. A bolus injection of 1.5% lidocaine with 1 : 200,000 epinephrine was given (15 μg total epinephrine). (Redrawn with permission from Huang, K.C.: Effect of intravenous epinephrine on heart rate as monitored with a computerized tachometer. Anesthesiology, *73*:A762, 1990.)

administered in conventional doses include those with any of the following conditions: unstable angina pectoris; recent (within 3 months) myocardial infarction or coronary artery bypass surgery; uncontrolled dysrhythmias, congestive heart failure, or hyperthyroidism; or uncontrolled severe hypertension.[47,48] These conditions, along with drug interactions that can lead to adverse outcomes, are discussed in Chapter 5.

When truly horrendous dosage errors are made, such as mistakenly injecting large amounts of 1:1,000 epinephrine instead of the 1:100,000 strength, all of the adrenergic vasoconstrictors produce alarming hypertensive responses with reflex bradycardia.[49] Death may result from myocardial infarction, ventricular fibrillation, cerebral hemorrhage, or pulmonary edema.

RESPIRATORY SYSTEM

Epinephrine is a potent relaxant of bronchial smooth muscle. The bronchodilation (β_2-receptor effect) and, to a lesser extent, the relief of mucosal congestion and inhibition of bronchial secretions (both α_1-receptor effects occurring with high doses of epinephrine) make the drug invaluable for treating asthmatic attacks and anaphylactic reactions. A β_2-mediated suppression of the release of inflammatory autacoids (e.g., histamine) by mast cells contributes to the therapeutic result. Epinephrine is also a respiratory stimulant, transiently increasing both the rate and the depth of respiration when large amounts of drug are injected. Neither norepinephrine nor levonordefrin share in the bronchodilating action of epinephrine to any degree.

By constricting the capacitance vessels of the systemic vasculature, epinephrine tends to redistribute the blood to the lungs and thus increase the blood pressure in the pulmonary circulation. This action is shared by all of the adrenergic vasoconstrictors. Although this shift is usually of no consequence at plasma concentrations relevant to regional anesthesia, massive doses of sympathomimetic amines can produce pulmonary edema that, as already pointed out, can be lethal.

GASTROINTESTINAL TRACT

The influences of adrenergic amines on the smooth muscle and secretory glands of the gastrointestinal tract are largely of heuristic interest in the present context, since these effects normally occur at dosages higher than those employed in regional anesthesia. Nevertheless, these drugs may diminish propulsive contractions of the intestinal wall and stimulate closure of the pyloric and ileocecal sphincters. Most secretory glands are inhibited indirectly by an α_1-receptor–mediated reduction in blood supply. Salivation is variably affected; large doses of epinephrine stimulate secretion of a saliva rich in amylase activity but small in volume.

GENITOURINARY SYSTEM

Epinephrine tends to inhibit urination by several mechanisms: contraction of the sphincter and trigone muscles and relaxation of the detrusor muscle of the bladder (see Table 3–3). Urine formation is essentially unimpaired even though the vasoconstrictors uniformly reduce renal blood flow in systemically active concentrations.

The effects of adrenergic agents on the uterus are complex and depend on menstrual phase and gestational state. During pregnancy, norepinephrine promotes uterine contraction, whereas epinephrine, at least in moderate doses, does the opposite. Because of its relative lack of effect on α_1 and β_2 adrenoceptors, levonordefrin presumably has little effect on uterine tone.

SKELETAL MUSCLE

As the "flight or fight" hormone, epinephrine prepares the body for vigorous physical activity.[9] As described elsewhere in this chapter, epinephrine shifts the blood supply from nonessential areas (at least insofar as physical exercise is concerned) to skeletal muscle and tissues (liver, fat) that provide the energy necessary for muscular exertion. Epinephrine also facilitates neuromuscular transmission by enhancing the release of acetylcholine. Both α and β effects appear to be involved in this effect.

Peak tension of fast-contracting motor fibers is increased by a direct action on muscle. More importantly, β_2-adrenoceptor stimulation of slow-contracting muscle shortens the contraction times of individual muscle fibers. A decrease in muscular force generated by maximum physiologic rates of nerve stimulation accompanies the failure of motor units to fuse fully in tetanic contraction. Tremor may result from the altered contraction of these muscles.

METABOLISM

The adrenergic amines influence a number of metabolic events throughout the body. In general, these influences serve to increase the availability of nutrients for cardiac and skeletal muscle metabolism. Epinephrine, in particular, elevates plasma glucose titers by several coordinated mechanisms[9,50–52]: (1) by enhancing glycogenolysis in the liver and other tissues, (2) by stimulating gluconeogenesis from lactic and amino acids, (3) by interfering with glucose uptake by various tissues, and (4) at high doses, by inhibiting the secretion of insulin. Lipolysis and fat metabolism are also affected by epinephrine-like drugs, resulting in elevated plasma titers of free fatty acids and, to a lesser extent, ketone bodies. Increased blood flow to the liver and fat supports the metabolic activation. Even without overt muscular activity, the various effects of epinephrine on

Table 3–4. **THRESHOLD PLASMA CONCENTRATIONS OF EPINEPHRINE REQUIRED FOR PHYSIOLOGIC CHANGE**

Response	*Epinephrine Conc.** *(pg/mL)*	*Intraoral Dose†* *(μg)*	*Cartridge Equivalent‡*
↑ Heart rate	50–100	20	1.0
↑ Plasma glycerol	75–125	30	1.5
↑ Systolic blood pressure	75–150	40	2.0
↓ Diastolic blood pressure	150–200	70	4.0
↑ Plasma glucose	150–200	70	4.0
↓ Insulin secretion	400–450	200	11.0

*Venous plasma concentrations. Data from Clutter, et al.[52]

†Dose of epinephrine injected intraorally (to the nearest 10 μg) that is estimated to yield the midrange concentration of epinephrine, assuming a basal epinephrine titer of 39 pg/mL and a dose-concentration relationship as defined in Figure 3–7.

‡Number of cartridges of 2% lidocaine with 1:100,000 epinephrine (to the nearest half cartridge) approximating the injected dose.

intermediary metabolism cause a 15% to 30% increase in oxygen consumption.

Table 3–4 records the minimum plasma concentrations required to elicit various metabolic changes according to Clutter et al.[52] Studies by Meechan and co-workers[53,54] demonstrated that glucose concentrations are elevated after local anesthesia was administered for dental procedures. Because of their inability to secrete insulin in response to the increased plasma glucose, patients with diabeties mellitus can exhibit pronounced hyperglycemia in response to epinephrine.[55]

Plasma potassium (K^+) concentrations are acutely decreased by epinephrine.[54,56] Through a β_2-dependent stimulation of skeletal muscle sodium (Na^+)-K^+ adenosine triphosphatase, K^+ is exchanged for intracellular Na^+.[56] While the effect is generally modest after doses used in dentistry, it is exaggerated in patients receiving kaliuretic diuretics (e.g., furosemide) and has been considered to be a potential cause of cardiac dysrhythmias in these patients as well as in individuals taking digitalis glycosides.[54]

CENTRAL NERVOUS SYSTEM

Overdosage or accidental intravascular injection of an adrenergic amine generally produces an array of subjective symptoms and observable signs normally attributed to the central nervous system. Such responses may include anxiety, restlessness, nausea, weakness, tremor, headache, and hyperventilation. Two facts indicate that these effects are not actually caused by a direct action of the drug on the brain. First, the low lipid solubility of the sympathomimetic vasoconstrictors tends to preclude significant entry into the central nervous system. Second, intracisternal or intraventricular injection (in essence, direct administration into the brain) of epinephrine causes sedation, quite the opposite of what the drug elicits peripherally. It appears, therefore, that most of the so-called central actions of the adrenergic vasoconstrictors are indirectly mediated via changes at the level of the peripheral nervous system resulting from alterations in cardiovascular status, metabolism, neuromuscular transmission, and the like.[9]

Absorption, Fate, and Excretion

The absorption of epinephrine, norepinephrine, and levonordefrin from intraoral injection sites is, of course, retarded by the drugs' vasoconstricting properties and may take several hours to reach completion. After intraoral injection of a single cartridge, peak plasma concentrations are usually observed within the first few minutes and then subside over the next 10 to 20 minutes. Larger doses produce similar peak times but a more extended duration. With large therapeutic doses administered subcutaneously to treat allergic reactions, systemic reactions become noticeable within several minutes, reach a peak between 10 and 30 minutes, and then subside. By comparison, the effects of epinephrine following intravenous bolus injection become maximal within 1 minute and last for only 5 to 10 minutes. Obviously, the body is very efficient in removing catecholamines from the bloodstream.

Figure 3–13 illustrates the fate of exogenously administered epinephrine.[21] Most of the drug is absorbed, distributed throughout the body, taken up by extraneuronal tissue, and inactivated by the enzyme catechol-O-methyltransferase (COMT). This cytoplasmic enzyme is found in

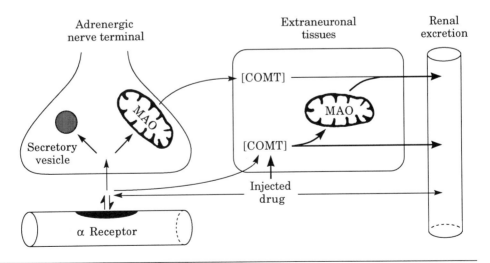

Figure 3–13. Distribution and fate of catecholamines injected into peripheral tissues. Dark arrows indicate the predominant pathways for epinephrine and norepinephrine. The fate of levonordefrin is modified by its resistance to monoamine oxidase (MAO) activity.

many tissues and is especially concentrated in the liver. The O-methylated product, metanephrine, is either excreted in the urine (mostly as the sulfate and glucuronide conjugates) or further metabolized (mostly in the liver) by the mitochondrial enzyme monoamine oxidase (MAO). The primary metabolite formed, 3-methoxy-4-hydroxymandelic acid (sometimes referred to as vanillylmandelic acid, or VMA), is then eliminated

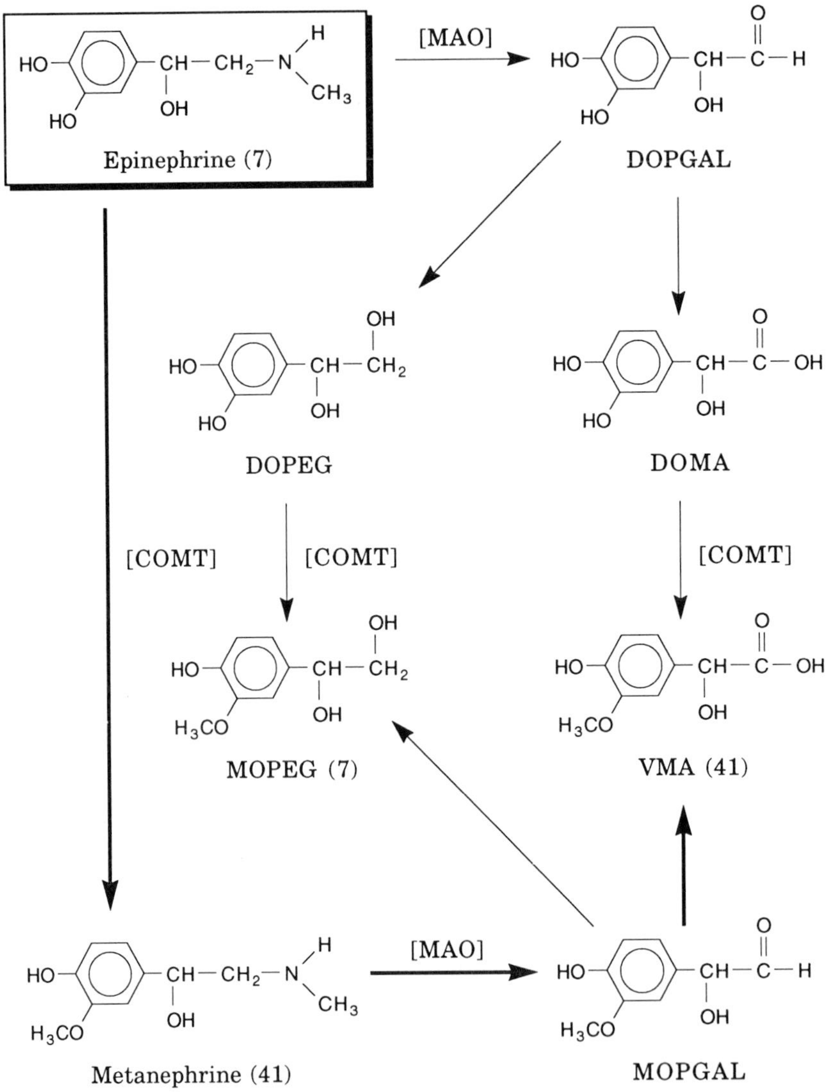

Figure 3–14.   Metabolism of epinephrine. Dark arrows indicate the predominant pathway. Values in parentheses are percentages recovered in the urine. MAO = monoamine oxidase; COMT = catechol-O-methyltransferase; DOPGAL = 3,4-dihydroxyphenylglycolaldehyde; DOPEG = 3,4-dihydroxyphenylethylene glycol; DOMA = 3,4-dihydroxymandelic acid; MOPEG = 3-methoxy-4-hydroxyphenylethylene glycol; VMA = 3-methoxy-4-hydroxymandelic acid; MOPGAL = 3-methoxy-4-hydroxyphenylglycolaldehyde. (Data from LaBrosse, E.H., Axelrod, J., et al., J. Clin. Invest., *40*:253–260, 1961.)

by the kidney. Although not shown in Figure 3–13, some epinephrine reaching the liver may be initially deaminated by MAO. Even then, most of the drug is subsequently converted to VMA.

The small amount of epinephrine that actually combines with receptors to elicit a pharmacologic response is subject to active transport into the adrenergic nerve terminals supplying the effector cells. Once taken up, epinephrine may be sequestered in secretory vesicles to be eventually released upon neural command, or it may be oxidized by intraneuronal MAO. The oxidized drug leaks out of the neuron and is further metabolized by COMT to yield VMA. Of an injected dose of epinephrine, approximately 40% is recovered in the urine as VMA, 40% as metanephrine, and small amounts (<10% each) as unchanged epinephrine and 3-methoxy-4-hydroxyphenylethylene glycol (Fig. 3–14).[57] The small amount (7%) unaccounted for in 2 days of testing represents other metabolites, unavoidable losses in urine collection, and possibly epinephrine stored within adrenergic nerve terminals.

The metabolic fate of norepinephrine is quite similar to that of epinephrine, with VMA and normetanephrine (the analogue of metanephrine) being the primary metabolites. With respect to levonordefrin, the methyl group on the α carbon (position ① in Fig. 3–3) protects the drug from oxidation by MAO. Therefore, inactivation by COMT is the only route of biotransformation available to it. Because MAO is not primarily responsible for terminating the action of catecholamines, however, the duration of systemic effects of levonordefrin is no greater than that of epinephrine.

Felypressin

Although the adrenergic amines are generally safe and effective as vasoconstrictors in regional anesthesia, they do have some drawbacks. All of the drugs can produce potentially dangerous cardiovascular effects and elicit disturbing subjective responses when high blood concentrations are obtained. In addition, certain drug interactions and disease states as described in Chapter 5 may limit or even contraindicate their use. For these reasons, nonsympathomimetic amine alternatives for vasoconstriction have been sought. Most attention has been focused on felypressin (Octapressin), the 2-phenylalanine-8-lysine analogue of antidiuretic hormone, or vasopressin (Fig. 3–15).

Felypressin is a direct stimulator of vascular smooth muscle. It binds to the V_1 receptor for antidiuretic hormone, which activates phospholipase C and initiates the cascade of intracellular events outlined in Figure 3–5 that lead to contraction.[58] Felypressin appears to act preferentially on the venous side of the microcirculation, but all parts of the vasculature can be affected by large doses.[59] Because felypressin has little or no direct effect on the myocardium and no influence on adrenergic nerve transmission, it may be safely given when dysrhythmia, uncontrolled

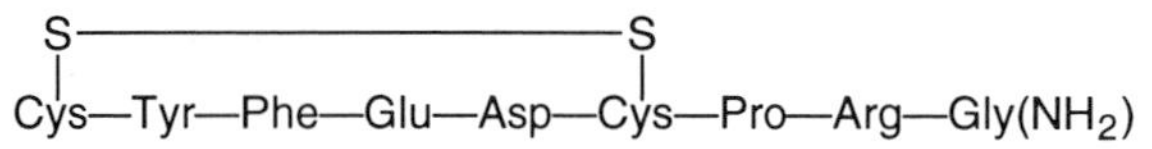

S————————————————S
| |
Cys—Tyr—Phe—Glu—Asp—Cys—Pro—Arg—Gly(NH$_2$)

Antidiuretic hormone (vasopressin)

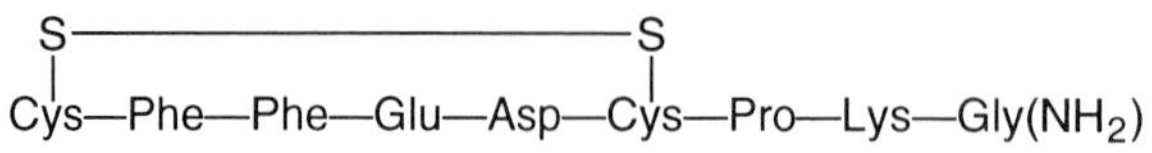

S————————————————S
| |
Cys—Phe—Phe—Glu—Asp—Cys—Pro—Lys—Gly(NH$_2$)

Felypressin (2-phe-8-lys-vasopressin)

Figure 3–15.   Structural formulas of antidiuretic hormone and felypressin. Cys = cysteine; Tyr = tyrosine; Phe = phenylalanine; Glu = glutamic acid; Asp = aspartic acid; Pro = proline; Arg = argenine; Gly = glycine; Lys = lysine.

hyperthyroidism, or concurrent medications precludes the use of epinephrine. In animal studies, felypressin has demonstrated an exceptionally wide margin of safety.[60] Felypressin is well tolerated by tissues and seems to lack the local tissue irritation sometimes caused by adrenergic amines.

Felypressin causes few systemic side effects. The peptide has some antidiuretic and oxytocic activity, the latter of which may preclude its use during pregnancy. With high doses of felypressin, facial pallor may result from constriction of cutaneous blood vessels, and coronary blood flow may also be impaired. Thus, the amount of felypressin administered to patients with ischemic heart disease should be limited to no more than five 1.8-mL cartridges of a 0.03 IU/mL solution (1 IU = 20 μg).

In Great Britain and other countries where felypressin is marketed (usually in combination with 3% prilocaine), the agent has compared favorably with epinephrine in regional anesthesia for restorative dentistry. Because felypressin is not very active in constricting arterioles, however, it is not nearly as effective as conventional vasoconstrictors in limiting hemorrhage at surgical sites.[61] Nevertheless, the distinctive properties of felypressin make it a useful addition to the anesthetic armamentarium of practitioners with access to the drug.

References

1. Berling, C.: Carbocain in local anaesthesia in the oral cavity: An experimental and clinical investigation comprising 1046 dental local anaesthesias. Odontol. Rev., 9:254–267, 1958.
2. Brown, G.: The influence of adrenaline, noradrenaline vasoconstrictors on the efficiency of lidocaine. J. Oral Ther. Pharmacol., 4:398–405, 1968.
3. Björn, H., and Huldt, S.: The efficiency of Xylocaine as a dental terminal anesthetic compared to that of procaine. Sven. Tandlak. Tidskr., 40:831–851, 1947.

4. Cannell, H., Walters, H., Beckett, A.H., and Saunders, A.: Circulating levels of lignocaine after peri-oral injections. Br. Dent. J., *138*:87–93, 1975.

5. Holroyd, S.V., and Requa-Clark, B.: Local anesthetics. *In* Holroyd, S.V., and Wynn, R.L., eds.: Clinical Pharmacology in Dental Practice, 3rd ed. St. Louis, C.V. Mosby Co., 1983.

6. Malamed, S.F.: Handbook of Local Anesthesia, 3rded. St. Louis, Mosby–Year Book, Inc., 1990.

7. Yagiela, J.A.: Vasoconstrictors: Their role in local anesthetic toxicity. J. Jpn. Dent. Soc. Anesthesiol., *21*:261–278, 1993.

8. Dhunér, K.-G.: Frequency of general side reactions after regional anaesthesia with mepivacaine with and without vasoconstrictors. Acta Anaesthesiol. Scand. Suppl., *48*:23–43, 1972.

9. Hoffman, B.B., and Lefkowitz, R.J.: Catecholamines and sympathomimetic drugs. *In* Gilman, A.G., Rall, T.W., Nies, A.S., and Taylor, P., eds.: Goodman and Gilman's The Pharmacological Basis of Therapeutics, 8th ed. New York, Pergamon Press, 1990.

10. Boakes, A.J., Laurence, D.R., Lovel, K.W., O'Neil, R., and Verrill, P.J.: Adverse reactions to local anaesthetic/vasoconstrictor preparations. Br. Dent. J., *133*:137–140, 1972.

11. Ferry, D.R., Henry, R.L., and Kern, M.J.: Epinephrine-induced myocardial infarction in a patient with angiographically normal coronary arteries. Am. Heart J., *111*:1193–1195, 1986.

12. Yagiela, J.A.: Death in a cardiac patient after local anesthesia with epinephrine. Orofac. Pain Manage., *1*(5):6, 1991.

13. Cowan, A.: Further clinical evaluation of prilocaine (Citanest), with and without epinephrine. Oral Surg. Oral Med. Oral Pathol., *26*:304–311, 1968.

14. Chilton, N.W.: Clinical evaluation of prilocaine hydrochloride 4% solution with and without epinephrine. J. Am. Dent. Assoc., *83*:149–154, 1971.

15. Epstein, S.: Clinical study of prilocaine with varying concentrations of epinephrine. J. Am. Dent. Assoc., *78*:85–90, 1969.

16. Ahlquist, R.P.: A study of the adrenotropic receptors. Am. J. Physiol., *153*:586–600, 1948.

17. Lands, A.M., Arnold, A., McAuliff, J.P., Luduena, F.P., and Braun, T.G., Jr.: Differentiation of receptor systems activated by sympathomimetic amines. Nature, *214*:597–598, 1967.

18. Langer, S.Z.: Presynaptic regulation of catecholamine release. Biochem. Pharmacol., *23*:1793–1800, 1974.

19. Ruffolo, R.R., Jr., Nichols, A.J., Stadel, J.M., and Hieble, J.P.: Structure and function of α-adrenoceptors. Pharmacol. Rev., *43*:475–505, 1991.

20. Ostrowski, J., Kjelsberg, M.A., Caron, M.G., and Lefkowitz, R.J.: Mutagenesis of the β_2-adrenergic receptor: How structure elucidates function. Annu. Rev. Pharmacol. Toxicol., *32*:167–183, 1992.

21. Lefkowitz, R.J., Hoffman, B.B., and Taylor, P.: Neurohumoral transmission: the autonomic and somatic motor nervous system. *In* Gilman, A.G., Rall, T.W., Nies, A.S., and Taylor, P., eds.: Goodman and Gilman's The Pharmacological Basis of Therapeutics, 8th ed. New York, Pergamon Press, 1990.

22. Dhunér, K.-G., and Lewis, D.H.: Effect of local anaesthetics and vasoconstrictors upon regional blood flow. Acta Anaesthesiol. Scand. Suppl., *23*:347–352, 1966.

23. Kim, S., Edwall, L., Trowbridge, H., and Chien, S.: Effects of local anesthetics on pulpal blood flow in dogs. J. Dent. Res., *63*:650–652, 1984.

24. Brodde, O.-E.: β_1- and β_2-adrenoceptors in the human heart: properties, function, and alterations in chronic heart failure. Pharmacol. Rev., *43*:204–241, 1991.

25. Cheraskin, E., and Prasertsuntarasai, T.: Use of epinephrine with local anesthesia in

hypertensive patients: I. Blood pressure and pulse rate observations in the waiting room. J. Am. Dent. Assoc., *55*:761–774, 1957.

26. Elliott, G.D., and Stein, E.: Oral surgery in patients with atherosclerotic heart disease: Benign effect of epinephrine in local anesthesia. JAMA, *227*:1403–1404, 1974.

27. Glover, J.: Vasoconstrictors in dental anaesthetics: Contraindication—fact or fallacy? Aust. Dent. J., *58*:65–69, 1968.

28. Nikki, P., Takki, S., and Jättel, A.: Effect of adrenaline infiltration on plasma catecholamines. Ann. Chir. Gynaecol., *62*:265–270, 1973.

29. Tolas, A.G., Pflug, A.E., and Halter, J.B.: Arterial plasma epinephrine concentrations and hemodynamic responses after dental injection of local anesthetic with epinephrine. J. Am. Dent. Assoc., *104*:41–43, 1982.

30. Yagiela, J.A.: Local anesthetics. *In* Dionne, R.A., and Phero, J.C., eds.: Management of Pain and Anxiety in Dental Practice. New York, Elsevier Science Publishing Co., 1991.

31. Goldstein, D.S., Dionne, R., Sweet, J., Gracely, R., Brewer, H.B., Jr., Gregg, R., and Keiser, H.R.: Circulatory, plasma catecholamine, cortisol, lipid, and psychological responses to a real-life stress (third molar extractions): Effects of diazepam sedation and inclusion of epinephrine with the local anesthetic. Psychosomat. Med., *44*:259–272, 1982.

32. Chernow, B., Balestrieri, F., Ferguson, C.D., Terezhalmy, G.T., Fletcher, J.R., and Lake, C.R.: Local dental anesthesia with epinephrine. Arch. Intern. Med., *143*:2141–2143, 1983.

33. Dionne, R.A., Goldstein, D.S., and Wirdzek, P.R.: Effects of diazepam premedication and epinephrine-containing local anesthetic on cardiovascular and plasma catecholamine responses in oral surgery. Anesth. Analg., *63*:640–646, 1984.

34. Cioffi, G.A., Chernow, B., Glahn, R.P., Terezhalmy, G.T., and Lake, C.R.: The hemodynamic and plasma catecholamine responses to routine restorative dental care. J. Am. Dent. Assoc., *111*:67–70, 1985.

35. Troullos, E.S., Goldstein, D.S., Hargreaves, K.M., and Dionne, R.A.: Plasma epinephrine levels and cardiovascular response to high administered doses of epinephrine in local anesthesia. Anesth. Prog., *34*:10–13, 1987.

36. Knoll-Köhler, E., Frie, A., Becker, J., and Ohlendorf, D.: Changes in plasma epinephrine concentrations after dental infiltration anesthesia with different doses of epinephrine. J. Dent. Res., *68*:1098–1101, 1989.

37. Sapira, J.D., and Bron, K.: Human epinephrine secretion: Direct measurement of the secretion of epinephrine from the human adrenal medulla. J. Clin. Endocrinol., *33*:436–447, 1971.

38. Lipp, M.D.W., Dick, W.F., Daubländer, M., Hornke, I., and Fuder, H.: Examination of the central-venous epinephrine level during local dental infiltration and block anesthesia using tritium-marked epinephrine as vasoconstrictor. Anesthesiology, *69*:A371, 1988.

39. Yagiela, J.A.: Epinephrine and the compromised heart. Orofac. Pain Manage., *1*(5):1–8, 1991.

40. Kopin, I.J.: Plasma levels of catecholamines and dopamine-β-hydroxylase. *In* Trendelenburg, U., and Weiner, N., eds.: Catecholamines. Handbook of Experimental Pharmacology. Vol. 90/II. Berlin, Springer-Verlag, 1989.

41. Kennedy, W.F., Jr., Bonica, J.J., Ward, R.J., Tolas, A.G., Martin, W.E., and Grinstein, A.: Cardiorespiratory effects of epinephrine when used in regional anesthesia. Acta Anaesthesiol. Scand. Suppl., *23*:320–333, 1966.

42. Robertson, V.J., Taylor, S.E., and Gage, T.W.: Quantitative and qualitative analysis of the pressor effects of levonordefrin. J. Cardiovasc. Pharmacol., *6*:929–935, 1984.

43. Huang, K.C.: Effect of intravenous epinephrine on heart rate as monitored with a computerized tachometer. Anesthesiology, *73*:A762, 1990.

44. Narchi, P., Mazoit, J.-X., Cohen, S., and Samii, K.: Heart rate response to an I.V. test dose of adrenaline and lignocaine with and without atropine pretreatment. Br. J. Anaesth., *66*:583–586, 1991.
45. Sung, B.H., Robinson, C., Thadani, U., Lee, R., and Wilson, M.F.: Effects of l-epinephrine on hemodynamics and cardiac function in coronary disease: Dose-response studies. Clin. Pharmacol. Ther., *43*:308–316, 1988.
46. Schechter, E., Wilson, M.F., and Kong, Y.-S.: Physiologic responses to epinephrine infusion: The basis for a new stress test for coronary artery disease. Am. Heart J., *105*:554–560, 1983.
47. Pérusse, R., Goulet, J.-P., and Turcotte, J.-Y.: contraindications to vasoconstrictors in dentistry: Part I. Oral Surg. Oral Med. Oral Pathol., *74*:679–686, 1992.
48. Pérusse, R., Goulet, J.-P., and Turcotte, J.-Y.: Contraindications to vasoconstrictors in dentistry: Part II. Oral Surg. Oral Med. Oral Pathol., *74*:687–691, 1992.
49. Campbell, R.L.: Cardiovascular effects of epinephrine overdose: Case report. Anesth. Prog., *24*:190–193, 1977.
50. Saccà, L., Vigorito, C., Cicala, M., Corso, G., and Sherwin, R.S.: Role of gluconeogenesis in epinephrine-stimulated hepatic glucose production in humans. Am. J. Physiol., *245*:E294–E302, 1983.
51. Hamburg, S., Hendler, R., Sherwin, R.S.: Influence of small increments of epinephrine on glucose tolerance in normal humans. Ann. Intern. Med., *93*:566–568, 1980.
52. Clutter, W.E., Bier, D.M., Shah, S.D., and Cryer, P.E.: Epinephrine plasma metabolic clearance rates and physiologic thresholds for metabolic and hemodynamic actions in man. J. Clin. Invest., *66*:94–101, 1980.
53. Meechan, J.G. The effects of dental local anaesthetics on blood glucose concentration in healthy volunteers and in patients having third molar surgery. Br. Dent. J., *170*:373–376, 1991.
54. Meechan, J.G., Thomson, C.W., Blair, G.S., and Rawlins, M.D.: The biochemical and haemodynamic effects of adrenaline in lignocaine local anaesthetic solutions in patients having third molar surgery under general anaesthesia. Br. J. Oral Maxillofac. Surg., *29*:263–268, 1991.
55. Berk, M.A., Clutter, W.E., Skor, D., Shah, S.D., Gingerich, R.P., Parvin, C.A., and Cryer, P.E.: Enhanced glycemic responsiveness to epinephrine in insulin-dependent diabetes mellitus is the result of the inability to secrete insulin. J. Clin. Invest., *75*:1842–1851, 1985.
56. Fellows, I.W., Bennett, T., and MacDonald, I.A.: The effect of adrenaline upon cardiovascular and metabolic functions in man. Clin. Sci., *69*:215–222, 1985.
57. LaBrosse, E.H., Axelrod, J., Kopin, I.J., and Kety, S.S.: Metabolism of 7-H^3-epinephrine-*d*-bitartrate in normal young men. J. Clin. Invest., *40*:253–260, 1961.
58. Hays, R.M.: Agents affecting the renal conservation of water. *In* Gilman, A.G., Rall, T.W., Nies, A.S., and Taylor, P., eds.: Goodman and Gilman's The Pharmacological Basis of Therapeutics, 8th ed. New York, Pergamon Press, 1990.
59. Altura, B.M., Hershey, S.G., and Zweifach, B.W.: Effects of a synthetic analogue of vasopressin on vascular smooth muscle. Proc. Soc. Exp. Biol. Med., *119*:258–261, 1965.
60. Åkerman, B.: On felypressin (Octapressin) as an adjunct to lidocaine and prilocaine—an experimental study in animals. Acta Pharmacol. Toxicol., *24*:377–388, 1966.
61. Newcomb, G.M., and Waite, I.M.: The effectiveness of two local analgesic preparations in reducing haemorrhage during periodontal surgery. J. Dent., *1*:37–42, 1972.

Clinical Preparations and Drug Selection

Since the discovery of cocaine anesthesia in 1884, a variety of local anesthetics have been formulated in an impressive array of concentrations and vasoconstrictor combinations for use in the oral cavity. Those local anesthetics in common use by dentists are discussed in this chapter, along with certain drugs and formulations that have potential application for nerve blockade. Many other agents have been used in the past that offer no particular benefit over the currently available drugs. These include such drugs as butacaine (Butyn), butethamine (Monocaine), and chloroprocaine (Nesacaine), and will not be discussed further.

Injectable Anesthetic Preparations

Local anesthetics intended for injection within the oral cavity are supplied in single-dose cartridges. Pyrogen-free distilled water serves as the local anesthetic vehicle, with sodium chloride added for osmotic balance. Local anesthetic solutions range in pH from under 3.0 to over 6.0; generally, preparations with vasoconstrictors are more acidic than are plain formulations. Small amounts of sodium hydroxide or hydrochloric acid are added to adjust the pH. Sodium metabisulfite or an equivalent antioxidant is included in solutions with adrenergic vasoconstrictors to help prevent vasoconstrictor breakdown. Intolerance to sulfites has occasionally complicated the use of local anesthetics; formulations containing these antioxidants should be used cautiously in asthmatic patients with a history of sensitivity to ingested or inhaled sulfites,[1] especially those with steroid-dependent asthma.[2] They should be avoided altogether in the rare patient with true allergy or documented sensitivity to injected sulfites.[3]

Finally, local anesthetics may contain antibacterial substances such as methylparaben. Useful for its antimicrobial action in multidose products, methylparaben serves no purpose in single-dose preparations, and its incorporation into local anesthetic cartridges has been discontinued in the United States. Methylparaben and related substances occasionally cause allergic reactions that can be confused with local anesthetic hyper-sensitivity.[4] Individuals reactive to one paraben generally show cross-sensitivity to others (e.g., propylparaben) as well as to closely related ester anesthetics.

PROCAINE HYDROCHLORIDE

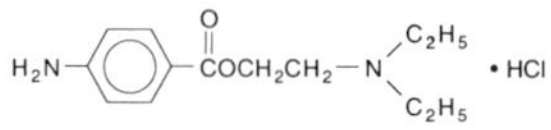

Chemical Name: 2-(diethylamino)ethyl *p*-aminobenzoate mono-hydrochloride
Trade Name: Novocain

Procaine, the ester derivative of *p*-aminobenzoic acid and diethylamino-ethanol, was the first local anesthetic to achieve widespread use for routine dental procedures and is considered the prototypical ester anes-thetic. Although still available in multidose vials for nerve blockade, it has been largely displaced by more effective, longer-acting, and less allergenic amide local anesthetics, such as lidocaine and mepivacaine.

Procaine is the least toxic injectable anesthetic used in dentistry (Table 4–1).[5-14] Conventional doses of procaine are rapidly hydrolyzed by plasma cholinesterase, as is shown in Figure 4–1.[15] Because procaine (and other ester local anesthetics) is inactivated by hydrolysis, toxic effects are generally associated with accidental intravascular injection,

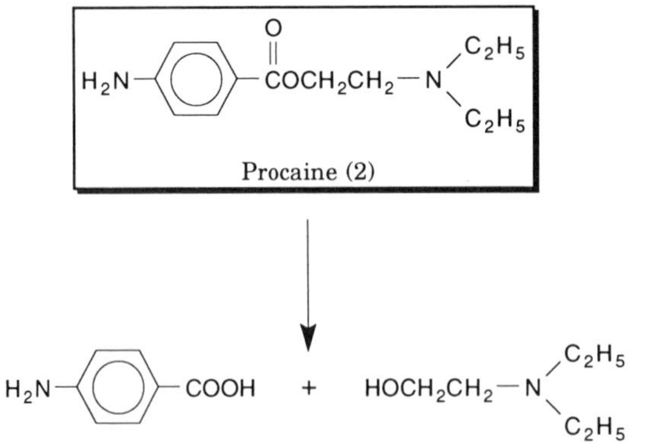

Procaine (2)

p-Aminobenzoic acid (79)   Diethylaminoethanol (29)

Figure 4–1.   Metabolism and excretion of procaine. Values in parentheses indicate the percentages of the dose found in the urine in the first 24 hours after intravenous administration. (Data from Brodie, B.B., Lief, P.A., and Poet, R.: J. Pharmacol. Exp. Ther. *94*:359–366, 1948.)

Table 4–1.   **MEDIAN LETHAL DOSE (LD50) MEASUREMENTS OF LOCAL ANESTHETICS IN RODENTS**

Formulation	Intravenous Injection in Rats (mg/kg)	Subcutaneous Injection in Mice (mg/kg)
Procaine	53	558
with 1 : 100,000 epinephrine	—	450
Lidocaine	25	217
with 1 : 100,000 epinephrine	14	207
Mepivacaine	29	265
with 1 : 20,000 levonordefrin	23	184
Prilocaine	39	619
with 1 : 200,000 epinephrine	34	438
Bupivacaine	6.5	62
with 1 : 200,000 epinephrine	3.7	95
Etidocaine	6.9	99
with 1 : 200,000 epinephrine	6.6	—
Articaine	24	—
with 1 : 100,000 epinephrine	11	—

Data from various sources.[5-14]

Table 4–2.   **AVERAGE DURATIONS OF LOCAL ANESTHESIA AFTER INTRAORAL INJECTION**

Preparation	Maxillary Infiltration		Inferior Alveolar Block	
	Pulpal Tissue	Soft Tissue	Pulpal Tissue	Soft Tissue
0.4% Propoxycaine HCl, 2% procaine HCl; 1 : 20,000 levonordefrin or 1 : 30,000 norepinephrine	40	145	60	175
2% Lidocaine HCl; 1 : 100,000 or 1 : 50,000 epinephrine	60	170	85	190
2% Mepivacaine HCl; 1 : 20,000 levonordefrin	50	130	75	185
3% Mepivacaine HCl	25	90	40	165
4% Prilocaine HCl	20	105	55	190
4% Prilocaine HCl; 1 : 200,000 epinephrine	40	140	60	220
0.5% Bupivacaine HCl; 1 : 200,000 epinephrine	40	340	240	440
1.5% Etidocaine HCl; 1 : 200,000 epinephrine	30	280	240	470
4% Articaine HCl; 1 : 200,000 or 1 : 100,000 epinephrine	60	170	90	220

Modified from Yagiela.[18]

Table 4–3.   **MAXIMUM RECOMMENDED DOSES OF LOCAL ANESTHETICS**

Drug	Trade Name	Maximum Dose (mg/kg)	Maximum Adult Dose (mg)
Propoxycaine/procaine	Ravocaine and Novocain	6.6*,†	—
Lidocaine	Alphacaine	4.5‡	300
	Lignospan	7.0 (4.5)†	500 (300)
	Lignospan Forte		
	Octocaine		
	Xylocaine		
Mepivacaine	Arestocaine	6.6 (4.5)	400 (300)
	Carbocaine		
	Isocaine		
	Polocaine		
	Scandonest		
Prilocaine	Citanest Plain	8.0 (6.0)	600 (400)
	Citanest Forte		
Bupivacaine	Marcaine	—	90†
Etidocaine	Duranest	8.0 (5.5)†	400
Articaine	Ultracaine D-S	7.0 (adult)	—
	Ultracaine D-S forte	5.0 (child)	—

Officially approved product information.[19-21] Values in parentheses are more conservative guidelines listed in Accepted Dental Therapeutics[22] *and/or the* USP Dispensing Information.[23]
* Combined anesthetic weight.
† With vasoconstrictor.
‡ Without vasoconstrictor.

except in the rare individual who lacks plasma cholinesterase activity (see Chapter 5).

Currently, 2% procaine is only available in a dental cartridge format in combination with 0.4% propoxycaine hydrochloride (described below) and either 1 : 20,000 (50 μg/mL) levonordefrin or norepinephrine bitartrate (equivalent to 1 : 30,000 [33 μg/mL] norepinephrine base) as the vasoconstrictor. Each milliliter of solution also contains 3 mg sodium chloride and up to 2 mg acetone sodium bisulfite. The addition of propoxycaine to the procaine solution increases the anesthetic's rate of onset, maximum efficacy, duration of action, and toxic potential.[16,17] Patients exhibiting an allergic response to other p-aminobenzoic acid esters will also exhibit cross-allergenicity to procaine and propoxycaine. Although not widely used, procaine with propoxycaine anesthesia is indicated for relatively short procedures, particularly in patients with a documented allergy to amide but not ester anesthetics. Onset of anesthesia normally occurs within 1 to 3 minutes after injection. Average expected durations of pulpal and soft tissue anesthesia for this and other injectable local anes-

Table 4–4. **MAXIMUM RECOMMENDED INJECTION VOLUMES
OF LOCAL ANESTHETICS**

Preparation	*Maximum Volume in mL/kg* (cartridges/kg)*	*Maximum Adult Volume in mL* (cartridges)*
0.4% Propoxycaine HCl, 2% procaine HCl; 1 : 20,000 levonordefrin or 1 : 30,000 norepinephrine	0.27 (0.15)	—
2% Lidocaine HCl	0.22 (0.12)	15.0 (8.3)
2% Lidocaine HCl; 1 : 100,000 or 1 : 50,000 epinephrine	0.35 (0.19)	25.0 (13.8)
3% Mepivacaine HCl	0.22 (0.12)	13.3 (7.3)
2% Mepivacaine HCl; 1 : 20,000 levonordefrin	0.33 (0.18)	20.0 (11.1)
4% Prilocaine HCl	0.20 (0.11)	15.0 (8.3)
4% Prilocaine HCl; 1 : 200,000 epinephrine	0.20 (0.11)	15.0 (8.3)
0.5% Bupivacaine HCl; 1 : 200,000 epinephrine†	—	18.0 (10.0)
1.5% Etidocaine HCl; 1 : 200,000 epinephrine	0.53 (0.29)	26.6 (14.7)
4% Articaine HCl; 1 : 200,000 or 1 : 100,000 epinephrine‡	0.17 (0.10) (adult) 0.12 (0.07) (child)	— —

* *Maximum volumes are calculated from the maximum recommended doses listed in Table 4–3. Except for articaine, the cartridge volume is 1.8 mL. All uneven values are truncated to avoid the possibility of exceeding maximum recommended doses.*

† *Bupivacaine is not recommended for children under the age of 12.*

‡ *Articaine is supplied in 1.7 mL cartridges. Separate dosage schedules are recommended for adults and for children 4 to 12 years of age.*

thetics are listed in Table 4–2.[18] The maximum dose recommendation, provided in Table 4–3,[19-23] is approximately equivalent to 0.27 mL/kg body weight, or 0.15 cartridges/kg body weight (Table 4–4). Because of a lack of information regarding the effects of this formulation on the developing fetus, it is classified by the Food and Drug Administration (FDA) in pregnancy category C (Table 4–5).[23]

PROPOXYCAINE HYDROCHLORIDE

$$H_2N-\text{(benzene ring)}-\overset{O}{\underset{OC_3H_7}{COCH_2CH_2}}-N\overset{C_2H_5}{\underset{C_2H_5}{}} \cdot HCl$$

Chemical Name: 2-(diethylamino)ethyl-4-amino-2-propoxybenzoate monohydrochloride
Trade Name: Ravocaine

The addition of a propoxy group to the ortho position on the aromatic ring of procaine yields propoxycaine, a local anesthetic approximately six times as potent as procaine. By intravenous injection, propoxycaine is eight times as toxic as procaine in mice. The pharmacologic effects, metabolic fate, and allergic potential are similar to those of procaine. The

Table 4–5. **PREGNANCY RISK CLASSIFICATION OF LOCAL ANESTHETICS**

Drug	*Pregnancy Category*	*Reason for Category Assignment*
Procaine/propoxycaine	C	Animal reproduction studies not done
Lidocaine	B	No fetal harm in rats with up to 6.6 times the maximum dose in humans
Mepivacaine	C	Animal reproduction studies not done
Prilocaine	B	No fetal harm with up to 30 times the maximum dose in humans
Bupivacaine	C	Embryocidal effect in rabbits and decreased pup survival in rats after 9 and 5 times the maximum recommended daily dose, respectively
Etidocaine	B	No fetal harm in rats or rabbits with up to 1.7 times the maximum dose in humans
Articaine	B*	No fetal harm in rats, rabbits, or cats with up to 3 times the maximum dose in humans

* *Estimated rank. Articaine has not been assigned a category by the Food and Drug Administration.*

clinical use of propoxycaine with procaine is described above. Propoxycaine is not available in any other formulation.

LIDOCAINE HYDROCHLORIDE

Chemical Name: 2-(diethylamino)-2′,6′-acetoxylidide monohydrochloride

Trade Names: Xylocaine, Alphacaine, Lignospan, Octocaine

Lidocaine, an aminoethylamide derivative of xylidine, was the first amide local anesthetic suitable for nerve block injection in dentistry.* It is approximately two times as potent and as toxic as procaine. When injected intraorally, lidocaine produces a greater depth of anesthesia, with a longer duration and affecting a larger area, than an equivalent amount of procaine.[24] As a result, lidocaine became the most popular local anesthetic agent available in a dental cartridge, and it is considered the prototypic amide agent. Lidocaine hydrochloride is available under a variety of trade names (Fig. 4–2); several manufacturers also market the drug by its nonproprietary (generic) designation (Fig. 4–3).

Lidocaine is available in North America in cartridges containing a 2% solution without vasoconstrictor or with 1 : 100,000 (10 μg/mL) or

* *Dibucaine, the first amide anesthetic to be introduced clinically (in 1930) is restricted because of its toxic potential to topical use in the United States but is widely used for spinal anesthesia in Europe, where it is known as cinchocaine.*

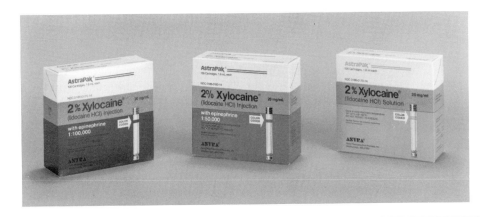

Figure 4–2.   Lidocaine hydrochloride marketed in dental cartridges by a trade name, Xylocaine. (Courtesy Astra Pharmaceutical Products, Inc., Westborough, Mass.)

1:50,000 (20 μg/mL) epinephrine (or its hydrochloride or bitartrate equivalent). The original formulation (Xylocaine, Astra) also contains 6 mg/mL sodium chloride and, in vasoconstrictor-containing preparations, 0.2 mg/mL citric acid and 0.5 mg/mL sodium metabisulfite. Some manufacturers use slightly different amounts of sodium chloride and other antioxidants, such as not more than 0.55 mg/mL sodium bisulfite or 1.2 mg/mL potassium metabisulfite with 0.25 mg/mL disodium edetate. Lido-

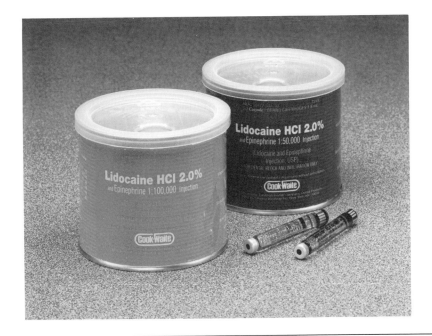

Figure 4–3.   Lidocaine hydrochloride marketed in dental cartridges by the nonproprietary name lidocaine HCl. (Courtesy Eastman Kodak Co., New York, N.Y.)

caine is also available outside the United States with 1 : 80,000 (12.5 μg/mL) epinephrine or with 1 : 25,000 (40 μg/mL) norepinephrine. Additionally, a recent European formulation of 2% lidocaine with both 1 : 50,000 epinephrine and 1 : 50,000 norepinephrine has been developed for "maximum anesthetic power." A 3% lidocaine with 1 : 25,000 norepinephrine preparation has also been marketed for the same purpose. Although these latter two preparations may improve pulpal anesthesia in selected patients, they substantially increase the risk of toxic reactions.

Lidocaine is probably the most versatile local anesthetic yet discovered. It has been injected by virtually every route available and has proved highly effective as a topical anesthetic (described below). The most commonly used formulation, 2% lidocaine with 1 : 100,000 epinephrine (or 1 : 80,000 in countries such as Great Britain, where it is known as lignocaine, and Japan), provides profound local anesthesia with acceptably low systemic toxicity and minimal allergic potential. Pulpal anesthesia occurs quickly and lasts sufficiently for most dental procedures to be completed without the need for reinjection.[25] Because of its potent vasodilatory property and inadequate duration of pulpal anesthesia, the plain solution is infrequently used in dentistry. The 1 : 50,000 strength of epinephrine, which provides no anesthetic advantage over the 1 : 100,000 concentration while increasing the risk of adverse cardiovascular responses, is best reserved for situations where specific benefit may accrue from its greater vasoconstrictor potential.[26] Indeed, some[27,28] but not all[29,30] investigators have argued that a more dilute, 1 : 200,000 (5 μg/mL) concentration of epinephrine is sufficient for most purposes and should be adopted as the standard.

In part because of its unique role in the management of ventricular dysrhythmias, more is known about the systemic actions and metabolic fate of lidocaine than of any other conventional local anesthetic. Indeed, much of the information in Chapter 2 is based on studies involving lidocaine. In contrast to other local anesthetics, lidocaine tends to produce a degree of sedation in subconvulsive doses, and even seizures caused by overdosage are often muted in magnitude compared to procaine. Convulsions typically occur in blood concentration above 10 μg/mL; however, they may develop at lower concentrations in especially sensitive patients. Peak blood concentrations after submucosal injection are reached in about 15 minutes; the presence of epinephrine can delay the attainment of peak values by an additional 5 to 15 minutes.[31-33] For 2% lidocaine, dose limits approved by the FDA permit the administration of up to a total of 15 mL without vasoconstrictor and 25 mL with 1 : 100,000 epinephrine (see Table 4–4) at any one time. While the 25-mL dosage limit also applies for 2% lidocaine with 1 : 50,000 epinephrine, this formulation is best used sparingly to avoid excessive administration of vasoconstrictor.

The metabolism and excretion of lidocaine are outlined in Figure 4–4.[34,35] (Factors that can influence the metabolism of lidocaine and other

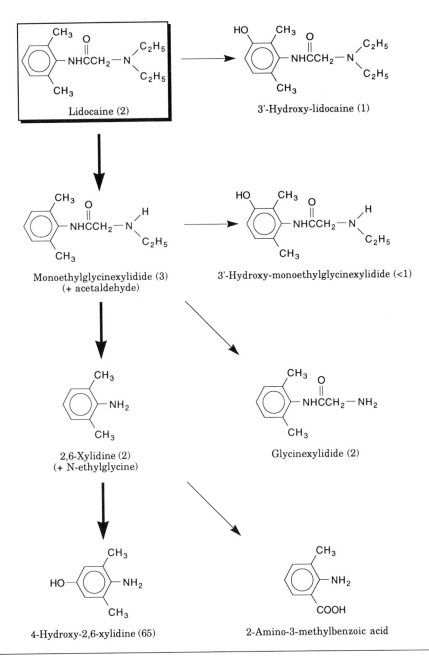

Figure 4–4.   Metabolism and excretion of lidocaine. Values in parentheses are the approximate percentages of the dose (free and conjugated) found in the urine in the first 24 hours after oral or intravenous administration. Several metabolic pathways are not shown, including the direct hydrolysis of lidocaine (to yield 2,6-xylidine and N,N-diethylglycine) and the oxidative cyclization of the amino terminus. (Data from Keenaghan, J.B., and Boyes, R.N.: J. Pharmacol. Exp. Ther. *180*:454–463, 1972; Mihaly, G.W., Moore, R.G., et al.: Eur. J. Clin. Pharmacol. *13*:143–152, 1978.)

amides are described in Chapter 5.) In contrast to procaine and other esters, lidocaine undergoes a complex pattern of metabolism catalyzed by a variety of hepatic enzymes. The initial primary metabolite, mono-ethylglycinexylidide, retains most of the pharmacologic efficacy of the parent drug. Hydrolysis of lidocaine (which accounts for about one-third of the drug[36]) or its deethylated derivatives by hepatic amidase activity inactivates the drug. However, 2,6-xylidine, which is produced by amide hydrolysis, can cause carcinoma and other tumors of the nasal cavity in rats given chronic daily doses greater than 50 mg/kg-day. There is no evidence that lidocaine is carcinogenic in man.

MEPIVACAINE HYDROCHLORIDE

Chemical Name: 1-methyl-2′,6′-pipecoloxylidide monohydro-chloride

Trade Names: Carbocaine, Arestocaine, Isocaine, Polocaine, Scandonest

Mepivacaine is an amide anesthetic product of xylidine and N-methylpi-pecolic acid. A 2% solution of mepivacaine is approximately equivalent to 2% lidocaine in potency and toxicity in animal studies. Mepivacaine has much less vasodilating activity than lidocaine, however, and thus can be reliably used without a vasoconstrictor for dental procedures of short duration. Mepivacaine shows little cross-allergenicity with lidocaine and none with ester anesthetics.

Mepivacaine is available as a 2% solution with 1:20,000 levonordefrin and as a 3% solution without vasoconstrictor. (In some countries 2% mepivacaine is combined with various strengths of epinephrine or norepi-nephrine.) Each milliliter of the 3% solution also contains 3 mg sodium chloride; 4 mg sodium chloride is added to the 2% strength along with not more than 2 mg acetone sodium bisulfite (original manufacturer) or with 1 mg sodium bisulfite or 0.5 mg sodium metabisulfite to protect the levonordefrin against oxidation.

Although individual studies vary somewhat, the preponderance of evidence indicates that 2% mepivacaine with 1:20,000 levonordefrin is almost therapeutically indistinguishable from 2% lidocaine with epineph-rine as an intraoral anesthetic.[37-39] As shown in Table 4–2, it may be somewhat shorter acting after supraperiosteal injection in the maxilla, but onset, efficacy, and duration of nerve block anesthesia are all comparable. Because of vasoconstrictor differences, the mepivacaine solution is less likely to cause cardiac palpitation than is lidocaine with epineph-rine, but it is more likely to increase blood pressure. As discussed in Chapter 5, there is a higher potential for interaction with tricyclic antide-pressants yet a lower risk with β-adrenergic blocking drugs.

The 3% solution of mepivacaine was the first local anesthetic without vasoconstrictor to rival traditional local anesthetic-vasoconstrictor products in effectiveness. Numerous studies have documented that the primary anesthetic difference between 3% mepivacaine and 2% lidocaine with 1 : 100,000 epinephrine is its shorter duration of action.[25,29,40,41] This difference is most pronounced after maxillary supraperiosteal injection, where both pulpal and soft tissue anesthesia are significantly abbreviated. The limited duration of pulpal anesthesia may explain why 3% mepivacaine is sometimes rated as slightly less effective than the lidocaine-epinephrine standard for maxillary anesthesia. Simply, the clinical procedure may take longer than the anesthesia lasts. For short procedures, however, 3% mepivacaine may be preferred. There are other potential advantages. Without a vasoconstrictor, 3% mepivacaine does not stimu-

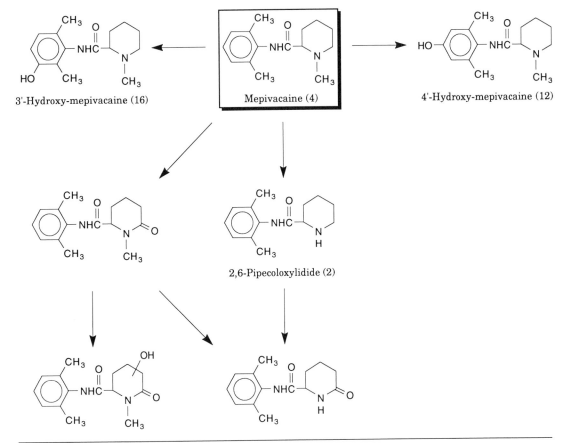

Figure 4–5. Metabolism and excretion of mepivacaine. Arrows between metabolites indicate possible metabolic pathways. Values in parentheses are the approximate percentages of the dose found in the urine (free and conjugated) in the first 24 to 30 hours after oral or intravenous administration. The three lactam metabolites (unlabeled, lower left) constitute no more than 10% of the total dose, but may give rise to further derivatives that have not been measured. (Data from Meffin, P., Long, G.J., and Thomas, J.: Clin. Pharmacol. Ther. *14*:218–225, 1973; Meffin, P., Robertson, A.V., et al.: Xenobiotica *3*:191–196, 1973; Tucker, G.T., and Mather, L.E. *In* Cousins, M.J., and Bridenbaugh, P.O., eds.: Neural Blockade in Clinical Anesthesia and Management of Pain, 2nd ed. Philadelphia, J.B. Lippincott Co., 1988.)

late the cardiovascular system significantly, and it can be used safely in patients taking medications that interact with adrenergic amines. The absence of sulfite preservatives minimizes the potential for allergic-like reactions. Finally, pain on injection is less, in part due to the higher pH of the solution.[42]

Mepivacaine does not have any unusual pharmacologic properties that differentiate it from other local anesthetics as described in Chapter 2. As outlined in Figure 4–5, mepivacaine is converted in the liver to a variety of metabolites.[43-45] The aromatic hydroxy compounds, which are largely excreted in the urine in conjugated form, retain significant pharmacologic activity. It appears that mepivacaine is at best a poor substrate for hepatic amidase enzymes. With a lower mean clearance rate and smaller volume of distribution than lidocaine (see Table 2–5), mepivacaine may tend to produce higher blood concentrations after intraoral injection that peak at 30 minutes before subsiding.[32,33] Intravenous infusion studies suggest, however, that patients may tolerate commensurately higher blood concentrations (e.g., up to 6 μg/mL) before toxic effects ensue.[46] Because the maximum recommended dose of mepivacaine is independent of vasoconstrictor content, 50% more volume of the 2% solution with levonordefrin can be administered than the 3% solution (see Table 4–4).

PRILOCAINE HYDROCHLORIDE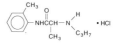

Chemical Name: 2-(propylamino)-o-propionotoluidine monohydrochloride
Trade Names: Citanest, Citanest Forte

Unlike other amide anesthetics, prilocaine is a secondary amino derivative of toluidine. The drug is somewhat less potent than lidocaine as an anesthetic and considerably less toxic after injection into peripheral tissues. As with mepivacaine, prilocaine produces less vasodilation than does lidocaine and can therefore be reliably used as a plain solution for short procedures. Prilocaine is similar to other amide local anesthetics in its relative freedom from allergic reactions.

Prilocaine is marketed in North America as a 4% solution with or without 1 : 200,000 epinephrine (as the bitartrate). Sodium metabisulfite (0.5 mg/mL) and citric acid (0.2 mg/mL) are included in the vasoconstrictor-containing formulation. In some countries, prilocaine (also called propitocaine) is available in a 3% concentration with 0.03 IU/mL felypressin (1 IU = 20 μg).

Prilocaine with epinephrine (Citanest Forte) provides anesthesia comparable in onset and efficacy[39,47-49] to that achieved with 2% lidocaine with 1 : 100,000 epinephrine. Pulpal anesthesia may be somewhat shorter in duration but is sufficient for most operative procedures. Removal of the vasoconstrictor causes no loss in activity after inferior alveolar nerve block. Anesthesia of the maxilla after supraperiosteal injection of 4% prilocaine alone (Citanest), however, is significantly shorter, with pulpal anesthesia lasting for as little as 10 minutes in some patients.[47-52] As with 3% mepivacaine, failure of anesthesia may occur because of the relatively evanescent action in maxillary teeth. The advantages to having no vasoconstrictor also apply.

Prilocaine is the least toxic amide anesthetic in current use, which permits its safe formulation as a 4% solution. It enjoys a significantly larger volume of distribution and greater clearance rate than xylidine-based anesthetics (see Table 2–5). Because the drug leaves the circulation rapidly, peak blood concentrations occur within 15 minutes after intraoral injection and are about half those achieved by similar doses of lidocaine or mepivacaine.[53] The metabolism of prilocaine is outlined in Figure 4–6.[45] Although the liver plays a major role in the biotransforma-

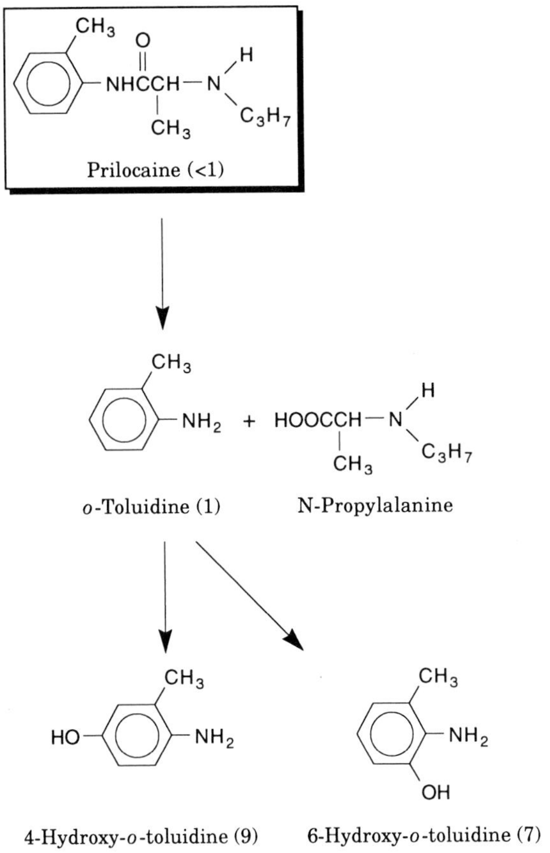

Figure 4–6. Metabolism and excretion of prilocaine. Values in parentheses are the percentages of the dose (free and conjugated) found in the urine in the first 24 hours after oral administration. (Data from Mather, L.E.: Studies in the Absorption, Distribution, Metabolism and Excretion of Drugs by Adult and Neonatal Humans [Thesis]. Sydney, University of Sydney, 1972.)

tion of prilocaine, clearance of prilocaine from the blood is significantly faster than its delivery to the liver via the bloodstream. Therefore, breakdown of the drug in other sites is predicted, with the kidneys and lungs being the most likely organs involved.[54,55] Perhaps because it is a secondary amine, hydrolysis of the amide bond is the major pathway for metabolism of the parent compound. Only a small percentage (<20%) of prilocaine has been recovered in the urine as the parent drug and its known metabolites.

The primary factor limiting the clinical use of prilocaine is methemoglobinemia, a side effect caused by its metabolite o-toluidine.[56,57] Hydroxylation reactions involving o-toluidine cause the oxidation of the iron (Fe) atom in hemoglobin from the Fe^{2+} to the Fe^{3+} state. The resulting methemoglobin is unable to transport oxygen and even impairs the ability of unaffected oxyhemoglobin to release its oxygen to the tissues. Although rarely seen at doses typically used for restorative dental care, clinically evident methemoglobinemia is regularly produced as the dose exceeds the maximum recommended limit of 8 mg/kg, and it may occur in lower doses in patients with congenital or acquired methemoglobinemia (see Chapter 5).

In animals studies, o-toluidine has shown some carcinogenic potential.[19] Positive results required the chronic oral administration of very large doses (≥150 mg/kg); there is no evidence of risk to humans from exposure to prilocaine administered for dental treatment. Even excessive doses of prilocaine in animals have not adversely affected reproductive outcomes (see Table 4–5).

BUPIVACAINE HYDROCHLORIDE

Chemical Name: 1-butyl-2′,6′-pipecoloxylidide monohydrochloride

Trade Name: Marcaine

Bupivacaine is the 1-butyl analogue of mepivacaine. The effects of this single substitution include a fourfold increase in potency and toxicity, a remarkable increase in the duration of nerve block anesthesia, and several qualitative changes in pharmacologic profile. A powerful vasodilator in the area of injection, bupivacaine is marketed for dental use in combination with epinephrine. The allergic potential of bupivacaine is presumably similar to that of other amide local anesthetics.

In dental cartridge form, bupivacaine is available as a 0.5% solution with 1 : 200,000 epinephrine (as the bitartrate). Sodium chloride is added for isotonicity, and the formulation also contains 0.5 mg/mL sodium metabisulfite, 0.001 mL/mL monothioglycerol, 2 mg/mL ascorbic acid, 0.0017 mL/mL 60% sodium lactate buffer, and 0.1 mg/mL edetate calcium disodium. The drug may have a slightly slower onset of action than clinical formulations of lidocaine, mepivacaine, or prilocaine,[58,59] a possible reflection of its greater degree of ionization at physiologic pH. Equally effective for nerve block, bupivacaine provides a duration of action several times longer than previously discussed agents.[58-61] Soft tissue anesthesia is likewise protracted after maxillary supraperiosteal injection; however, compared to 2% lidocaine with 1:100,000 epinephrine, anesthesia of the teeth is less widespread and of shorter duration.[62] The extremely high lipid:buffer partition coefficient of bupivacaine so favors absorption by local tissues that little free drug is available for distribution to the superior dental plexus supplying the teeth. Decreased delivery of drug to the superior dental plexus after supraperiosteal injection may also contribute to a slower onset of pulpal anesthesia in the maxilla.

Bupivacaine is infrequently used for routine restorative dentistry. Its greatest application is in surgery, where the prolonged duration of action after nerve block anesthesia furnishes postoperative analgesia of 5 to 6 hours in the maxilla and 7 to 8 hours in the mandible. An independent measure of the effectiveness of this approach is the significant decrease in the number of postoperative analgesic doses taken by patients given bupivacaine.[63,64]

As discussed in Chapter 2, bupivacaine is noted for its ability to produce use-dependent block. This attribute may help explain the drug's selective effectiveness as an analgesic (it blocks small nociceptive fibers at concentrations that leave large motor fibers functional), as well as its propensity for producing cardiac abnormalities in overdose. Whereas bupivacaine has been responsible for life-threatening reactions, including cardiovascular collapse, in medicine,[65,66] serious toxic reactions are exceedingly unlikely after intraoral injections, for the following reasons. First, the maximum recommended dose of bupivacaine in dentistry, 90 mg, is much less than the 225-mg limit approved for nondental use. With 9 mg per dental cartridge, ten cartridges can be given to the adult patient and still reach only 40% of the maximum dose for such nondental uses as brachial plexus block and epidural block. Although blood concentrations of bupivacaine after intraoral injection have not been reported, existing evidence with other drugs suggests that the peak concentration would not be especially high after intraoral injection.[31-33,45,53] A second feature favoring safety in dentistry is the dental cartridge unit dose. Since it is unlikely that the contents of any given cartridge would be accidentally injected directly into the bloodstream, the potential for intravascular administration of multiple cartridges leading to systemic toxicity seems especially remote. Finally, there is a strong tendency not to use bupivacaine in pediatric patients because of the desire to avoid prolonged soft tissue anesthesia (and the potential for self-injury) and because the agent has not been approved for use in children under the age of 12. This aversion removes the population at greatest risk of local anesthetic overdose. Systemic effects of bupivacaine become noticeable at venous

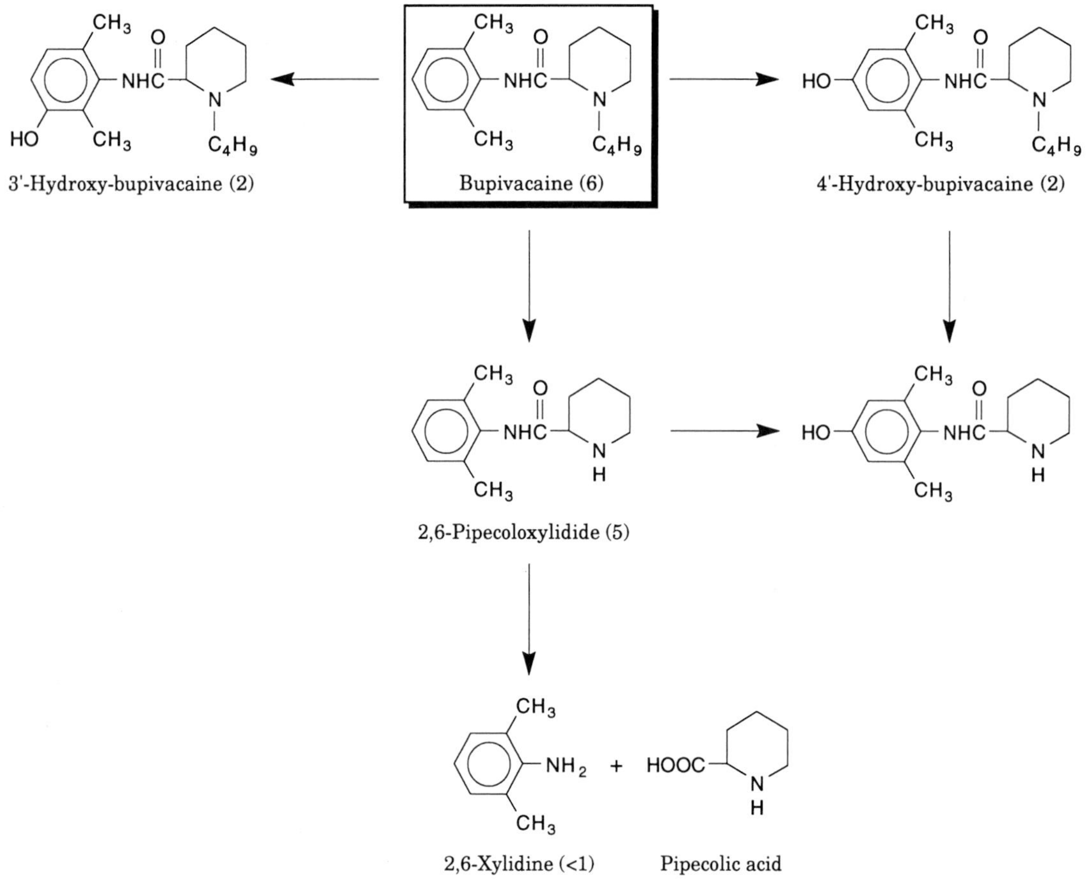

Figure 4–7. Metabolism and excretion of bupivacaine. Values in parentheses are the percentages of the dose (free and conjugated) found in the urine in the first 24 hours after intravenous administration. (Data from Reynolds, F.: Br. J. Anaesth. *43*:33–36, 1971; Tucker, G.T., and Mather, L.E. *In* Cousins, M.J., and Bridenbaugh, P.O., eds.: Neural Blockade in Clinical Anesthesia and Management of Pain, 2nd ed. Philadelphia, J.B. Lippincott Co., 1988.)

plasma concentrations of 2 μg/mL[45,46]; convulsions and other serious sequellae occur at concentrations above 4 μg/mL.[67] Fetal toxicity has been observed in several animal models after large daily doses of bupivacaine (see Table 4–5); there is no evidence of harm in humans with normal clinical exposure to the drug.

Hepatic clearance of bupivacaine is relatively low, yielding a terminal half-life ($t_{1/2}$) of 162 minutes, compared to 96 minutes for lidocaine. Figure 4–7 presents the known metabolites of bupivacaine and their 24-hour recovery from urine.[45,68] As is the case with mepivacaine, bupivacaine is apparently resistant to amide hydrolysis in humans.

ETIDOCAINE HYDROCHLORIDE

Chemical Name: 2-(ethylpropylamino)-2′,6′-butyroxylidide
monohydrochloride

Trade Name: Duranest

Etidocaine is a highly lipophilic homologue of lidocaine in which one of the ethyl groups on the amino terminus is replaced with a propyl substitution and an ethyl moiety is added to the intermediate carbon atom. In preclinical studies, the drug proved similar to bupivacaine in potency and duration of action. Its toxicity is equivalent in animals to bupivacaine after intravascular bolus injection but is relatively less with other modes of administration because of its faster removal from the bloodstream through redistribution and metabolism. The drug shares with bupivacaine a predisposition for causing cardiac dysrhythmias in toxic doses. It is believed to be equivalent to other amide local anesthetics in its near total freedom from allergic reactions.

Etidocaine is available in dental cartridges as a 1.5% solution with 1 : 200,000 epinephrine (as the bitartrate). Sodium chloride (6.2 mg/mL), sodium metabisulfite (0.5 mg/mL), and citric acid (0.2 mg/mL) are also included for osmotic balance and protection of the vasoconstrictor against oxidation.

Clinical trials of the marketed solution of etidocaine have largely focused on its use in oral and periodontal surgery.[69–72] The etidocaine formulation is as rapidly acting and effective as 2% lidocaine with 1 : 100,000 epinephrine for nerve block anesthesia, but anesthesia of the maxillary teeth may be slightly delayed, slightly less reliable, and of shorter duration after supraperiosteal injection.[62,70] Soft tissue anesthesia in the area of infiltration, however, is pronounced and prolonged. The primary benefit of using etidocaine, as with bupivacaine, is the remarkable duration of postoperative analgesia obtained. Although discomfort after surgery may begin to be felt approximately 2 hours before all sensations of local anesthesia have dissipated, the pain-free interval is still 2 to 3 hours longer on average than that afforded by the standard lidocaine anesthetic. In addition, less postoperative pain may be experienced during the first 24 hours after surgery[73]; patients taking analgesics ‘‘as needed’’ start later and take fewer doses overall.[72,73] The primary disadvantage of the etidocaine preparation is increased bleeding during surgery. Because intraoperative hemorrhage was not mentioned as a problem in trials of 1% etidocaine with 1 : 200,000 epinephrine,[74,75] it is believed the heightened vasodilatory activity of the 1.5% formulation overcomes the local ischemic effect of the vasoconstrictor. Bupivacaine (0.5%) with 1 : 200,000 epinephrine provides the same duration of postoperative analgesia without causing extra blood loss during surgery.

The pharmacologic effects of etidocaine are similar to those of bupivacaine. Thus, use-dependent block and cardiac toxicity are more prominent than with lidocaine, its closest relative structurally. Etidocaine is exceptional in that it anesthetizes motor fibers as readily as it does the smaller sensory neurons. Therefore, while etidocaine appears as potent as bupivacaine in blocking compound action potentials experimentally, it must be used in a higher concentration clinically (e.g., 1.5% vs. 0.5%) to achieve the same degree of pain relief. Equally as toxic as bupivacaine after intravascular injection, a single cartridge of 1.5% etidocaine injected intravascularly is theoretically more toxic than a similar volume of any other anesthetic used in dentistry. The danger of extravascular injection is tempered by the drug's large volume of distribution, which reflects its ability to avoid high blood concentrations by being sequestered in peripheral tissues. With a maximum recommended total dose of 400 mg in the adult patient (see Table 4–3), a maximum dose of 8 mg/kg was determined by the manufacturer based on a weight of 50 kg (instead of the 70 kg normally used). The net effect is that a significantly higher volume of etidocaine can be injected than any other dental anesthetic without exceeding the recommended limit in patients weighing 50 kg or less. Animal data (see Table 4–1) suggest that this limit may have a lower margin of safety than analogous doses recommended for other agents.

No measurements have been reported of blood concentrations achieved after intraoral injection of etidocaine. The majority of studies in medicine indicate that concentrations are significantly less than those associated with identical doses of bupivacaine.[45] Because the threshold concentrations for systemic toxicity are comparable, larger doses of etidocaine can be safely administered.[76] Animal studies have detected no fetal toxicity after large daily doses given throughout pregnancy (see Table 4–5).

The hepatic clearance of etidocaine is at least as fast as that of lidocaine (see Table 2–5). However, because of its large volume of distribution, etidocaine has a terminal elimination $t_{1/2}$ equivalent to bupivacaine. Over 20 metabolites of etidocaine have been discovered. Figure 4–8 illustrates the primary metabolites recovered from the urine.[77,78]

ARTICAINE HYDROCHLORIDE

Chemical Name: 3-propylamino-propionylamino-2-carbomethoxy-4-methylthiophene monohydrochloride

Trade Names: Ultracaine D-S, Ultracaine D-S forte

Articaine is an analogue of prilocaine in which the benzene moiety is replaced with a thiophene ring. Less lipid soluble than lidocaine, articaine is nevertheless more potent in blocking nerve conduction in the frog sciatic nerve.[79] The drug is similar to lidocaine in toxicity after rapid

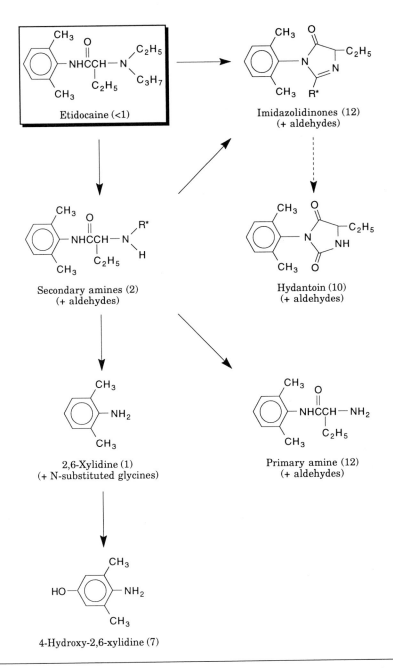

Figure 4–8. Metabolism and excretion of etidocaine. Values in parentheses are the approximate percentages of the dose found in the urine in the first 24 to 48 hours after epidural administration (including conjugated metabolites). Not shown are the 3′- and 4′-hydroxy derivatives of etidocaine and its N-dealkylated metabolites. R* = methyl or ethyl group. (Data from Morgan, D.J., Smyth, M.P., et al.: Xenobiotica 7:365–375, 1977; Morgan, D.J., Cousins, M.J., et al.: Eur. J. Clin. Pharmacol. *12*:359–365, 1977.)

intravascular injection but is less toxic by other modes of administration. Allergic reactions to articaine are rare.

Articaine is available in Canada and Europe as a 4% solution with 1 : 200,000 epinephrine (Ultracaine D-S) and with 1 : 100,000 epinephrine (Ultracaine D-S forte). Sodium chloride (1 mg/mL) and sodium metabisulfite (0.5 mg/mL) are included for osmotic balance and to protect the epinephrine against oxidation. Articaine is the only injectable dental anesthetic marketed in Canada that contains methylparaben (1 mg/mL). Should the drug become available in the United States, this antibacterial but potentially allergenic agent will be removed from the formulation.

Because articaine is a potent vasodilator (roughly comparable to lidocaine), it must be used in conjunction with a vasoconstrictor for intraoral anesthesia. Combined with epinephrine, articaine is a highly effective local anesthetic. Several early studies[80,81] reported the 4% solution with 1 : 200,000 epinephrine to be equal or superior to 2% lidocaine with 1 : 100,000 epinephrine in anesthetic effectiveness, whereas several more recent trials have found the formulation equivalent to standard anesthetic preparations in both onset and efficacy.[82-84] The duration of action of 4% articaine with 1 : 200,000 epinephrine is comparable in the maxilla, and presumably in the mandible, to that of 2% lidocaine with 1 : 100,000 epinephrine. The 1 : 100,000 epinephrine version of 4% articaine has not been well studied. Although one might expect a longer duration of action because of the increased vasoconstrictor content, no published evidence supports this supposition.[85] Open-label studies suggest that the 1 : 100,000 formulation may be more effective for certain uses, such as supraperiosteal injection for mandibular molar restorations in children.[86]

Articaine enjoys a reputation for spreading through tissues well, even being able to provide palatal anesthesia after buccal infiltration in the maxilla and pulpal anesthesia after buccal infiltration in the mandible. Indeed, claims have been made that simple maxillary extractions can be accomplished in children without the use of palatal injections.[87] Properly controlled clinical trials have failed to substantiate such benefits.[88,89] However, these studies have shown 4% articaine with 1 : 200,000 epinephrine to produce pulpal anesthesia in the mandible in 60% to 65% of adult subjects, in comparison to 50% to 55% of subjects receiving 4% prilocaine with 1 : 200,000 epinephrine. Further research will be required to determine what advantages, if any, articaine enjoys over other local anesthetic formulations.

Relatively little information on the pharmacology of articaine has been published. Pharmacologic and toxic effects are qualitatively similar to those of other amide local anesthetics. Articaine has caused methemoglobinemia after intravenous regional anesthesia, but not after injection for dental anesthesia. Although articaine has not been assigned a pregnancy risk category by the FDA, animal studies have not revealed any embryotoxic or teratogenic effects. Approximately 67% of articaine is bound to plasma proteins.[90]

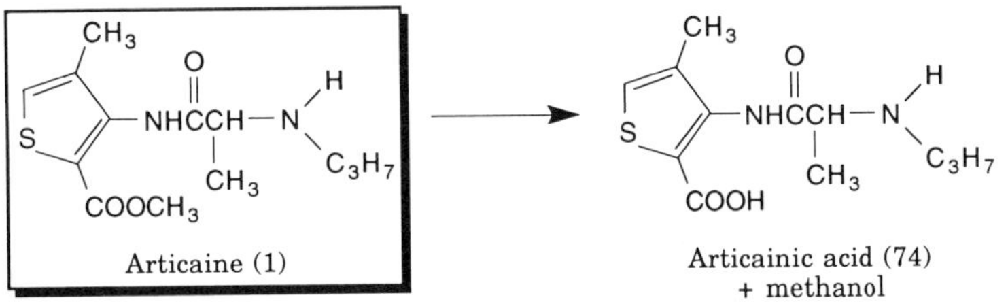

Figure 4–9. Metabolism and excretion of articaine. Values in parentheses are the percentages of the dose (free and conjugated) found in the urine in the first 36 hours after epidural administration. (Data from van Oss, G.E.C.J.M., Vree, T.B., et al.: Eur. J. Anaesthesiol. 6:49–56, 1989.)

The metabolic fate of articaine is unusual for an amide anesthetic (Fig. 4–9).[90] The thiophene ring and carbomethoxy side chain protect the amide linkage from hepatic amidase activity. Instead, the ester side chain is hydrolyzed by plasma and hepatic esterases. The product, articainic acid, is believed to be essentially devoid of pharmacologic effect.[91] The $t_{1/2}$ of articaine in blood at body temperature is about 75 minutes[92]; however, the concomitant processes of absorption and distribution of articaine after parenteral injection contribute to the removal of over 90% of the drug from the bloodstream quickly (apparent $t_{1/2}$ of about 35 minutes) and the remainder at a slower rate ($t_{1/2}$ of 2.3 hours). Articainic acid is excreted in the urine as both the free metabolite and its glucuronide conjugate. Small amounts of articaine (<5%) appear unchanged in the urine.

DRUG SELECTION

The selection of a local anesthetic for intraoral injection must include considerations of efficacy, safety, and individual patient and operative needs. Over the years, manufacturers sensitive to market forces and medicolegal concerns have replaced clearly inferior products with local anesthetics that reliably produce effective anesthesia and little toxicity when administered carefully in recommended doses. The continued availability of multiple drugs and drug formulations is prima facie evidence that no single product is a clear choice for all clinical situations.

Historically, the introduction of lidocaine with epinephrine in 1948 marked a signal advance in the development of local anesthesia. The 2% concentration with 1:100,000 epinephrine proved superior to, and eventually replaced, all previous injectable anesthetics for dental use. As yet, no agent subsequently introduced has been demonstrated to be better for routine clinical use. Several agents, however, are comparable to lidocaine with epinephrine, and others have properties that make them especially useful for special circumstances.

Duration of Action

The standard lidocaine with epinephrine formulation provides a clinical duration of anesthesia suitable for most dental procedures. Agents with similar durations of action (and equivalent onsets and efficacies) include 2% mepivacaine with 1:20,000 levonordefrin, 4% prilocaine with 1:200,000 epinephrine, and 4% articaine with epinephrine (see Table 4–2). For a short procedure involving the maxillary arch, 3% mepivacaine or 4% prilocaine without vasoconstrictor may be preferred because of their significantly shorter durations of action. Because the duration of pulpal anesthesia with these solutions may be as short as 10 minutes in some patients,[41,52] inadequate pain control may result if the clinician mistimes the procedure. Less advantage is gained by omitting the vasoconstrictor in the mandible, as the duration of soft tissue anesthesia after inferior alveolar nerve block is reduced only by 10% to 15%.

For very long procedures or for pain relief that persists for hours after surgery, 0.5% bupivacaine with 1:200,000 epinephrine or 1.5% etidocaine with 1:200,000 epinephrine may be selected. When either of these formulations is used in concert with a nonsteroidal antiinflammatory agent such as flurbiprofen, postoperative analgesia superior to the traditional regimen of an intermediate-acting local anesthetic (e.g., lidocaine with epinephrine) and postoperative opioid-containing analgesic (e.g., acetaminophen with codeine) can be obtained.[93] Fewer postoperative side effects, such as drowsiness and nausea, may also occur. Two caveats should be noted, however. First, the duration and even the effectiveness of pulpal anesthesia after supraperiosteal injection of these agents are inferior with respect to lidocaine with epinephrine.[62] Second, some patients may find the extended duration of soft tissue anesthesia unpleasant, especially if they are not forewarned that they may feel numb for up to 12 hours.[71,94]

Vasoconstrictor Intolerance

As is discussed in Chapter 5, the normal use of adrenergic vasoconstrictors is restricted in several groups of patients. A simple solution to this problem is to administer local anesthetics without vasoconstrictors: 3% mepivacaine or 4% prilocaine. However, when the duration of action of these agents is insufficient for the procedure, and the use of epinephrine is not absolutely contraindicated, formulations containing 1:200,000 epinephrine may be preferred. Of course, complex procedures requiring an extended duration of anesthesia are usually not appropriate for those few patients who cannot be given any epinephrine whatsoever (e.g., the patient with unstable cardiac dysrhythmias).

Dosage Considerations

Multiple cartridges are injected for pain control and surgical hemostasis during appointments involving all four quadrants. In this situation, lidocaine with epinephrine and mepivacaine with levonordefrin provide the greatest volumes of anesthetic that can be administered while still remaining within the recommended dosage limits (see Table 4–4). Should a long-acting formulation be desired, etidocaine with epinephrine provides the same advantage.

Dosage considerations and the use of vasoconstrictor-free anesthetics in children require special comment. Many dentists use 3% mepivacaine in young children on the assumption that a shorter duration of soft tissue anesthesia will reduce the incidence of self-inflicted lip, tongue, and cheek trauma. There are no studies documenting a decreased incidence of traumatic cheilitis when plain solutions are used. Even theoretically, these benefits are dubious, as most tissues at risk (e.g., the lower lip) are anesthetized by nerve block anesthesia in which there is little difference in the duration of anesthesia between plain solutions and vasoconstrictor-containing anesthetics.

Of much greater concern is the issue of anesthetic toxicity in the young child.[95,96] Two cartridges of 3% mepivacaine or 4% prilocaine, for example, exceed the maximum recommended dose in a 15-kg child, whereas the same volume of 2% lidocaine with 1:100,000 epinephrine does not. Because the safety margin in small children is so low, it is beneficial to employ a preparation containing a vasoconstrictor that reduces the dosage of local anesthetic required for an equivalent analgesic effect.

Surgical Hemostasis

Adrenergic vasoconstrictors are of considerable value when control of bleeding is required intraoperatively. For convenience, local anesthetics with vasoconstrictors are infiltrated for hemostasis even when local anesthesia has already been obtained. The amount of bleeding generally is inversely related to the vasoconstrictor concentration in the preparation. Thus, infiltration of 2% lidocaine with 1:50,000 epinephrine decreases bleeding during periodontal surgery to less than half that recorded for a similar volume of 2% lidocaine with 1:100,000 epinephrine.[26] In turn, local infiltration of 2% lidocaine with 1:80,000 to 1:100,000 epinephrine reduces blood loss by a factor of two to three when compared to 3% mepivacaine[97] or no injection.[98] The influence of the local anesthetic itself on bleeding is observed in the greater hemorrhage associated with 1.5% etidocaine with 1:200,000 epinephrine than with other anesthetic formulations containing the same concentration of vasoconstrictor. Indeed, it is predicted[99] that epinephrine would produce better surgical hemostasis and at lower concentrations if administered by itself.

The use of vasoconstrictors for hemorrhage control during surgery must be tempered with an appreciation of their potential liabilities. Although epinephrine restricts blood loss intraoperatively, increased bleeding may occur postoperatively.[97] In addition, postoperative pain may be increased and wound healing delayed.[97,100] These effects occur because adrenergic vasoconstrictors cause local ischemia, acidosis, and accumulation of inflammatory mediators. The possibility of systemic reactions also suggests that vasoconstrictors for hemostasis should be infiltrated only as needed and not merely by habit.

Unusual Drug Sensitivity

Allergic and allergic-like reactions occasionally modify drug selection. Obviously, if a patient claims an allergy to one drug, an alternative agent should be selected. Perhaps the only specific indication for use of the ester-based propoxycaine and procaine formulation is in the rare patient who may be allergic to multiple amide anesthetics but is tolerant of esters. Unusual sensitivity to sulfites may rule out the use of vasoconstrictor-containing formulations, as described previously. Recommendations for drug selection in patients with specific congenital or acquired medical conditions are detailed in Chapter 5.

Topical Anesthetic Preparations

Topical anesthetics (Fig. 4–10) are used in the oral cavity to provide soft tissue anesthesia for a variety of reasons, including pain relief from den-

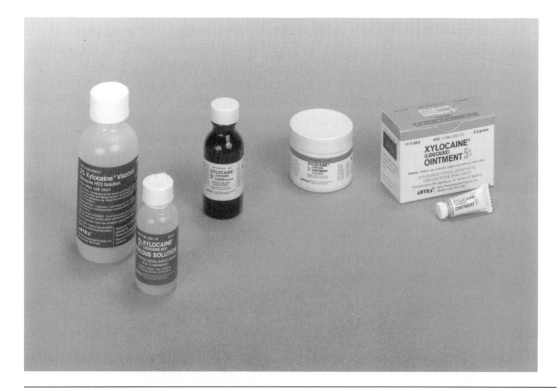

Figure 4–10.   Topical anesthetic preparations of lidocaine. (Courtesy Astra Pharmaceutical Products, Inc., Westborough, Mass.)

tal procedures (e.g., needle insertion, orthodontic band placement, and gingival curettage) and from acute infections, inflammatory conditions, ulcerations, or wounds. Topical anesthetics are also helpful in obtunding the pain and gagging some patients experience while having radiographs or impressions taken. Finally, topical anesthetics may be combined with other ointments in postsurgical dressings for the management of alveolar osteitis (dry socket).

Formulations marketed as pressurized sprays can produce widespread surface anesthesia. Such preparations are potentially hazardous, however, and only products with metered valve dispensers (Fig. 4–11) to help

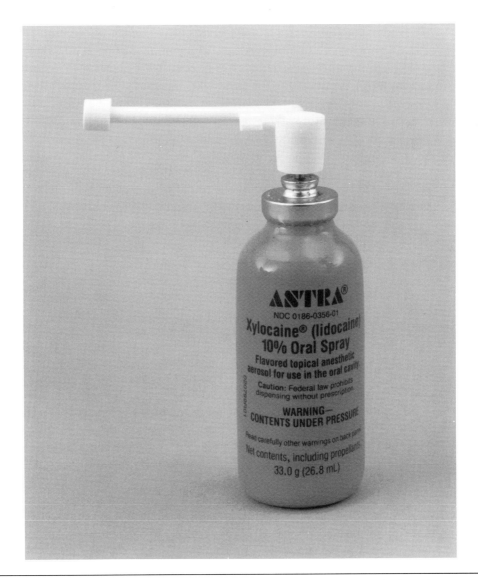

Figure 4–11.   Metered spray preparation of lidocaine. (Courtesy Astra Pharmaceutical Products, Inc., Westborough, Mass.)

prevent inadvertent overdosage should be employed. Topical liquids, which avoid the possibility of aerosol inhalation, may also be used for anesthetic coverage of large surface areas. Nonaqueous or viscous preparations are suitable for most other procedures and are safer for use on abraded or lacerated tissues. Common local anesthetic vehicles include ethanol, glycerin, lanolin, petrolatum, mineral oil, sodium carboxymethylcellulose, propylene glycol, and polyethylene glycol. Other ingredients may include benzalkonium chloride, clove oil, dimethylethyl ammonium bromide, eugenol, gelatin, hydroxyquinoline sulfate, pectin, and various propellants, flavorings, and coloring agents.

Local anesthetics intended for topical use are selected for their ability to penetrate the oral mucosa and reach the free nerve endings supplying the tissue. Often, local anesthetics effective for nerve block or infiltration anesthesia are unsuitable for surface application. In all cases, the concentration of the anesthetic drug needed for effective diffusion through the mucosa is much higher than that of injectable preparations. Vasoconstrictors cannot easily penetrate the intact oral mucosa and therefore are not used in topical anesthetic preparations. Systemic uptake can be rapid if the drug is highly lipid soluble and spread over a large surface area.

The rate of onset varies considerably among topical agents, ranging from as little as 30 seconds up to 10 minutes. The duration of surface anesthesia tends to be short and the depth of submucosal anesthesia limited. Removal of the agent by rinsing quickly causes cessation of anesthesia.

BENZOCAINE

$$H_2N-\!\!\!\left\langle\bigcirc\right\rangle\!\!\!-\overset{\overset{\displaystyle O}{\|}}{C}OCH_2CH_3$$

Chemical Name: ethyl *p*-aminobenzoate
Trade Names: Americaine, Anbesol, Benzodent, Gingicaine, Hurricaine, Kank-a, Numzident, Orabase-O, Orajel, Rid-A-Pain, Tanac, Topex, Topicale, Xylonor, ZilaDent (and in Cetacaine)

Benzocaine, otherwise referred to as ethyl aminobenzoate, is a derivative of procaine in which the diethylamino terminus is missing. Poorly soluble in aqueous fluid, benzocaine tends to remain at the site of application and is not readily absorbed into the systemic circulation.

Depending on the specific formulation and manufacturer, benzocaine is available as a 6% to 20% concentration in a liquid, gel, ointment, or spray. It is also incorporated in lower concentrations in surgical dressing medicaments. The most commonly used formulation for topical anesthesia prior to local anesthetic injection is the 20% strength in a polyethylene glycol base. Various flavoring and coloring agents are added to improve patient acceptance of the gel. Benzocaine is frequently formulated in combination with other agents, such as chlorobutanol or tetracaine.

At the 20% strength, benzocaine can produce surface mucosal anesthesia in 30 seconds.[101] The depth and intensity of the anesthesia, however, require several minutes for full development. Although 20% benzocaine significantly lessens the pain of needle insertion into the alveolar mucosa[102] and causes numbness of the tongue, no effect on the palatal mucosa is observed.[103] Once established, anesthesia normally dissipates over the next 5 to 15 minutes.

Benzocaine, particularly with prolonged or repeated use, may occasionally cause allergic sensitization. Although systemic toxic reactions to benzocaine are almost nonexistent, methemoglobinemia has occasionally been reported, usually in small children given large doses.[104,105] Inspiration of aerosolized benzocaine greatly increases the chances for methemoglobinemia.[106]

TETRACAINE HYDROCHLORIDE

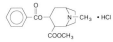

Chemical Name: 2-(dimethylamino)ethyl-4-butylaminobenzoate hydrochloride
Trade Names: Pontocaine, Supracaine (and in Cetacaine)

Tetracaine is an ester derivative of *p*-aminobenzoic acid in which a butyl chain replaces one of the hydrogens on the *p*-amino group and confers increased lipid solubility and anesthetic potency when compared to procaine. In fact, tetracaine is the most potent (and toxic) topical anesthetic available for dental use. Concentrations from 0.2% to 2% have been used in spray, liquid, and ointment formulations. A common preparation combines 2% tetracaine with 14% benzocaine, 2% butylaminobenzoate, 0.5% benzalkonium chloride, and 0.005% cetyldimethylethyl ammonium bromide in a liquid or metered spray.

Anesthesia normally begins within 2 minutes of application and may last for 20 minutes to 1 hour. Because absorption of tetracaine from mucous membranes is unusually fast, especially from the respiratory tree,[107] no more than 20 mg (1 mL of a 2% solution) should be administered at any one time to a healthy adult. Failure to restrict administration, as can easily occur with unmetered sprays, has led to multiple fatalities.[108] Tetracaine is metabolized by plasma esterase, but at a slower rate than procaine.

COCAINE HYDROCHLORIDE

Chemical Name: methyl 3β-hydroxy-1αH,5αH-tropan-2β-carboxylate ester benzoate hydrochloride

Cocaine, an ester derivative of benzoic acid and ecgonine methyl ester, is the only naturally occurring local anesthetic. Of great historical significance as the first effective local anesthetic, cocaine currently is much more prominent as a substance of abuse than as a therapeutic agent. Although cocaine has been superseded by more reliable and less toxic agents for parenteral injection, it remains a clinically acceptable topical anesthetic when used in concentrations from 1% to 10%. Onset of anesthesia after application of a 4% solution on the tongue occurs within several minutes and persists for 10 minutes.[101] Higher concentrations work faster and longer but are more likely to cause undesirable side effects.

Cocaine is the only local anesthetic with intrinsic vasoconstrictor activity after topical application. It is, therefore, a drug of choice for surface anesthesia of mucous membranes when hemostasis is needed. Cocaine is most commonly used by plastic surgeons for intranasal operations and by some anesthesiologists before nasal intubation.[109] For the latter use, combinations of lidocaine with phenylephrine have proved therapeutically equivalent.[110]

Despite its vasoconstrictive potential, cocaine is absorbed in sufficient concentrations to produce acute toxicity in doses above 1 mg/kg. Peak blood concentrations occur within 30 minutes of topical application and can remain elevated for hours if the drug is not removed from the site of application. Cocaine is metabolized primarily by plasma and hepatic esterases, with a $t_{1/2}$ of 1 hour. Nonenzymatic hydrolysis yielding benzoylecgonine may also occur, as can hepatic oxidation.

The ability of cocaine to potentiate the action of adrenergic amines, which gives the drug its vasoconstrictor action, also accounts for its unique abuse potential and toxic profile. Cocaine inhibits the active reuptake of biogenic amine neurotransmitters back into presynaptic nerve terminals. Norepinephrine released by sympathetic neurons supplying vascular smooth muscle can then achieve a higher concentration and stimulate more vasoconstrictive α receptors. In addition, cocaine may augment neurotransmitter release by blocking presynaptic autoregulation, and may increase tissue responses directly through a postsynaptic mechanism.[109] Potentiation of dopaminergic transmission in the brain is believed to be responsible for the euphoria produced by the drug. Central activation and peripheral potentiation of sympathetic neuronal activity combine to stimulate the cardiovascular system. In sensitive individuals, dysrhythmias, myocardial infarction, and sudden death may occur even without preexisting heart disease.[111] Because of its many liabilities and its status as a controlled substance (Schedule II in the United States), cocaine is best reserved for situations where it is clearly superior to other topical anesthetics.

LIDOCAINE AND LIDOCAINE HYDROCHLORIDE

Chemical Name: 2-(diethylamino)-2′,6′-acetoxylidide (monohydrochloride)

Trade Names: Xylocaine, Alphacaine, Octocaine

Lidocaine is currently the only amide anesthetic formulated for topical use in the oral cavity and the only anesthetic also used for intraoral injection (as described previously). Preparations designed for dental use include a 2% and 5% gel, 2% viscous solution, 4% and 5% liquid, 5% ointment, and 10% aerosol spray. Anesthesia typically begins within 1 to 2 minutes, but peak effects may take up to 5 minutes. The duration of action is approximately 15 minutes. The ointment and spray preparations use lidocaine base; the others use the hydrochloride salt and generally include methylparaben as a preservative.

The 5% ointment commonly applied to reduce needle pain contains lidocaine (base form) in polyethylene and propylene glycols. Versions of the product specifically marketed for intraoral use are flavored with sodium saccharin, peppermint oil, and spearmint oil. The 5% ointment is at least as effective as 20% benzocaine for providing anesthesia of the alveolar mucosa[102]; however, it is not as fast acting and should be left on the mucosa for 3 minutes before needle insertion. As with benzocaine, soft tissue anesthesia of the hard palate is unobtainable.[103]

In contrast to tetracaine and cocaine, absorption of lidocaine after topical application is not especially rapid. Peak blood concentrations are similar to those achieved by peripheral nerve blocks,[107] and this is reflected in the maximum recommended dose of 4.5 mg/kg (up to a total dose of 300 mg) for topical lidocaine hydrochloride.[19] Comparable values for lidocaine base are 3.6 mg/kg and 250 mg.[19]

DYCLONINE HYDROCHLORIDE

Chemical Name: 4'-butoxy-3-piperidinopropiophenone hydrochloride

Trade Name: Dyclone

Dyclonine hydrochloride is a unique local anesthetic in which the aromatic and amino ends of the molecule are connected by a ketone linkage. It is used solely for topical anesthesia because it is only slightly soluble in water and irritating to tissues on injection. Dyclonine is available in 0.5% and 1% solutions. Other constituents include 3 mg/mL chlorobutanol and sodium chloride for isotonicity; the pH is adjusted to 4 (±1) with hydrochloric acid.

Surface anesthesia usually begins after 2 minutes but may be delayed for up to 10 minutes. It persists for about 30 minutes. Studies comparing dyclonine to other topical anesthetics for dental uses have not been performed; however, it compares favorably with other drugs for surface anesthesia of the tongue.[101] The maximum recommended dose is 300 mg. Smaller doses are recommended for children, debilitated adults, and for use on heavily abraded mucosa. Allergic reactions are uncommon.

CHLOROBUTANOL

$$H_3C-\underset{\underset{OH}{|}}{\overset{\overset{CH_3}{|}}{C}}-CCl_3$$

Chemical Name: 1,1,1-trichloro-2-methyl-2-propanol

Chlorobutanol is an aliphatic compound structurally unrelated to typical local anesthetics. Chlorobutanol has weak anesthetic properties and is employed in combination with other agents. The drug is used primarily in obtundent dressings to relieve symptoms of acute pulpitis and postextraction wound pain. It is also used as a preservative in aqueous solutions of more powerful anesthetics (e.g., benzocaine and dyclonine).

New and Experimental Agents

Although currently marketed local anesthetic preparations are highly effective and reasonably safe when used properly, none are 100% effective or perfectly nontoxic. Thus, the search for new local anesthetics and improved formulations of existing agents continues.

pH STRATEGIES

Numerous attempts have been made to enhance regional anesthesia by capitalizing on the influence of pH. Alkalization of the anesthetic solution theoretically should increase local anesthetic activity by promoting tissue penetration and nerve uptake. Although it has been shown in vitro that alkalization enhances nerve block, clinical results have been mixed, as extracellular fluid in tissues often has enough buffering capacity to negate differences in local anesthetic pH soon after injection. Although adding sodium bicarbonate to neutralize the acidic pH of commercial lidocaine with epinephrine may increase the rate of onset,[112] the therapeutic benefit of this practice in dentistry is insufficient to warrant its routine use.

An alternative approach to modifying drug distribution is through the addition of carbon dioxide. Carbonation of a local anesthetic solution can increase the rate of onset and sometimes the profundity of anesthesia in vitro. Presumably, the injected carbon dioxide diffuses into the nerve trunk, where it lowers the internal pH and concentrates local anesthetic activity by ion trapping.[113] The hydrocarbonate form of the local anesthetic may also penetrate the nerve sheath better, if only because of the higher pH of the solution. In addition, carbon dioxide may act directly on the nerve membrane to increase local anesthetic efficacy.[114] The clinical benefits of carbonated local anesthetics, however, are unclear. In dentistry, no anesthetic difference of any kind was observed between lidocaine hydrocarbonate and lidocaine hydrochloride (both with 1 : 100,000 epinephrine) after inferior alveolar nerve block.[115]

DEPOT FORMULATIONS

The addition of dextran to local anesthetic solutions has been used clinically as a means of increasing the duration of regional anesthesia. Dextran is a complex polysaccharide used clinically as a plasma expander. It was originally believed that dextran formed complexes with local anesthetics, slowing their absorption and removal from the injection site. However, a reported lack of effectiveness during maxillary infiltration[116] and the realization that reported "successes" were merely the result of injecting alkaline material[117] has limited further interest.

The concept of slow-release or "depot" forms of local anesthetics continues to drive research because of the potential benefits such agents would provide in the treatment of postoperative pain. Three depot strategies under current investigation use lipid-based vehicles to retard the release of anesthetic at the injection site. The first involves the radiocontrast medium iophendylate. When tetracaine was prepared in iophendylate versus 10% glucose for spinal anesthesia in rabbits, the duration of motor block was increased by a factor of three.[118] The relative safety of lipid agents like iophendylate represents an advance over substances such as peanut oil that were once used in dentistry for similar purposes and led to cases of blindness after accidental intraarterial injection.

Liposomes are artificial microspheres composed generally of a single lipid bilayer surrounding an aqueous central compartment. Modification of liposome formation to yield a multilamellar structure has been used to provide a vehicle for the epidural injection of bupivacaine.[119] Absorption of bupivacaine from the injection site was greatly slowed and yielded constant blood concentrations for 3 days, raising the hope of reduced systemic toxicity and prolonged duration of effect.

A further modification of the basic liposome is the Liposphere drug delivery system. In this case, microspheres are made of an inner hydrophobic core covered by an outer layer of phospholipid. When bupivacaine is included in the core matrix, it diffuses out over a 2-day period. Subcutaneous injection of the 2% bupivacaine lipospheres can produce anesthesia that is as profound as that afforded by 0.5% bupivacaine with 1:200,000 epinephrine but lasts six times longer.[120] More research, of course, will be required before this or any of these depot strategies can be approved for clinical use.

NEW AND EXPERIMENTAL DRUGS

New local anesthetics continue to be derived from existing agents. In addition, drugs with structures unrelated to existing agents are being studied in the hope of developing clinically useful agents with novel antinociceptive properties.

Ropivacaine is a structural analogue of mepivacaine and bupivacaine (Fig. 4–12). It is unique as a local anesthetic in that the drug is prepared

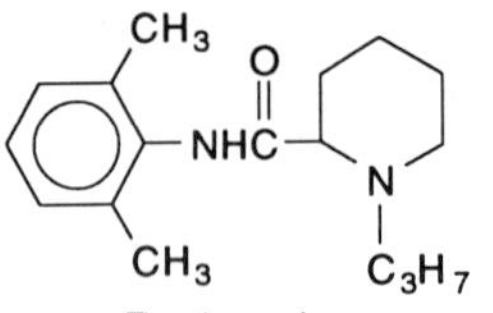

Ropivacaine

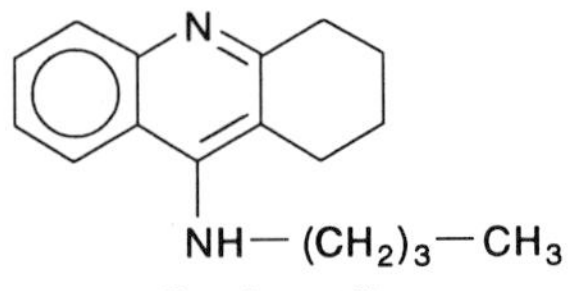

Centbucridine

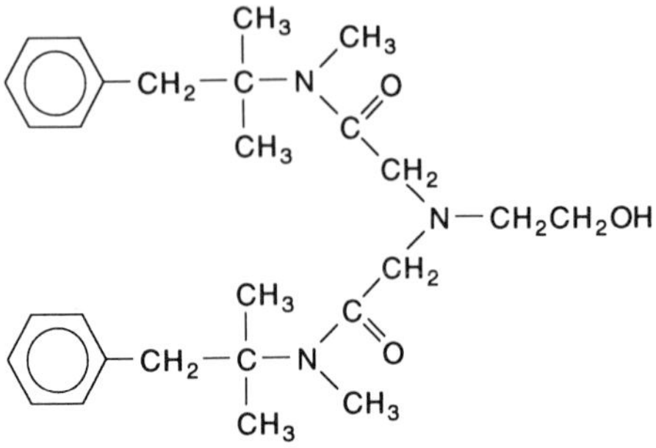

Oxethazaine

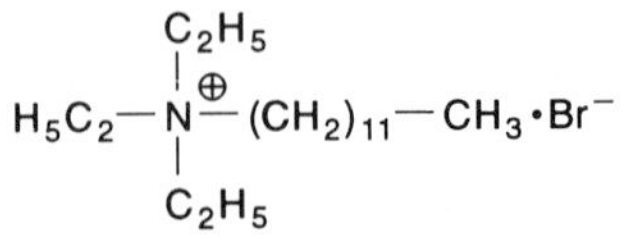

Triethyldodecyl ammonium bromide

Figure 4–12. Structural formulas of several new and experimental drugs with local anesthetic activity.

as a single stereoisomer instead of the usual racemic mixture. This difference may explain the relative lack of cardiodepressant activity of ropivacaine compared to bupivacaine despite the fact that the drugs are equivalent in anesthetic potency and central nervous system toxicity.[121] Most clinical experience with ropivacaine has been gained during epidural anesthesia. Comparisons of 0.5% ropivacaine and 0.5% bupivacaine document that the two formulations are equivalent in onset and degree of nerve block but that ropivacaine may have a 20% shorter duration of action.[122] Although ropivacaine use has yet to be reported in dentistry, it is likely that the drug's reduced cardiac toxicity will permit it to compete successfully for the niche of long-acting anesthetics currently occupied by bupivacaine and etidocaine.

EMLA, the acronym for "eutectic mixture of local anesthetics," is a topical anesthetic approved for dermal anesthesia before venipuncture and minor surgical procedures. The combination of equal amounts of lidocaine and prilocaine produces a liquid at room temperature that is easily emulsified and prepared in the form of a cream. When applied under an occlusive dressing, the cream, containing 2.5% lidocaine base and 2.5% prilocaine base, can penetrate the intact skin and render needle insertion pain free.[123] Although this formulation has not been optimized for intraoral use, it is at least as effective as 5% lidocaine ointment when applied to alveolar mucosa.[124] When placed under an adhesive bandage for 5 minutes, EMLA significantly relieved the discomfort of palatal injections.[125] It is anticipated that a version of this highly active anesthetic agent will be developed specifically for intraoral use.

Centbucridine and oxethazaine are representative of local anesthetics with unusual molecular structures (see Fig. 4–12). Centbucridine is a quinoline derivative discovered in India. A potent drug, 0.5% centbucridine is clinically equivalent to 2% lidocaine.[126] In contrast to lidocaine, centbucridine in overdose is a true central nervous system stimulant. Oxethazaine is a bis-acetamide derivative. Although its anesthetic properties have long been recognized (since 1962), and the agent has found clinical application as a topical anesthetic for hiatal hernia and gastric ulceration, its effectiveness for intraoral anesthesia has only recently been examined. At a 0.1% concentration, oxethazaine without epinephrine provided anesthesia for minor oral surgery (i.e., exodontia or apicoectomy) comparable to that of 2% lidocaine with 1:80,000 epinephrine.[127] Because oxethazaine retains activity in an acidic environment, it may be very useful in patients with acute pulpitis or periapical abscess.

Some drugs are of scientific interest because they have proved useful in elucidating possible new mechanisms for peripheral nerve blockade. For example, the naturally occurring biotoxins tetrodotoxin (in the puffer fish) and saxitoxin (in dinoflagellates) are highly specific blockers of sodium channels. Properly diluted, these extremely potent drugs can effect prolonged spinal anesthesia (subarachnoid block). Although poor lipid solubility limits the clinical potential of these agents for peripheral nerve block, tetrodotoxin has been shown in animals to act synergistically with conventional agents, increasing the duration of anesthesia up to sixfold.[128]

Tetraethylammonium (TEA) is an investigational drug used to selectively block potassium (K^+) channels. TEA also selectively potentiates the blockade by lidocaine of nerve fibers dependent on K^+ efflux for repolarization.[129] In mammals, C fibers constitute this population of neurons. Sodium (Na^+) channels, dependent on repolarization for recovery, remain in the inactivated state, which effectively increases local anesthetic binding. Other drugs that have been shown to enhance preferentially local anesthetic blockade of C fibers, albeit through different mechanisms, include veratridine,[130] a steroidal alkaloid once used to treat hypertension, and clonidine,[131] an α_2-adrenergic receptor agonist currently used for the same purpose. Research in this area will continue, as the selective inhibition of nociceptive C fibers obviously holds enormous potential for the management of chronic pain.

A final observation of interest involves derivatives of TEA in which one of the ethyl groups is replaced by a longer alkyl chain. In one study, the duration of anesthesia of the rat infraorbital nerve increased exponentially from 1 hour to 16 days as the alkyl substitution was increased up to 12 carbons in length (see Fig. 4–12).[132] Onset of anesthesia also decreased by a factor of six. There was no electron microscopic evidence of neuronal toxicity, and the mechanism of action underlying this protracted anesthesia remains unknown.

References

1. Simon, R.A.: Sulfite sensitivity. Ann. Allergy *56*:281–288, 1986.
2. Bush, R.K., Taylor, S.L., Holden, K., Nordlee, J.A., and Busse, W.W.: Prevalence of sensitivity to sulfiting agents in asthmatic patients. Am. J. Med. *81*:816–820, 1986.
3. Schwartz, H.J., Gilbert, I.A., Lenner, K.A., Sher, T.H., and McFadden, E.R., Jr.: Metabisulfite sensitivity and local dental anesthesia. Ann. Allergy *62*:83–86, 1989.
4. Luebke, N.H., and Walker, J.A.: Discussion of sensitivity to preservatives in anesthetics. J. Am. Dent. Assoc. *97*:656–657, 1978.
5. Bilger, P.A.L., Yagiela, J.A., Hardin, R.L., and Hunt, L.M.: Measurement of physiologic responses to local anesthetics in unanesthetized rats. J. Dent. Res. *60*(A):463, 1981.
6. Remely, L., and Yagiela J.A.: Effects of vasoconstrictors on local anesthetic toxicity. J. Dent. Res. *64*:307, 1985.
7. Ultracaine® DS, Ultracaine® DS Forte (Articaine Hydrochloride with Epinephrine) Injection: Summary of Product Information. Montreal, Hoechst-Roussel Canada, Inc., 1991.
8. Luduena, F.P., Hoppe, J.O., Coulston, F., and Drobeck, H.P.: The pharmacology and toxicology of mepivacaine, a new local anesthetic. Toxicol. Appl. Pharmacol. *2*:295–315, 1960.
9. Avant, W.E., and Weatherby, J.H.: Effects of epinephrine on toxicities of several local anesthetic agents. Proc. Soc. Exp. Biol. Med. *103*:353–356, 1960.
10. Åström, A., Persson N.H., and Örtengren, B.: The effect of adrenaline on the toxicities and absorptions of L 67 (Citanest®) and some other local anaesthetics studied in mice and rabbits. Acta Pharmacol. Toxicol. *21*:161–171, 1964.
11. Åkerman, B.: On felypressin (Octapressin®) as an adjunct to lidocaine and prilocaine—an experimental study in animals. Acta Pharmacol. Toxicol. *24*:377–388, 1966.
12. Henn, F., and Brattsand, R.: Some pharmacological and toxicological properties of a new long-acting local analgesic, LAC-43 (Marcaine®), in comparison with mepivacaine and tetracaine. Acta Anaesthesiol. Scand. Suppl. *21*:9–30, 1966.
13. Adams, H.J., Kronberg, G.H., and Takman, B.H.: Local anesthetic activity and acute toxicity of (±)-2-(*N*-ethylpropylamino)-2′, 6′-butyroxylidide, a new long-acting agent. J. Pharm. Sci. *61*:1829–1831, 1972.
14. de Jong, R.H., and Bonin, J.D.: Deaths from local anesthetic-induced convulsions in mice. Anesth. Analg. *59*:401–405, 1980.
15. Brodie, B.B., Lief, P.A., and Poet, R.: The fate of procaine in man following its intravenous administration and methods for the estimation of procaine and diethylaminoethanol. J. Pharmacol. Exp. Ther. *94*:359–366, 1948.
16. Dobbs, E.C., DeVier, C.W., Jr., and Rapoport, L.: A new local anesthetic agent. J. Am. Dent. Assoc. *49*:409–413, 1954.
17. Tainter, M.L., Wessinger, G.D., and Lee, J.W.: New local anesthetic solutions containing propoxycaine. J. Am. Dent. Assoc. *51*:19–27, 1955.
18. Yagiela, J.A.: Local anesthetics.: *In* Dionne, R.A., and Phero, J.C., eds.: Management of Pain and Anxiety in Dental Practice. New York, Elsevier Science Publishing Co., 1991.
19. Prescribing Information—Dental. Westborough, Mass., Astra Pharmaceutical Products, Inc., 1990.
20. Kodak Dental Products: Catalog and Reference Guide. Rochester, N.Y., Eastman Kodak Co., 1991.
21. Ultracaine® D-S Ultracaine® D-S Forte. Montreal, Hoechst-Roussel Canada, Inc.
22. Council on Dental Therapeutics of the American Dental Association: Accepted Dental Therapeutics, ed. 40. Chicago, American Dental Association, 1984.

23. USP Dispensing Information, ed. 13. Rockville, Md., United States Pharmacopeial Convention, Inc., 1993.

24. Björn, H.: A survey of recently introduced drugs for local anaesthesia. Odontol. Rev. 7:305–353, 1956.

25. Cowan, A.: Minimum dosage technique in the clinical comparison of representative modern local anesthetic agents. J. Dent. Res. *43*:1228–1249, 1964.

26. Buckley, J.A., Ciancio, S.G., and McMullen, J.A.: Efficacy of epinephrine concentration in local anesthesia during periodontal surgery. J. Periodontol. *55*:653–657, 1984.

27. Keesling, G.R., and Hinds, E.C.: Optimal concentration of epinephrine in lidocaine solutions. J. Am. Dent. Assoc. *54*:338–340, 1963.

28. Gangarosa, L.P., and Halik, F.J.: A clinical evaluation of local anaesthetic solutions containing graded epinephrine concentrations. Arch. Oral Biol. *12*:611–621, 1967.

29. Berling, C.: Carbocain in local anaesthesia in the oral cavity: An experimental and clinical investigation comprising 1046 dental local anaesthesias. Odontol. Rev. *9*:254–267, 1958.

30. Fink, B.R., Aasheim, G.M., and Levy, B.A.: Neural pharmacokinetics of epinephrine. Anesthesiology *48*:263–266, 1978.

31. Cannell, H., and Beckett, A.H.: Peri-oral injections of local anæsthetic into defined sites. Br. Dent. J. *139*:242–244, 1975.

32. Goebel, W.M., Allen, G., and Randall, F.: Comparative circulating serum levels of mepivacaine with levo-nordefrin and lidocaine with epinephrine. Anesth. Prog. *26*:93–97, 1979.

33. Goebel, W.M., Allen, G., and Randall, F.: Comparative circulating serum levels of 2 per cent mepivacaine and 2 per cent lidocaine. Br. Dent. J. *148*:261–264, 1980.

34. Keenaghan, J.B., and Boyes, R.N.: The tissue distribution, metabolism and excretion of lidocaine in rats, guinea pigs, dogs, and man. J. Pharmacol. Exp. Ther. *180*:454–463, 1972.

35. Mihaly, G.W., Moore, R.G., Thomas, J., Triggs, E.J., Thomas, D., and Shanks, C.A.: The pharmacokinetics and metabolism of the aniline local anaesthetics in neonates. 1. Lignocaine. Eur. J. Clin. Pharmacol. *13*:143–152, 1978.

36. Nelson, S.D., Garland, W.A., Breck, G.D., and Trager W.F.: Quantification of lidocaine and several metabolites utilizing chemical-ionization mass spectrometry and stable isotope labelling. J. Pharm. Sci. *66*:1180–1190, 1977.

37. Dobbs, E.C., and Ross, E.C.: The new local anesthetic Carbocaine. N. Y. State Dent. J. *27*:453–457, 1961.

38. Stibbs, G.D., and Korn, J.H.: An evaluation of the local anesthetic, mepivacaine hydrochloride, in operative dentistry. J. Prosthet. Dent. *14*:355–364, 1964.

39. Hinkley, S.A., Reader, A., Beck, M., and Meyers, W.J.: An evaluation of 4% prilocaine with 1 : 200,000 epinephrine and 2% mepivacaine with 1 : 20,000 levonordefrin compared with 2% lidocaine with 1 : 100,000 epinephrine for inferior alveolar nerve block. Anesth. Prog. *38*:84–89, 1991.

40. Mumford, J.M., and Geddes, I.C.: Trial of Carbocaine in conservative dentistry. Br. Dent. J. *110*:92–94, 1961.

41. Petersen, J.K., Lück, H., Kristensen, F., and Mikkelsen, L.: A comparison of four commonly used local analgesics. Int. J. Oral Surg. *6*:51–59, 1977.

42. Oikarinen, V.J., Ylipaavalniemi, P., and Evers, H.: Pain and temperature sensations related to local analgesia. Int. J. Oral Surg. *4*:121–156, 1975.

43. Meffin, P., Long, G.J., and Thomas, J.: Clearance and metabolism of mepivacaine in the human neonate. Clin. Pharmacol. Ther. *14*:218–225, 1973.

44. Meffin, P., Robertson, A.V., Thomas, J., and Winkler, J.: Neutral metabolites of mepivacaine in humans. Xenobiotica *3*:191–196, 1973.

45. Tucker, G.T., and Mather, L.E.: Properties, absorption, and disposition of local anesthetic agents. *In* Cousins, M.J., and Bridenbaugh, P.O., eds.: Neural Blockade

in Clinical Anesthesia and Management of Pain, ed. 2. Philadelphia, J.B. Lippincott Co., 1988.

46. Jorfeldt, L., Löfström, B., Pernow, B., Persson, B., Wahren, J., and Widman, B.: The effect of local anaesthetics on the central circulation and respiration in man and dog. Acta Anaesthesiol. Scand. *12*:153–169, 1968.

47. Cowan, A.: Further clinical evaluation of prilocaine (Citanest), with and without epinephrine. Oral Surg. Oral Med. Oral Pathol. *26*:304–311, 1968.

48. Epstein, S.: Clinical study of prilocaine with varying concentrations of epinephrine. J. Am. Dent. Assoc. *78*:85–90, 1969.

49. Chilton, N.W.: Clinical evaluation of prilocaine hydrochloride 4% solution with or without epinephrine. J. Am. Dent. Assoc. *83*:149–154, 1971.

50. Berling, C., and Björn, H.: L 67—a new local anaesthetic of anilide type: Experimental determination of its efficacy in dental plexus anaesthesia in man. Sver. Tandlakarforb. Tidn. *52*:511–522, 1960.

51. Cowan, A.: Comparison of two ultrashort duration anesthetic agents. J. Dent. Res. *44*:13–19, 1965.

52. Brown, G., and Ward, N.L.: Prilocaine and lignocaine plus adrenaline: A clinical comparison. Br. Dent. J. *126*:557–562, 1969.

53. Cannell, H., and Whelpton, R.: Systemic uptake of prilocaine after injection of various formulations of the drug. Br. Dent. J. *160*:47–49, 1986.

54. Åkerman, B., Åström, A., Ross, S., and Telč, A.: Studies on the absorption, distribution and metabolism of labelled prilocaine and lidocaine in some animal species. Acta Pharmacol. Toxicol. *24*:389–403, 1966.

55. Arthur, G.R., Scott, D.H.T., Boyes, R.N., and Scott D.B.: Pharmacokinetic and clinical pharmacological studies with mepivacaine and prilocaine. Br. J. Anaesth. *51*:481–485, 1979.

56. Warren, R.E., Van de Mark, T.B., and Weinberg, S.: Methemoglobinemia induced by high doses of prilocaine. Oral Surg. Oral Med. Oral Pathol. *37*:866–871, 1974.

57. Klos, C.P., and Hays, G.L.: Prilocaine-induced methemoglobinemia in a child with Shwachman syndrome. J. Oral Maxillofac. Surg. *43*:621–623, 1985.

58. Nespeca, J.A.: Clinical trials with bupivacaine in oral surgery. Oral Surg. Oral Med. Oral Pathol. *42*:301–307, 1976.

59. Pricco, D.F.: An evalution of bupivacaine for regional nerve block in oral surgery. J. Oral Surg. *35*:126–129, 1977.

60. Laskin, J.L., Wallace, W.R., and deLeo, B.: Use of bupivacaine hydrochloride in oral surgery: A clinical study. J. Oral Surg. *35*:25–29, 1977.

61. Chapman, P.J., and Gordon Macleod, A.W.: A clinical study of bupivacaine for mandibular anesthesia in oral surgery. Anesth. Prog. *32*:69–72, 1985.

62. Danielsson, K., Evers, H., and Nordenram, Å.: Long-acting local anesthetics in oral surgery: An experimental evaluation of bupivacaine and etidocaine for oral infiltration anesthesia. Anesth. Prog. *32*:65–68, 1985.

63. Trieger, N., and Gillen, G.H.: Bupivacaine anesthesia and post-operative analgesia in oral surgery. Anesth. Prog. *26*:20–23, 1979.

64. Linden, E.T., Abrams, H., Matheny, J., Kaplan, A.L., Kopczyk, R.A., and Jasper, S.J., Jr.: A comparison of postoperative pain experience following periodontal surgery using two local anesthetic agents. J. Periodontol. *57*:637–642, 1986.

65. Moore, D.C., Bridenbaugh, L.D., Thompson, G.E., Balfour, R.I., and Horton, W.G.: Bupivacaine: A review of 11,080 cases. Anesth. Analg. *57*:42–53, 1978.

66. Albright, G.A.: Cardiac arrest following regional anesthesia with etidocaine or bupivacaine. Anesthesiology *51*:285–287, 1979.

67. Moore, D.C., Balfour, R.I., and Fitzgibbons, D.: Convulsive arterial plasma levels of bupivacaine and the response to diazepam therapy. Anesthesiology *50*:454–456, 1979.

68. Reynolds, F.: Metabolism and excretion of bupivacaine in man: A comparison with mepivacaine. Br. J. Anaesth. *43*:33–36, 1971.

69. Giovannitti, J.A., and Bennett, C.R.: The effectiveness of 1.5% etidocaine HCl with epinephrine 1 : 200,000 and 2% lidocaine HCl with epinephrine 1 : 100,000 in oral surgery: A clinical comparison. J. Am. Dent. Assoc. *107*:616–618, 1983.

70. Sisk, A.L., Dionne, R.A., and Wirdzek, P.R.: Evaluation of etidocaine hydrochloride for local anesthesia and postoperative pain control in oral surgery. J. Oral Maxillofac. Surg. *42*:84–88, 1984.

71. Danielsson, K., Evers, H., Holmlund, A., Kjellman, O., Nordenram, Å., and Persson, N.-E.: Long-acting local anaesthetics in oral surgery: Clinical evaluation of bupivacaine and etidocaine for mandibular nerve block. Int. J. Oral Maxillofac. Surg. *15*:119–126, 1986.

72. Crout, R.J., Koraido, G., and Moore, P.A.: A clinical trial of long-acting local anesthetics for periodontal surgery. Anesth. Prog. *37*:194–198, 1990.

73. Donoghue, R., Doberenz, K., and Jacobsen, P.L.: Etidocaine hydrochloride in surgical procedures: Effects on postoperative analgesia. J. Am. Dent. Assoc. *120*:429–434, 1990.

74. Laskin, J.L.: Use of etidocaine hydrochloride in oral surgery: A clinical study. J. Oral Surg. *36*:863–865, 1978.

75. Jensen, O.T., Upton, L.G., Hayward, J.R., and Sweet, R.B.: Advantages of long-acting local anesthesia using etidocaine hydrochloride. J. Oral Surg. *39*:350–353, 1981.

76. Covino, B.G.: Clinical pharmacology of local anesthetic agents. *In* Cousins, M.J., and Bridenbaugh, P.O., eds.: Neural Blockade in Clinical Anesthesia and Management of Pain, ed. 2. Philadelphia, J.B. Lippincott Co., 1988.

77. Morgan, D.J., Smyth, M.P., Thomas, J., and Vine, J.: Cyclic metabolites of etidocaine in humans. Xenobiotica *7*:365–375, 1977.

78. Morgan, D.J., Cousins, M.J., McQuillan, D., and Thomas, J.: Disposition and placental transfer of etidocaine in pregnancy. Eur. J. Clin. Pharmacol. *13*:359–365, 1977.

79. Borchard, U., and Drouin, H.: Carticaine: Action of the local anesthetic on myelinated nerve fibres. Eur. J. Pharmacol. *62*:73–79, 1980.

80. Winther, J.E., and Nathalang, B.: Effectivity of a new local analgesic Hoe 40 045. Scand. J. Dent. Res. *80*:272–278, 1972.

81. Ferger, P., and Marxkors, R.: Ein neues Anästhetikum in der zahnärztlichen Prosthetik. Dtsch. Zahnarztl. Z. *28*:87–89, 1973.

82. Donaldson, D., James-Perdok, L., Craig, B.J., Derkson, G.D., and Richardson, A.S.: A comparison of Ultracaine® DS (articaine HCl) and Citanest® Forte (prilocaine HCl) in maxillary infiltration and mandibular nerve block. J. Can. Dent. Assoc. *53*:38–42, 1987.

83. Wright, G.Z., Weinberger, S.J., Marti, R., and Plotzke, O.: The effectiveness of infiltration anesthesia in the mandibular primary molar region. Pediatr. Dent. *13*:278–283, 1991.

84. Knoll-Köhler, E., and Rupprecht, S.: Articaine for local anaesthesia in dentistry: A lidocaine controlled double blind cross-over study. Eur. J. Pain *13*:59–63, 1992.

85. Lemay, H., Albert, G., Hélie, P., Dufour, L., Gagnon, P., Payant, L., and Laliberté, R.: Ultracaine in conventional operative dentistry. J. Can. Dent. Assoc. *50*:703–708, 1984.

86. Dudkiewicz, A., Schwartz, S., and Laliberté, R.: Effectiveness of mandibular infiltration in children using the local anesthetic Ultracaine® (articaine hydrochloride). J. Can. Dent. Assoc. *53*:29–31, 1987.

87. Malamed, S.F.: Handbook of Local Anesthesia, ed. 3. St. Louis, Mosby–Year Book, Inc., 1990.

88. Haas, D.A., Harper, D.G., Saso, M.A., and Young, E.R.: Comparison of articaine and prilocaine anesthesia by infiltration in maxillary and mandibular arches. Anesth. Prog. *37*:230–237, 1990.

89. Haas, D.A., Harper, D.G., Saso, M.A., and Young, E.R.: Lack of differential effect by Ultracaine™ (articaine) and Citanest™ (prilocaine) in infiltration anesthesia. J. Can. Dent. Assoc. *57*:217–223, 1991.

90. van Oss, G.E.C.J.M., Vree, T.B., Baars, A.M., Termond, E.F.S., and Booij, L.H.D.J.: Pharmacokinetics, metabolism, and renal excretion of articaine and its metabolite articainic acid in patients after epidural administration. Eur. J. Anaesthesiol. *6*:49–56, 1989.

91. van Oss, G.E.C.J.M., Vree, T.B., Baars, A.M., Termond, E.F.S., and Booij, L.H.D.J.: Clinical effects and pharmacokinetics of articainic acid in one volunteer after intravenous administration. Pharm. Weekbl. (Sci.) *10*:284–286, 1988.

92. Vree, T.B., Baars, A.M., van Oss, G.E.C.J.M., and Booij, L.H.D.J.: High-performance liquid chromatography and preliminary pharmacokinetics of articaine and its 2-carboxy metabolite in human serum and urine. J. Chromatogr. *424*:440–444, 1988.

93. Dionne, R.A., Wirdzek, P.R., Fox, P.C., and Dubner, R.: Suppression of postoperative pain by the combination of a nonsteroidal anti-inflammatory drug, flurbiprofen, and a long-acting local anesthetic, etidocaine. J. Am. Dent. Assoc. *108*:598–601, 1984.

94. Moore, P.A., and Dunsky, J.L.: Bupivacaine anesthesia—a clinical trial for endodontic therapy. Oral Surg. Oral Med. Oral Pathol. *55*:176–179, 1983.

95. Berquist, H.C.: The danger of mepivacaine 3% toxicity in children. J. Calif. Dent. Assoc. *3*(9):13, 1975.

96. Hersh, E.V., Helpin, M.L., and Evans, O.B.: Local anesthetic mortality: Report of case. ASDC J. Dent. Child. *58*:489–491, 1991.

97. Sveen, K.: Effect of the addition of a vasoconstrictor to local anesthetic solution on operative and postoperative bleeding, analgesia and wound healing. Int. J. Oral Surg. *8*:301–306, 1979.

98. Hecht, A., and App, G.R.: Blood volume lost during gingivectomy using two different anesthetic techniques. J. Periodontol. *45*:9–12, 1974.

99. Ueda, W., Hirakawa, M., and Mori, K.: Acceleration of epinephrine absorption by lidocaine. Anesthesiology *63*:717–720, 1985.

100. Skoglund, L.A., and Jorkjend, L.: Postoperative pain experience after gingivectomies using different combinations of local anaesthetic agents and periodontal dressings. J. Clin. Periodontol. *18*:204–209, 1991.

101. Adriani, J., Zepernick, R., Arens, J., and Authement, E.: The comparative potency and effectiveness of topical anesthetics in man. Clin. Pharmacol. Ther. *5*:49–62, 1964.

102. Rosivack, R.G., Koenigsberg, S.R., and Maxwell, K.C.: An analysis of the effectiveness of two topical anesthetics. Anesth. Prog. *37*:290–292, 1990.

103. Gill, C.J., and Orr, D.L., II: A double-blind crossover comparison of topical anesthetics. J. Am. Dent. Assoc. *98*:213–214, 1979.

104. Kellett, P.B., and Copeland, C.S.: Methemoglobinemia associated with benzocaine-containing lubricant. Anesthesiology *59*:463–464, 1983.

105. Anderson, S.T., Hajduczek, J., and Barker, S.J.: Benzocaine-induced methemoglobinemia in an adult: Accuracy of pulse oximetry with methemoglobinemia. Anesth. Analg. *67*:1099–1101, 1988.

106. Barker, S.J., Tremper, K.K., Hyatt, J., and Zaccari, J.: Effects of methemoglobinemia on pulse oximetry and mixed venous oximetry. Anesthesiology *67*:A171, 1987.

107. Åström, A., and Persson, N.H.: The toxicity of some local anesthetics after application on different mucous membranes and its relation to anesthetic action on the nasal mucosa of the rabbit. J. Pharmacol. Exp. Ther. *132*:87–90, 1961.

108. Adriani, J., and Campbell, B.: Fatalities following the topical application of local anesthetics to mucous membranes. J.A.M.A. *162*:1527–1530, 1956.

109. Fleming, J.A., Byck, R., and Barash, P.G.: Pharmacology and therapeutic applications of cocaine. Anesthesiology *73*:518–531, 1990.

110. Gross, J.B., Hartigan, M.L., and Schaffer, D.W.: A suitable substitute for 4% cocaine before blind nasotracheal intubation: 3% lidocaine–0.25% phenylephrine nasal spray. Anesth. Analg. *63*:915–918, 1984.

111. Lathers, C.M., Tyau, L.S.Y., Spino, M.M., and Agarwal, I.: Cocaine-induced seizures, arrhythmias, and sudden death. J. Clin. Pharmacol. *28*:584–593, 1988.

112. DiFazio C.A., Carron, H., Grosslight, K.R., Moscicki, J.C., Bolding, W.R., and Johns, R.A.: Comparison of pH-adjusted lidocaine solutions for epidural anesthesia. Anesth. Analg. *65*:760–764, 1986.

113. Catchlove, R.F.H.: Potentiation of two different local anaesthetics by carbon dioxide. Br. J. Anaesth. *45*:471–474, 1973.

114. Bokesch, P.M., Raymond, S.A., and Strichartz, G.R.: Dependence of lidocaine potency on pH and Pco_2. Anesth. Analg. *66*:9–17, 1987.

115. Chaney, MA., Kerby, R., Reader, A., Beck, F.M., Meyers, W.J., and Weaver, J.: An evaluation of lidocaine hydrocarbonate compared with lidocaine hydrochloride for inferior alveolar nerve block. Anesth. Prog. *38*:212–216, 1991.

116. Åberg, G., Friberger, P., and Sydnes, G.: Studies on the duration of local anaesthesia: A possible mechanism for the prolonging effect of dextran on the duration of infiltration anaesthesia. Acta Pharmacol. Toxicol. *42*:88–92, 1978.

117. Rosenblatt, R.M.: Dextran is not a potent local anesthetic adjuvant. Anesthesiology *55*:480–481, 1981.

118. Langerman, L., Golomb, E., and Benita, S.: Spinal anesthesia: Significant prolongation of the pharmacologic effect of tetracaine with lipid solution of the agent. Anesthesiology *74*:105–107, 1991.

119. Legros, F., Luo, H., Bourgeois, P., Lafont, N., and Boogaerts, J.: Influence of different liposomal formulations on pharmacokinetics of encapsulated bupivacain. Anesthesiology *73*:A851, 1990.

120. Hersh, E.V., Maniar, M., Green, M., and Cooper, S.A.: Anesthetic activity of the Lipospheres Bupivacaine Delivery System in the rat. Anesth. Prog. *39*:197–200, 1992.

121. Moller, R.A., and Covino, B.G.: Effect of progesterone on the cardiac electrophysiologic alterations produced by ropivacaine and bupivacaine. Anesthesiology *77*:735–741, 1992.

122. Brown, D.L., Carpenter, R.L., and Thompson, G.E.: Comparison of 0.5% ropivacaine and 0.5% bupivacaine for epidural anesthesia in patients undergoing lower-extremity surgery. Anesthesiology *72*:633–636, 1990.

123. Evers, H., von Dardel, O., Juhlin, L., Ohlsén, L., and Vinnars, E.: Dermal effects of compositions based on the eutectic mixture of lignocaine and prilocaine (EMLA): Studies in volunteers. Br. J. Anaesth. *57*:997–1005, 1985.

124. Holst, A., and Evers, H.: Experimental studies of new topical anaesthetics on the oral mucosa. Swed. Dent. J. *9*:185–191, 1985.

125. Svensson, P., and Petersen, J.K.: Anesthetic effect of EMLA occluded with Orahesive Oral Bandages on oral mucosa. Anesth. Prog. *39*:79–82, 1992.

126. Samsi, A.B., Bhalerao, R.A., Shah, S.C., Mody, B.B., Paul, T., and Satoskar, R.S.: Evaluation of centbucridine as a local anesthetic. Anesth. Analg. *62*:109–111, 1983.

127. Brennan, P.A., and Langdon, J.D.: A preliminary report using oxethazaine—a potential new dental local anesthetic. Br. J. Oral Maxillofac. Surg. *28*:26–28, 1990.

128. Adams, H.J., Blair, M.R., Jr., and Takman, B.H.: The local anesthetic activity of tetrodotoxin alone and in combination with vasoconstrictors and local anesthetics. Anesth. Analg. *55*:568–573, 1976.

129. Drachman, D., and Strichartz, G.: Potassium channel blockers potentiate impulse inhibition by local anesthetics. Anesthesiology 75:1051–1061, 1991.
130. Schneider, M., Datta, S., and Strichartz, G.: A preferential inhibition of impulses in C-fibers of the rabbit vagus nerve by veratridine, an activator of sodium channels. Anesthesiology 74:270–280, 1991.
131. Gaumann, D.M., Brunet, P.C., and Jirounek, P.: Clonidine enhances the effects of lidocaine on C-fiber action potential. Anesth. Analg. 74:719–725, 1992.
132. Scurlock, J.E., and Curtis, B.M.: Tetraethylammonium derivatives: Ultralong-acting local anesthetics? Anesthesiology 54:265–269, 1981.

Patient Evaluation

Local anesthesia intended for regional pain control can be administered to almost anyone. This assertion is particularly true regarding anesthesia of the oral cavity, in which the amount injected is typically modest compared with anesthetic dosages employed elsewhere in the body. Nevertheless, an accurate preanesthetic evaluation of each patient is necessary in order to identify the rare individual who should not receive regional anesthesia under any circumstances or patients who need some special modification of technique, dosage, or drug selection.

The preanesthetic evaluation should include an adequate medical history and, when appropriate, a physical examination. In case of severe ongoing disease, appropriate consultation is strongly recommended to help estimate the patient's functional reserve and identify specific treatment limitations.

General Physical State

A major consideration in the preanesthetic evaluation is whether the patient has sufficient functional reserve to undergo the proposed procedure. The stress of injection coupled with a subsequent restorative or surgical procedure may occasionally precipitate serious complications in the severely compromised patient.

One of the simplest, most convenient, and most easily remembered methods of assessing the general physical state of a patient is through the classification scheme adopted by the American Society of Anesthesiologists.[1] As described in Table 5–1, this system groups patients into five categories on the basis of overall health. As a general rule, individuals who are in class 1 or 2 can receive routine care, including the use of local anesthetics. However, some limitations in either the complexity or duration of treatment rendered per appointment may be desirable with individuals in class 2. In addition, some form of anxiety control is often

Table 5–1.   **AMERICAN SOCIETY OF ANESTHESIOLOGISTS (ASA) PHYSICAL STATUS CLASSIFICATION**

ASA Class*	Patient Description	Clinical Examples	Clinical Management
1	A normally healthy patient	No organic, physiologic, biochemical, or psychiatric disturbances; treatment is for localized disorder	Routine care
2	A patient with mild systemic disease	Controlled essential hypertension, pronounced obesity, psychiatric disturbance	Routine care, but procedural stress and length of appointment limited
3	A patient with severe systemic disease that is nonincapacitating	Severe diabetes mellitus, congestive heart failure, chronic obstructive pulmonary disease	Strict limitation of complex procedures; careful control of procedural stress
4	A patient with an incapacitating systemic disease that is a constant threat to life	Acute myocardial infarction; advanced pulmonary, cardiac, hepatic, or renal insufficiency	Emergency or palliative care, usually in a hospital
5	A moribund patient who is not expected to live 24 hours with or without operation	Uncontrolled massive internal bleeding; rapidly progressing cardiac insufficiency with renal failure	Emergency life support only

* Emergency cases are designated by the addition of the letter E to the classification number.

appropriate for patients who are apprehensive about intraoral injections or the proposed treatment. Class 3 patients may also receive local anesthetics, but procedural stress should be strictly limited. Consideration should be given to ensuring proper rest the night before the procedure, limiting the amount of work to be performed, and affording effective postoperative medication, if needed.[2] Vital signs should be monitored during the procedure as necessary. Class 4 patients should, in many instances, receive emergency care only, and often within the confines of a hospital. When elective procedures are indicated, hospitalization is recommended. Routine care is proscribed in class 5 patients.

Specific Questions Relevant to Evaluating a Patient for Local Anesthesia

Besides assessment of the global health of a patient, it is important that attention be paid during the preanesthetic evaluation to several specific disorders that may influence either drug selection or anesthetic technique. These conditions relate not only to the patient's health, but to his or her genetic background and concurrent medication use. The following are questions typically found in medical history forms that help address this need.

- *Have you been a patient in the hospital during the past 2 years?*
- *Have you been under recent medical treatment?*
- *Are you on a special diet?*

These questions in some respects ask the same query in different ways so that the clinician can obtain information that the patient may have forgotten about or thinks is unimportant to treatment.

Overall health assessment is valuable in determining a patient's ability to cope with procedural stress, including that induced by local anesthetic administration. Many patients are unfamiliar with a specific diagnosis or its significance. If a patient indicates recent medical management and cannot provide adequate details or is unsophisticated about them, identifying the treating physician and his or her specialty is often helpful in defining significant conditions. Some patients underestimate their problems, others magnify them. Finally, many individuals intentionally leave out critical information because they fear not being treated (i.e., people with hepatitis B, acquired immune deficiency syndrome [AIDS], AIDS-related condition [ARC], or recreational drug use) or simply feel it is unimportant for receiving dental treatment. Under these circumstances, communicating with the treating physician will often identify conditions, attitudes, and problems not well delineated in a self-administered health history and which may explain difficult behavior patterns, unusual responses to medications, habitual use of drugs, and so forth.

- *Have you taken any medicine or drugs in the past 2 years?*

This question can also provide the clinician with information about general health. A patient who denies cardiac disease may reveal the use of a medication normally prescribed for cardiovascular disorders. In like fashion, regular use of corticosteroids is commonly associated with immune disorders, organ transplantation, connective tissue disease, cancer, or various minor dermatologic conditions. Thus, the specific importance of medication use is principally related to the medical diagnosis attached to it.

Local anesthetics may potentially interact with a variety of therapeutic agents. Most of these interactions are primarily of heuristic interest and are seen only in the laboratory or perhaps in patients who have taken excessive doses or in whom other atypical factors are present. However, a few interactions may occur in routine clinical practice and should be taken into account when anesthetic preparations are selected.

An important adverse drug interaction involving local anesthetics, and one of the first to be identified, is inhibition of the antibacterial action of sulfonamides by procaine. Sulfonamides exert a bacteriostatic effect against susceptible bacteria by competitively antagonizing the incorporation of *p*-aminobenzoic acid (PABA) into folic acid. Procaine and related esters can yield sufficient PABA upon hydrolysis to overcome the sulfonamide block, particularly in the area of injection. Although the sulfonamides have largely been replaced by other antibiotics, sulfamethoxazole marketed in combination with the nonsulfonamide trimethoprim (Bactrim, Septra) is used for urinary tract and middle ear infections and occasionally for other antimicrobial therapy. Ester anesthetics normally should not be administered to patients receiving sulfonamides alone or in combination with other agents.

Because amide anesthetics are biotransformed in the liver, potential interactions may occur with other drugs that influence hepatic metabolism. The H_2 antihistamine cimetidine, for instance, impairs the metabolism of lidocaine, presumably by competing with the local anesthetic for binding to hepatic oxidative enzymes. Alternative H_2-receptor blockers, such as ranitidine and famotidine, are not substrates for these enzymes and do not impair lidocaine clearance. The β-adrenergic blocking drugs propranolol and metoprolol, however, share this effect of cimetidine on lidocaine breakdown. In addition, by decreasing hepatic blood flow, they interfere with the delivery of lidocaine to the liver for biotransformation. While these drugs are unlikely to increase significantly the toxicity of local anesthetics administered within single recommended doses, they have proved dangerous in patients receiving lidocaine by continuous infusion and dictate caution regarding the reinjection of local anesthetics during prolonged procedures.

Most drug interactions involving local anesthetics are related not to the local anesthetics themselves but to the vasoconstrictors included in the preparations. For example, a local anesthetic with epinephrine used either to supplement general anesthesia or to enhance hemostasis should be administered with caution in patients anesthetized with any general anesthetic that sensitizes the heart to catecholamines. No more than 100 μg of epinephrine, corresponding to 10 mL of a 1 : 100,000 solution, is recommended within a 10-minute period when halothane is used for general anesthesia.[3] Although halothane is less popular today than it once was, primarily owing to the introduction of less arrhythmogenic anesthetics, it is still a drug of choice in children and continues to be used in selected circumstances, particularly by oral surgeons in outpatient settings. Table 5–2 summarizes maximum recommended doses of epinephrine, levonordefrin, and norepinephrine (contained in local anesthetics)

Table 5–2. **MAXIMUM RECOMMENDED DOSES OF VASOCONSTRICTORS IN PATIENTS RECEIVING INHALATION GENERAL ANESTHESIA**

	Halothane *(Fluothane)*	*Enflurane* *(Ethrane)*	*Isoflurane* *(Forane)*
Epinephrine (mg)*			
10 min	0.10	0.10	0.30
60 min	0.30	0.30	0.90
Levonordefrin (mg)†			
10 min	0.32	0.32	—
60 min	0.96	0.96	—
Norepinephrine (mg)‡			
10 min	0.10	0.10	0.30
60 min	0.30	0.30	0.90

* *1/100,000 solution = 0.01 mg/mL.*
† *1/20,000 solution = 0.05 mg/mL.*
‡ *1/30,000 solution = 0.033 mg/mL.*

when used with the three most commonly utilized inhalation general anesthetics.

Another interaction of clinical note is the potentiation of amine vasoconstrictors by guanethidine (Ismelin), and other adrenergic neuronal blocking agents employed in the treatment of hypertension. Guanethidine prevents the release of norepinephrine from sympathetic nerves. With time, effector organs become "supersensitive" to direct-acting sympathomimetic amines, and administration of local anesthetics with epinephrine or related drugs may then lead to exaggerated changes in blood pressure and/or cardiac rhythm, particularly if the solution is unintentionally injected into the bloodstream.

Other drugs with antiadrenergic activity that may interact with epinephrine-like drugs are the α- and β-receptor antagonists. Drugs with significant α-adrenergic blocking activity, including several antihypertensive agents (e.g., prazosin) and antipsychotic medications (e.g., chlorpromazine), competitively inhibit the systemic vasoconstricting actions of epinephrine. Should epinephrine be administered during an emergency to treat hypotension caused by one of these agents, the vasoconstricting action of epinephrine would be blocked, and the blood pressure would fall even further because of the unopposed actions of epinephrine on vasodilatory β_2 receptors (see Chapter 3). There is no evidence, however, of a clinically significant interaction between epinephrine and α blockers in normotensive patients. Norepinephrine and levonordefrin, neither of which possess strong β_2 activity, show no such interaction in either circumstance.

Nonselective β-blocking drugs cause the reverse interaction with epinephrine. In the sensitive patient, inhibition of epinephrine binding to β_2

receptors reveals the systemic α-agonistic effect of the vasoconstrictor. Exaggerated hypertensive responses coupled with reflex bradycardia can develop. The interaction has not been observed in patients taking cardioselective β_1 agonists and is less likely to occur with norepinephrine and levonordefrin. If a local anesthetic with epinephrine is to be injected in a patient taking propranolol or another nonselective β blocker, small volumes (e.g., 1-mL amounts of the 1:100,000 epinephrine concentration) should initially be administered and blood pressure measurements taken 5 minutes later. In this manner, the hyperreactor can be identified before a large, potentially dangerous dose is administered.

The most publicized interactions involving local anesthetic solutions are those of vasoconstrictors and certain drugs used in the management of psychologic depression.[4] Depression is a frequent diagnosis in modern society, and several of the tricyclic antidepressants listed in Table 5–3 remain among the more commonly prescribed drugs. Tricyclic agents accentuate the effects of norepinephrine and other amines by blocking their uptake into sympathetic nerve terminals. Exogenously administered drugs and endogenously released catecholamines are similarly affected. When norepinephrine is used as a vasoconstrictor, dangerous elevations of systolic blood pressure have been reported. With respect to epinephrine, only modest changes in blood pressure usually occur, but

Table 5–3.   **TRICYCLIC ANTIDEPRESSANTS: NONPROPRIETARY AND TRADE NAMES***

Amitriptyline	Imipramine
Amitid	Antipress
Amitril	Imavate
Elavil	Janimine
Endep	Norfranil
Etrafon†	Pramine
Limbitrol‡	Presamine
Triavil†	Tofranil
Amoxapine	Maprotiline§
Asendin	Ludiomil
Clomipramine	Nortriptyline
Anafranil	Aventyl
Desipramine	Pamelor
Norpramin	Protriptyline
Pertofrane	Vivactil
Doxepin	Trimipramine
Adapin	Surmontil
Sinequan	

* Salt designations excluded.
† In combination with perphenazine.
‡ In combination with chlordiazepoxide.
§ A tetracyclic antidepressant with similar pharmacologic actions.

the chances that cardiac irregularities will develop are enhanced. Inasmuch as epinephrine is potentiated by a factor of two to four, careful administration in commensurately reduced doses is permissible. Norepinephrine and levonordefrin should be avoided completely, however, because they are more greatly influenced, a reflection of their normally more avid uptake by sympathetic neurons.

Less frequently used in the treatment of depression are the monoamine oxidase (MAO) inhibitors, including isocarboxazid (Marplan), tranylcypromine (Parnate), and phenelzine (Nardil). Despite statements and advertisements to the contrary, local anesthetics with catecholamine vasoconstrictors can be used without special reservation in patients taking MAO inhibitors.[5,6] The actions of exogenously administered epinephrine, norepinephrine, and levonordefrin are primarily terminated by the enzyme catechol-O-methyltransferase and by uptake into sympathetic nerve terminals; inhibition of MAO has little effect on the disposition of these drugs.

- *Are you allergic to (i.e., have itching, rash, swelling of hands, eyes, or feet) or made sick by penicillin, aspirin, codeine, or any other drugs or medications?*

Local anesthetics rarely cause allergic reactions. Nevertheless, patients often claim allergy to one or more anesthetic agents. When a history of local anesthetic allergy is obtained, the patient should be carefully questioned to rule out the possibility of misinformation or misdiagnosis. Access to relevant hospital records or direct contact with clinicians involved in the alleged allergic response is also very helpful in this regard. If the episode in question is consistent with drug allergy, every effort should be made to identify the preparation. (This task may be difficult, since patients often do not remember which drugs are involved and tend to view all "caine" anesthetics as one.)

In the vast majority of instances, individuals yield histories compatible with anxiety responses (e.g., syncope, mild nausea) or toxic reactions (e.g., local irritation, drowsiness).[7] Although special care, such as preoperative sedation, may be indicated in some of these patients to avoid future untoward responses, usually no special precaution is necessary with respect to drug allergy.

When a patient has a well-documented history of local anesthetic allergy and the specific agent is known, an unrelated anesthetic should be chosen. Unfortunately, drug selection is complicated by the fact that cross-reactivity between different anesthetic formulations may occur. Most commonly used ester anesthetics are derivatives of PABA, and antibodies or immunocompetent cells directed against the PABA moiety on one drug may react with the same group on another.

Although cross-reactivity between PABA esters (e.g., procaine) and amide anesthetics (e.g., lidocaine) does not occur, many amide anesthetic solutions contain methylparaben, a preservative structurally re-

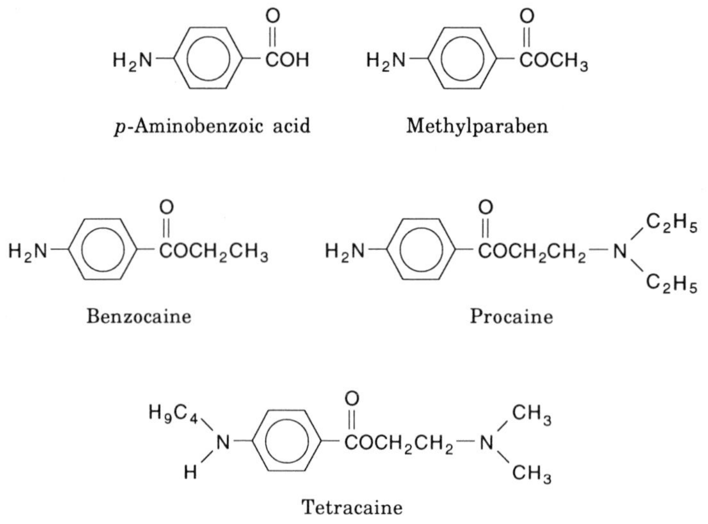

Figure 5–1. Molecular similarity between *p*-aminobenzoic acid, methylparaben, and certain ester local anesthetics.

lated to PABA (Fig. 5–1).[8,9] In addition to eliciting allergic responses in patients sensitized to PABA, methylparaben may also serve as the initial antigenic stimulant, especially as it is widely used in many prescription and over-the-counter medicines, dermatologic creams and ointments, suntan oils, toothpastes, and even some foods. Because of this potential for allergic response, U.S. manufacturers removed methylparaben from amide local anesthetic solutions contained in dental cartridges. However, the preservative remains part of anesthetic solutions contained in reusable multidose vials used by some dentists and most physicians and is present in articaine cartridges marketed in Canada.

As discussed in Chapter 4, local anesthetics with adrenergic vasoconstrictors include a sulfite antioxidant, usually sodium metabisulfite, acetone sodium bisulfite, or sodium or potassium bisulfite. Patients who are truly allergic to sulfites should not receive local anesthetics that contain them (i.e., preparations with vasoconstrictors). More commonly, a history of intolerance to ingested or inhaled sulfites is obtained. Careful questioning often reveals which of these individuals have received local anesthetics with vasoconstrictors previously without incident and who may be so reactive that even the small amounts in local anesthetic solutions should be avoided.

On occasion, the clinician will be faced with a presumptive case of local anesthetic allergy in which the drug or drugs involved cannot be positively identified.[10] One of several options, none of which are ideal, must then be chosen for managing the patient. The clinician may elect to forgo regional anesthesia entirely and rely on some other modality, such as electrical analgesia or nitrous oxide sedation/analgesia, for pain control. Although suitable for some patients requiring nonsurgical treatment, this approach is by no means universally acceptable, and in certain instances can make the procedure barely tolerable for both patient and clinician. Alternatively, an antihistamine with local anesthetic activity (for example, 1% diphenhydramine) may be used in place of a conventional anesthetic. Here, too, pain relief is not consistent in all patients, and diphenhydramine can be irritating to tissues. Indeed, use of the more concentrated 5% solution (50 mg/mL) may cause tissue sloughing and prolonged paresthesia.

In an emergency, the clinician may decide to employ an amide preparation without preservatives. Mepivacaine without vasoconstrictor is a good choice. This approach does entail a small risk that the patient may actually be allergic to mepivacaine, but, in view of the paucity of documented cases of allergy to amides and the fact that many patients have never been exposed to mepivacaine, the risk is often worth taking in patients whose supposed allergic manifestations were mild and occurred some time ago.

A final approach for the patient with presumed allergy to local anesthetics is sensitivity testing. Although not recommended for the uninitiated, intradermal testing has long been employed for assessing local anesthetic allergy. To be valid, however, the testing must be conducted properly (with appropriate controls, preservatives, and pure drugs), and even then, interpretation can be difficult. Although intradermal testing has been criticized, largely because of false-positive reactions,[11] no instance of an immediate allergic response to a drug administered for regional anesthesia has ever been reported in a patient with a negative intradermal test for that agent followed by a negative intraoral challenge injection. Therefore, a negative intradermal response gives assurance that the anesthetic in question may be used with a reasonable degree of confidence.[7]

- *Do you have or have you ever had a heart murmur, rheumatic fever, congenital heart lesion, artificial heart valve, heart surgery, or an artificial joint?*

These questions are significant because selected anesthesia techniques and subsequent restorative or surgical treatment cause transient bacteremia. Although the number of microbes that normally gain access to the bloodstream is small and of little consequence to most patients, some individuals are at risk of developing serious infection.

Rheumatic fever is known to cause cardiac valvular damage, which provides a nidus for bacteria to lodge and proliferate. Rheumatic fever is not exclusive in that effect however, as various acquired and congenital cardiac disorders are equally dangerous in this regard. The end result is bacterial endocarditis, a life-threatening systemic bacterial infection that is best prevented when possible, rather than treated after its establishment. Surgical manipulation is especially important as a source of bacteremia, but even restorative treatment has been implicated in bacteremia and endocarditis. For this reason, the American Heart Association has recommended antibiotic prophylaxis for all patients susceptible to bacterial endocarditis in whom oral procedures are likely to cause gingival or muscosal bleeding (including periodontal ligament injection). Inasmuch as viridans streptococci are most commonly associated with endocarditis following dental treatment, the prophylactic use of amoxicillin or alternative chemotherapeutic agents effective against gram-positive microorganisms is indicated. Periodically, the American Heart Association publishes updated guidelines for managing patients subject to bacterial endocarditis.[12]

In addition to their use in patients with cardiac disorders, prophylactic antibiotics have been advocated for patients with kidney disease (e.g., renal obstruction, transplants) or with orthopedic prosthesis (e.g., total joint replacement).[13] Because prophylactic requirements for these patients differ, and no unified opinion exists as to the most correct prophylactic drug regimen, it may be helpful to obtain appropriate consultation prior to initiating specific chemotherapeutic coverage.

- *Have you had heart failure, heart disease or a heart attack, angina pectoris, high blood pressure, a heart pacemaker, or heart surgery?*
- *Have you ever had chest pain or shortness of breath with walking?*
- *Have you ever had swollen ankles?*
- *Do you wake up short of breath or use two pillows to sleep?*

These questions all relate to cardiovascular disorders. Most local anesthetic agents are well tolerated by patients with cardiac or vascular disease, provided that care is exercised in limiting procedural stress and pain. A major point of controversy, however, is the use of vasoconstrictors, particularly epinephrine, in conjunction with local anesthetics. The American Heart Association has stated that the typical concentrations of vasoconstrictors contained in local anesthetics are not contraindicated in patients with cardiovascular disease so long as preliminary aspiration is practiced, the agent is injected slowly, and the smallest effective dose is administered.[14] With regard to the maximum permissible amount for any given session, a special committee of the New York Heart Association recommended in 1954 that no more than 0.2 mg of epinephrine be used in any form (Table 5–4).[15] This determination was colored, however, by the unavailability at that time of local anesthetics effective without vasoconstrictors.

In support of these official determinations are several studies that have shown that inclusion of vasoconstrictors in local anesthetic solutions does not statistically increase the incidence of adverse effects in cardiovascular patients.[6,16] However, there have been reported instances of electrocardiographic alterations and precipitous changes in cardiovascular function following administration of local anesthetics containing vasoconstrictors.[17,18] In addition, the possibility exists of unintentional intra-

Table 5–4. **MAXIMAL CONCENTRATIONS AND DOSAGES OF VASOCONSTRICTORS CONTAINED IN LOCAL ANESTHETICS**

Drug	Concentration, mg/mL (parts/thousand)*	Maximal Recommended Dose, mg (mL)†
Epinephrine	0.02 (1 : 50,000)	0.20 (10)
	0.01 (1 : 100,000)	0.20 (20)
	0.005 (1 : 200,000)	0.20 (40)
Levonordefrin	0.05 (1 : 20,000)	1.00 (20)
Norepinephrine	0.033 (1 : 30,000)	0.33 (10)

* *Epinephrine 1 : 50,000 should be reserved for local infiltration when hemostasis is required.*

† *Maximal dose for epinephrine as recommended by the New York Heart Association.[15] Values for levonordefrin and norepinephrine are unofficial estimates.*

vascular injection (even with aspiration), and the American Heart Association now believes that restriction of epinephrine in regional anesthesia is desirable in patients with ischemic heart disease.[19] Finally, compelling data indicate that the use of local anesthetics containing epinephrine leads to significant increases in plasma epinephrine levels.[20-22] Concomitant with this is the potential in certain patients for substantial elevations in systolic blood pressure, heart rate, and rate–pressure product, although healthy young adults do not normally demonstrate clinically significant changes in these parameters. Therefore, it would seem prudent to minimize or avoid the use of sympathomimetics when possible in patients with moderate to severe cardiovascular disease. Patients who would tolerate tachycardia or increased blood pressure poorly, such as those with congestive heart failure or severe uncontrolled hypertension, normally should not receive such agents. Also, patients with a history of cardiac dysrhythmias are at risk for vasoconstrictor-induced dysrhythmias. However, balancing this view is one that adequate anesthesia must also be achieved, and poor pain control can cause undesired cardiovascular changes. Thus, a sometimes difficult judgment must be made as to when and how much vasoconstrictor should be used.

- *Have you ever had thyroid disease, taken cortisone, had chemotherapy or rheumatism?*

Two endocrine conditions, hyperthyroidism and adrenocortical insufficiency, pose potential difficulties for individuals requiring regional anesthesia. Hyperthyroidism (Graves' disease) predisposes patients to certain forms of cardiac dysfunction if overproduction of thyroid hormone is not controlled by drugs or surgery. Local anesthetics containing epinephrine or related vasoconstrictors that stimulate the heart are generally contraindicated because these patients may be extremely sensitive to the arrhythmogenic actions of such drugs. Furthermore, regardless of anesthesia, routine elective treatment is best delayed when overt manifestations of thyrotoxicosis (i.e., tachycardia, hypertension, anxiety, and insomnia) are present until chemotherapeutic suppression of the hyperthyroidism has been completed. Patients receiving appropriate thyroid supplements to replace thyroid function lost by virtue of disease, surgery, or radiation treatment may receive adrenergic drugs.

Adrenocortical insufficiency (Addison's disease) is not a contraindication to regional anesthesia per se, but signifies potential intolerance to any major procedural stress. Adrenal hypofunction can arise from a number of causes, including primary adrenocortical disease, surgical adrenalectomy, or therapeutic use of corticosteroids in the treatment of various rheumatologic, immunologic, dermatologic, or malignant disorders.

During the 1950s, there were several reports of postoperative circulatory collapse and death in patients previously taking corticosteroid therapy.[23,24] Subsequently it was described that certain anesthetic agents, and the surgery itself, caused the adrenal cortex to increase secretion of cortisol commensurate with the degree of procedural stress the patient was subjected to. Since long-term exposure to exogenous corticosteroids as part of a therapeutic regimen suppresses this stress response, most anesthesiologists have advocated and used corticosteroid supplementation preoperatively in order to prevent peripheral vascular collapse, shock, and cardiac arrest. Reported dosage protocols of steroids vary, and indeed some authors have questioned the need for such supplementation in selected situations.[25] However, the critical issue is the degree of procedural stress a patient with hypoadrenalism (endogenous or exogenous) is subjected to. A small quantity of local anesthetic given during a typical oral injection, followed by a relatively benign restorative dental procedure in an otherwise healthy, cooperative adult, is not likely to provoke enough stress to require supplementary steroids. By contrast, a very frightened, uncooperative patient or one who has a painful submandibular cellulitis requiring substantial quantities of anesthetic and invasive, uncomfortable oral surgery under emergency conditions is an individual who should receive corticosteroid supplementation before any treatment is initiated. Although the exogenous use of corticosteroids is known to adversely affect wound healing and spread of infection, short-term preoperative supplementation seems to be associated with minimal risk. Therefore, if the clinician is uncertain whether the patient needs corticosteroid supplementation, it is probably useful to use a lower dose supplemental regimen (Tables 5–5 and 5–6). In very complex cases, tapering regimens may be justified, and consultation with the practitioner responsible for management of the patient's corticosteroid therapy would undoubtedly be useful.

> • *Have you ever had any excessive bleeding requiring special treatment, or hemophilia, or do you bruise easily?*

It is beyond the scope of this text to describe the various bleeding and clotting disorders that have been encountered. However, it is important to recognize that injecting a local anesthetic can be hazardous, particu-

Table 5–5. CORTICOSTEROID SUPPLEMENTATION FOR PATIENTS WITH ADRENAL INSUFFICIENCY

Anticipated Condition	*Clinical Examples*	*Dose*
Moderate stress	Multiple or complex restorative, periodontal, or oral surgical procedures requiring multiquadrant anesthesia	2 to 4 times daily dose
Severe stress	Major oral surgery, general anesthesia, severe infection, trauma	4 to 8 times daily dose

larly if the patient's affliction is severe. The following is offered as a general guide[26]: *Infiltration anesthesia utilizing small amounts of solution, administered very gently and slowly with small-gauge needles, is permissible. Block anesthesia in areas where there is significant risk of damaging blood vessels (e.g., inferior alveolar nerve block, posterior superior alveolar nerve block) is contraindicated unless the patient has received replacement therapy.*

Frequently, specific clotting factors, such as factor VIII for classic hemophilia, are used in replacement therapy to elevate the missing factor to at least 30% of the normal plasma titer. Alternative regimens employing aminocaproic acid or desmopressin (DDAVP) have become popular in recent years. Assuming the patient has no endogenous inhibitor of the factor or other contraindication that would nullify the replacement therapy, block injections may then be performed as in a normal individual. Of course, extra care, gentle technique, and slow administration are desirable. If a positive aspirate is obtained during the injection, replacement therapy should be maintained for 36 to 48 hours.

Anticoagulant treatment with drugs such as warfarin (Coumadin) represents an acquired form of hemophilia. However, as long as the pro-

Table 5–6. FREQUENTLY USED GLUCOCORTICOIDS

Drug	*Potency*	*Equivalent Dose (mg)*
Short-acting		
Cortisone	0.8	25
Hydrocortisone (cortisol)	1	20
Intermediate-acting		
Methylprednisolone	5	4
Prednisolone	4	5
Prednisone	4	5
Triamcinolone	5	4
Long-acting		
Betamethasone	25	0.75
Dexamethasone	25	0.75

thrombin time is maintained within 1½ to 2 times control, routine regional anesthesia may be performed.[27] Some clinicians have been using periodontal ligament injections in place of nerve blocks for local anesthesia in patients with congenital or acquired hemorrhagic disorders. Experience seems to indicate satisfactory results with this approach for restorative procedures on individual teeth.

- *Have you ever had hepatitis B (serum), yellow jaundice, liver disease, ARC or AIDS, HIV antibody, blood transfusions, or drug addiction?*

Lidocaine and other amides are largely degraded in the liver, and interruption of their metabolism may permit toxic amounts of drug to accumulate in the systemic circulation. Although switching to an ester may seem appropriate for patients with advanced hepatic disease, it must be recognized that the liver is responsible for the synthesis of pseudocholinesterase and that no benefit in drug safety will be gained. Fortunately, even patients with acute hepatitis or pronounced cirrhosis of the liver can usually metabolize amide anesthetics at a rate adequate for the dosages conventionally administered in the oral cavity. Ambulatory patients with hepatic disease but without documented intolerance to amide anesthetics may therefore be given regional anesthesia without undue concern.

Concerning the issue of AIDS and patient groups known to be at high risk for infection with human immunodeficiency virus, the routine use of local anesthetics for dental treatment is both practical and safe, provided that adequate infection control measures are taken to protect the clinician and assistants. The routine use of a mask, rubber gloves, eye protection, and precautions against an accidental needle stick is mandatory. Moreover, the arbitrary refusal of care to such patients is unethical, unnecessary, and ignores the fact that patients within such risk groups are frequently unaware of their infection (especially early), often are not easily identifiable, and sometimes deliberately hide such information from the practitioner because of prior experience with uninformed health care personnel. Therefore, clinicians must assume that they will encounter and treat such patients in practice, whether or not the patients are specifically identified as at risk. Ergo, protective measures should be taken in caring for all patients.

- *Do you have any disease, condition, or problem not listed in the history?*
- *Are you pregnant?*

Although it is widely recognized that certain drugs or procedures administered during pregnancy constitute a potential hazard to the fetus, clinical experience suggests that there is little added danger in using local anesthetics during pregnancy. Pregnancy risk categories of individual agents are outlined in Chapter 4.

- *Have you had a bad experience in a dental office?*
- *Do you feel very nervous about dental treatment?*
- *Have you received psychiatric treatment? Are you very anxious?*

Psychologic disorders vary widely in both cause and effect and often are of little importance with regard to the use of local anesthetics or the delivery of dental care. However, a significant minority of patients express great anxiety or fear of dental treatment. Others do so indirectly, usually with statements such as "Novocain never works," or "nobody can make me numb." Although failure to achieve local anesthesia can occur despite the best of technique, it is rare, and most patients expressing such comments are acutely anxious about dental care. Often it is not possible to treat such patients without dealing with their odontophobia. Gentle technique and adequate amounts of local anesthetics frequently are insufficient to correct such patients' fear and permit satisfactory treatment. In such instances the use of specific psychologic intervention or pharmacologic control of anxiety in the form of nitrous oxide–oxygen sedation, parenteral sedation, or even ultralight general anesthesia may be required for adequate patient management.

Metabolic Disorders

PSEUDOCHOLINESTERASE DEFICIENCY

Certain uncommon genetic or acquired alterations in enzyme activity can influence regional anesthesia. Procaine and its congeners are metabolized by cholinesterase enzymes in the plasma and, to a lesser extent, in the liver. Some individuals (one in 3,000) have very low titers of plasma pseudocholinesterase activity and are intolerant to large doses of local ester anesthetics. Because the enzyme responsible for hydrolysis of procaine is also necessary for inactivation of succinylcholine (a neuromuscular blocking drug used to facilitate endotracheal intubation), patients with a history of prolonged apnea following general anesthesia in which succinylcholine was administered should be suspected of having a possible pseudocholinesterase deficiency until proved otherwise. However, nonester (amide) local anesthetics can be safely used in such patients.

MALIGNANT HYPERTHERMIA

In the early 1960s, Denborough and co-workers[28] described a potentially fatal syndrome provoked by certain anesthetic and adjunctive drugs. It is currently referred to as malignant hyperthermia or malignant hyperpyrexia. Its occurrence is estimated to be one case per 12,000 to 40,000 general anesthetic administrations, but its true incidence in the general population is unknown. Many patients with the trait are never identified, as it may occur only after the administration of several anesthetics or only when certain anesthetic agents are utilized (particularly halothane and succinylcholine). The disease runs in families, and some variants at least are transmitted in an autosomal dominant manner. Besides general anesthesia, infections, exercise, muscle injury, and stress have been reported to provoke this or similar syndromes. Nonfulminant or mild cases have been described and apparently are often overlooked or misdiagnosed as other diseases. Symptoms variably include tachycardia, generalized muscle contraction, rapid elevation of body temperature, cardiac dysrhythmias, metabolic acidosis, disseminated intravascular coagulopathy, and, if a fulminant case is untreated, death. Although the triggering ability of specific general anesthetics is well recognized, the ability of certain local anesthetics to trigger this response has been controversial. It has been experimentally documented in vitro that lidocaine and other amide anesthetics augment caffeine-stimulated muscle contracture, whereas ester anesthetics such as procaine and tetracaine do not. Because of these theoretical findings and the overwhelming nature of the disturbance, some authors have recommended that only ester-type local anesthetics be used in patients suspected of having the malignant hyperthermia trait.[29] Other clinicians, fearful of provoking such an attack, have even denied dental or surgical care to patients with such a trait. Alternatively, hospital admission with extensive (and expensive) monitoring has been utilized even for routine dental care with local anesthesia to protect the patient (and doctor) against the chance occurrence of this condition. More recently, however, this issue has been under critical discussion, as there are in fact *no documented cases* in the medical or dental literature (over the past 25 years) supporting the concept of amide anesthetics triggering malignant hyperthermia. Indeed, recent papers have indicated safe use of lidocaine, prilocaine, and bupivacaine for regional anesthesia in patients known to have the malignant hyperthermia trait[30,31]; the lack of malignant hyperthermia occurring in a European study of 300,000 regional anesthetics using lidocaine[32]; and no known reports of malignant hyperthermia triggered in dental patients receiving amide anesthetics. Finally, in animal studies, pigs susceptible to malignant hyperthermia were deliberately administered large (toxic) volumes of lidocaine intravenously without triggering any hyperthermic response.[33,34] For these reasons, unusual precautions, including excessive monitoring, hospitalization, the exclusive use of ester anesthetics (procaine, etc.), and so on are unnecessary, and the routine use of lidocaine or other commonly available amide anesthetics is both safe and acceptable.

METHEMOGLOBINEMIA

A very few patients have a hereditary condition in which they are exquisitely sensitive to *o*-toluidine, a compound formed by the metabolic hydrolysis of prilocaine and which oxidizes hemoglobin to methemoglobin. In normal unaffected individuals very large doses of prilocaine (>8 mg/kg) may lead to a sufficient accumulation of methemoglobin (3 to 5 g/100 mL) in the blood to cause a patient to appear cyanotic and the blood to take on a brownish hue. However, in patients without significant cardiovascular or pulmonary disease, this circumstance is usually well tolerated. On the other hand, patients with hereditary methemoglobinemia are very sensitive to *small* doses of prilocaine and become intolerant to the formation of excessive quantities of methemoglobin. Because of this, and the ready availability of alternative local anesthetics, prilocaine should not be used where hereditary methemoglobinemia is suspected.

References

1. Owens, D.W., Felts, J.A., and Spitznagel, E.L., Jr.: ASA physical status classifications: A study of consistency of ratings. Anesthesiology, *49*:239–243, 1978.
2. McCarthy, F.M., and Malamed, S.F.: Physical evaluation system to determine medical risk and indicated dental therapy modifications. J. Am. Dent. Assoc., *99*:181–184, 1979.
3. Katz, R.L., Matteo, R.S., and Papper, E.M.: The injection of epinephrine during general anesthesia with halogenated hydrocarbons and cyclopropane in man: 2. Halothane. Anesthesiology, *23*:597–600, 1962.
4. Boakes, A.J., Laurence, D.R., Teoh, P.C., Barar, F. S. K., Benedikter, L. T., and Prichard, B. N. C.: Interactions between sympathomimetic amines and antidepressant agents in man. Br. Med. J., *1*:311–315, 1973.
5. Newcomb, G.M.: Contraindications to the use of catecholamine vasoconstrictors in dental local analgesics. N.Z. Dent. J., *69*:25–30, 1973.
6. Verrill, P.J.: Adverse reactions to local anaesthetics and vasoconstrictor drugs. Practitioner, *214*:380–387, 1975.
7. Arora, S., and Aldrete, J.A.: Investigation of possible allergy to local anesthetic drugs: Correlation of intradermal and intramuscular injections. Anesth. Rev., *3*:13–16, 1976.
8. Lampe, K.: Allergic hypersensitivity to local anesthetics. J.A.M.A., *247*:2155, 1982.
9. Luebke, N.H., and Walker, J.A.: Discussion of sensitivity to preservatives in anesthetics. J. Am. Dent. Assoc., *97*:656–657, 1978.
10. Aldrete, J.A., and Johnson, D.A.: Allergy to local anesthetics. J.A.M.A., *207*:356–357, 1969.
11. Fisher, M.McD.: Intradermal testing in the diagnosis of acute anaphylaxis during anaesthesia—results of five years experience. Anaesth. Intensive Care, *7*:58–61, 1979.
12. Dajani, A.S., Bisno, A.L., Chung, K.J., et al.: Prevention of bacterial endocarditis: Recommendations by the American Heart Association. J.A.M.A., *264*:2919–2922, 1990.
13. Zallen, R.D., and Black, S.L.: Antibiotic therapy in oral and maxillofacial surgery. J. Oral. Surg., *34*:349–351, 1976.
14. Management of dental problems in patients with cardiovascular disease: Report of a working conference jointly sponsored by the American Dental Association and American Heart Association. J. Am. Dent. Assoc., *68*:333–342, 1964.
15. Use of epinephrine in connection with procaine in dental procedures: Report of the Special Committee of the New York Heart Association, Inc. on the Use of Epineph-

rine in Connection with Procaine in Dental Procedures. J. Am. Dent. Assoc., *50*:108, 1955.

16. Boakes, A.J., Laurence, D.R., Lovel, K.W., O'Neil, R., and Verrill, P.J.: Adverse reactions to local anæsthetic/vasoconstrictor preparations: A study of the cardiovascular responses to Xylestesin and Hostacain-with-Noradrenaline. Br. Dent. J., *133*:137–140, 1972.

17. Aellig, W.H., Laurence, D.R., O'Neill, R., and Verrill, P.J.: Cardiac effects of adrenaline and felypressin as vasoconstrictors in local anaesthesia for oral surgery under diazepam sedation. Br. J. Anaesth., *42*:174–176, 1970.

18. Lilienthal, B.: Cardiovascular responses to intraosseous injections of prilocaine containing vasoconstrictors. Oral Surg. Oral Med. Oral Pathol., *42*:552–558, 1976.

19. Kaplan, E.L., ed.: Cardiovascular Disease in Dental Practice. Dallas, American Heart Association, 1986.

20. Cotton, B.R., Henderson, H.P., Achola, K.J., and Smith, G.: Changes in plasma catecholamine concentrations following infiltration with large volumes of local anaesthetic solution containing adrenaline. Br. J. Anaesth., *58*:593–597, 1986.

21. Tolas, A.G., Pflug, A.E., and Halter, J.B.: Arterial plasma epinephrine concentrations and hemodynamic responses after dental injection of local anesthetic with epinephrine. J. Am. Dent. Assoc., *10*:41–43, 1982.

22. Chernow, B., Balestrieri, F., Ferguson, C.D., Terezhalmy, G.T., Fletcher, J.R., and Lake, C.R.: Local dental anesthesia with epinephrine: Minimal effects on the sympathetic nervous system or on hemodynamic variables. Arch. Intern. Med., *143*:2141–2143, 1983.

23. Fraser, C.G., Preuss, F.S., and Bigford, W.D.: Adrenal atrophy and irreversible shock associated with cortisone therapy. J.A.M.A., *149*:1542–1543, 1952.

24. Lewis, L., Robinson, R.F., Yee, J., Hacken, L.A., and Eisen, G.: Fatal adrenal cortical insufficiency precipitated by surgery during prolonged continuous cortisone treatment. Ann. Intern. Med., *39*:116–126, 1953.

25. Weatherill, D., and Spence, A.A.: Anaesthesia and disorders of the adrenal cortex. Br. J. Anaesth., *56*:741–749, 1984.

26. Evans, B.E., and Aledort, L.M.: Hemophilia and dental treatment. J. Am. Dent. Assoc., *96*:827–834, 1978.

27. Glasser, S.P.: The problems of patients with cardiovascular disease undergoing dental treatment. J. Am. Dent. Assoc., *94*:1158–1162, 1977.

28. Denborough, M.A., Forster, J.F., Lovell, R.R., Maplestone, P.A., and Villiers, J.D.: Anaesthetic deaths in a family. Br. J. Anaesth., *34*:395–396, 1962.

29. Malamed, S.F.: Handbook of Local Anesthesia, 2nd ed. St. Louis, C.V. Mosby Co., 1986.

30. Gielen, M., and Viering, W.: 3-in-1 lumbar plexus block for muscle biopsy in malignant hyperthermia patients: Amide local anaesthetics may be used safely. Acta Anaesthesiol. Scand., *30*:581–583, 1986.

31. Paasuke, R.T., and Brownell, A.K.W.: Amine local anaesthetics and malignant hyperthermia (editorial). Can. Anaesth. Soc. J., *33*:126–129, 1986.

32. Ording, H.: Incidence of malignant hyperthermia in Denmark. Anesth. Analg., *64*:700–704, 1985.

33. Harrison, G.G., and Morrell, D.F.: Response of swine to IV infusion of lignocaine and bupivacaine. Br. J. Anaesth., *42*:385–387, 1980.

34. Wingard, D.W., and Bobko, S.: Failure of lidocaine to trigger porcine malignant hyperthermia. Anesth. Analg., *58*:99–103, 1979.

Chapter 6

Anesthetic Equipment

The safe and effective administration of a local anesthetic depends to a large extent on the armamentarium used during injection. When handled correctly, the single-dose anesthetic cartridge, disposable hypodermic needle, and the sterile aspirating syringe combine to ensure accurate placement of the local anesthetic solution without risk to the patient of cross-infection or intravascular injection. Although outmoded instruments and supplies such as nonaspirating syringes and reusable needles are occasionally employed by some, the use of such antiquated equipment is not the current standard of care. The basic instruments required for the use of local anesthetics in dentistry are syringes, anesthetic cartridges, and needles. Additionally, technical developments have added special devices such as needleless jet injectors and syringes specifically designed for periodontal ligament anesthesia.

Syringes

There are many different types of syringes available on the market. However, there are certain criteria for syringes established by the Council on Dental Materials and Devices of the American Dental Association.[1,2] These include:

1. They must be durable and able to withstand repeated sterilization without damage. (If the unit is disposable, it should be packaged in a sterile container.)
2. They should be capable of accepting a variety of cartridges and needles of different manufacture and permit repeated use.
3. They should be inexpensive, self-contained, lightweight, and simple to use with one hand.
4. They should provide for effective aspiration and be constructed so that blood may be easily observed in the cartridge.

It is accepted that aspiration prior to injecting a local anesthetic is extremely important to reduce the risk of inadvertent intravascular injections.

The most satisfactory and widely used syringe for intraoral anesthesia is the metallic aspirating cartridge syringe. Cook Laboratories introduced the cartridge syringe in 1921. A major improvement occurred 36 years later with the addition of an aspirating plunger. This engaged the rubber stopper of the anesthetic cartridge with a harpoon or hook, thus allowing the induction of negative pressure within the cartridge by pulling back the stopper. The style of aspirating syringe varies with the manufacturer, but most are made of chrome-plated brass or stainless steel (Fig. 6–1). Recently, nonmetallic syringes have also been marketed, including both single-use and reusable styles (Fig. 6–2). Personal preference dictates whether to use a syringe with finger and thumb rings or one with ringless finger grips.

Syringes are manufactured with different-sized thumb rings to accommodate different hand sizes. This is important, since small-handed operators have difficulty in retracting the plunger of harpoon-type syringes when using too large a thumb ring and may dislodge the needle from the target area when attempting to do so.

The newest variant of the cartridge syringe is the "self-aspirating" syringe.[3-7] This device has a flat plunger designed solely to depress the stopper, with no ability to retract it. Instead, aspiration is achieved by a metallic sleeve surrounding the needle and resting on the cartridge dia-

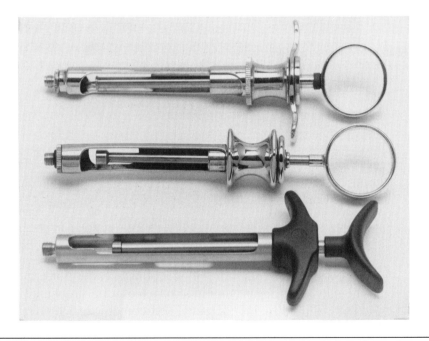

Figure 6–1.   Three different styles of metallic aspirating syringes. Note the absence of a hook or harpoon in the two lower syringes, indicating that they are self-aspirating types.

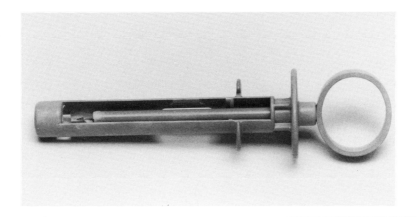

Figure 6–2.   Nonmetallic reusable aspirating syringe.

phragm. When pressure is applied to the plunger, the whole cartridge moves forward, causing the diaphragm to be pushed inward by the sleeve. When the plunger is released the cartridge and the diaphragm spring back to their original position, providing a negative pressure within the cartridge sufficient for aspiration.

An alternative method for aspirating with this syringe uses a thumb disk that, when depressed, pushes the cartridge forward and causes the diaphragm to be depressed. Because the thumb disk acts directly on the cartridge casing, it is capable of approximately twice the negative pressure induced by the plunger shaft. However, it can be awkward to use.

Routine maintenance of reusable syringes entails thorough cleaning and sterilization after use on each patient. After repeated autoclaving, the syringe should be dismantled and lubricated with a light oil at all threaded joints and where the piston contacts the thumb ring and guide bearings (Fig. 6–3).

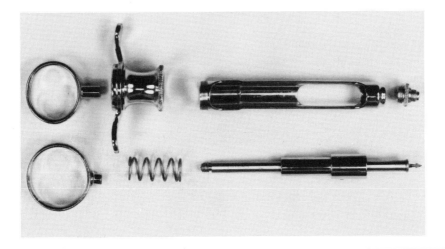

Figure 6–3.   Metallic cartridge syringe dismantled for cleaning and oiling of threaded parts.

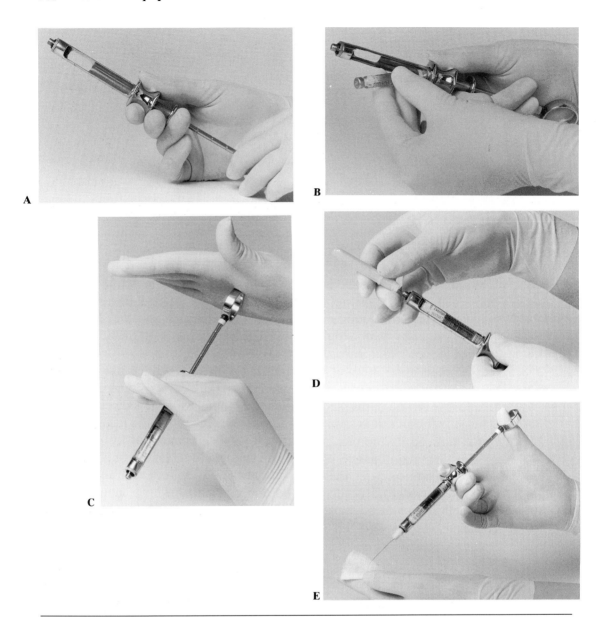

Figure 6–4. Steps in preparing the anesthetic syringe for injection. **A.** Retracting the syringe piston. **B.** Inserting the anesthetic cartridge. **C.** Inserting the harpoon into the cartridge stopper (using a harpoon-style syringe). **D.** Needle attachment. **E.** Freeing the stopper by expressing a small amount of anesthetic.

Figure 6–4 demonstrates the correct steps involved in inserting and removing a cartridge in a sideloading harpoon syringe. After the piston is retracted, the anesthetic cartridge is inserted plunger end first. The harpoon is then engaged by pushing down on the piston firmly. Alternatively, a *gentle* tap can be used to seat the harpoon (excessive force may cause the cartridge to shatter). Also, as a precaution, the barrel of the syringe can be covered by the supporting hand. If the needle has been

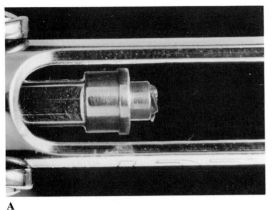 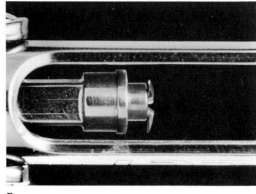

A   B

Figure 6–5.   Aspirating feature of the articaine syringe. **A**. Engaging blades of the plunger in the retracted position. **B**. Engaging blades fully extended.

previously attached, this step causes anesthetic fluid to be expressed. Note that if the syringe is self-aspirating, this latter step is unnecessary. When attaching the needle, the cartridge diaphragm is punctured in the center, and one or two drops of anesthetic is expressed in order to free the plunger, which may initially adhere to the glass. If this step is omitted, there may be a sudden painful surge of local anesthetic into the tissues when the injection is started. The fully loaded syringe is now ready for use. To remove an empty cartridge, the plunger is fully retracted and the cartridge pushed out. A second cartridge may then be inserted, with care taken to ensure proper needle puncture of the diaphragm.

Subsequent cartridges may be loaded into the same syringe and needle for use on the same patient, but *under no circumstances should any needle or cartridge be used on more than one patient.*

The recent introduction of articaine to North America requires the use of a special type of aspirating syringe. The piston of this syringe is capped by three retractable blades (Fig. 6–5). During loading, it is placed into the silicone stopper of the cartridge, which has a recess designed to fit the end of the piston. When a control wheel on the handle of the syringe is turned, the three blades are extended to engage the plunger and permit aspiration.

Although single-use disposable plastic syringes with presterilized needle–cartridge assemblies have been marketed, the reusable plastic syringe (see Fig. 6–2) has proved to be more popular. These may be sterilized either by autoclaving or by using chemicals but are only recommended for use with disposable needles having plastic hubs. Gas and spring-loaded syringes have also been produced and allow for smooth injections but are relatively expensive, and some designs have no aspirating mechanism and therefore are not recommended.

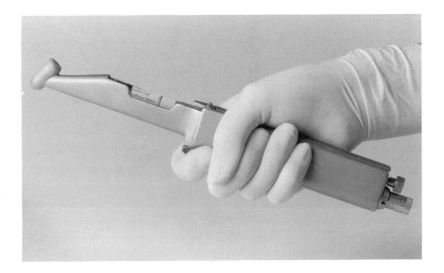

Figure 6–6.   Loaded jet injector.

JET INJECTOR

A syringe that dispenses with needles altogether is the jet injector (Fig. 6–6). With this device, the release of a mechanically activated spring forces 0.05 to 0.2 mL of anesthetic solution under high pressure through a very small orifice into the mucosa. The head of the jet injector through which the local anesthetic solution is propelled is covered with a removable hood that can be sterilized separately from the rest of the device.

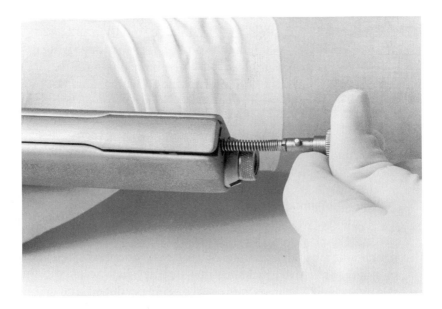

Figure 6–7.   Spring loading of jet injector.

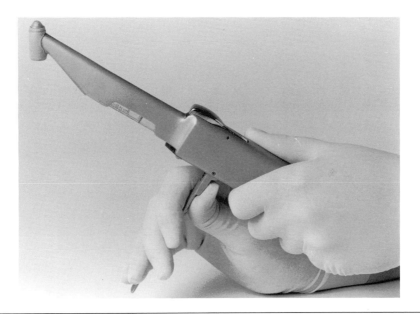

Figure 6–8.   Priming of jet injector.

After the cartridge is inserted, the jet injector is spring loaded (Fig. 6–7) and primed (Fig. 6–8). The depth of penetration can be adjusted to accommodate the anesthetic technique being attempted (Fig. 6–9).

The tip of the jet injector is then placed against the mucosa over the

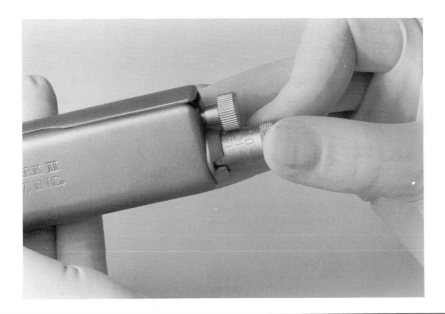

Figure 6–9.   Adjusting force of anesthetic penetration.

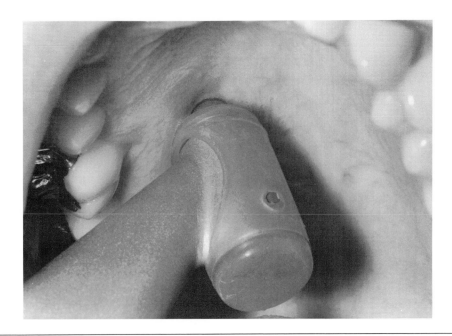

Figure 6–10.   Clinical placement of jet injector for palatine injection. Note removable hood covering injector head.

area to be anesthetized and the trigger pulled (Fig. 6–10). An area of tissue blanching is produced at the site of the injection.

The original design of the jet injector produced an alarming, explosive sound during use, but recent devices produce only a muffled sound. The injection itself is surprisingly pain free and ideal for greater palatine or nasopalatine injections, which are particularly uncomfortable anesthetic procedures. In general, its success rate appears to be much better in children than in adults, in whom the jet injector is often used only for preliminary anesthesia prior to needle insertion. In this regard, a major drawback is the device's high cost for a technique that is used infrequently or as a supplement.

PERIODONTAL LIGAMENT SYRINGE

This type of syringe is designed specifically for the periodontal ligament injection technique.[8] Although there are several types available, they normally have two common characteristics: (1) they are designed to administer measured dosages of 0.2 mL of anesthetic, and (2) they are very expensive. During use of these devices, considerable pressure builds up within the cartridge when the local anesthetic solution is injected into the periodontal membrane. It is possible for anesthetic cartridges to shatter under this force. Recently, to address this problem, the barrel of these

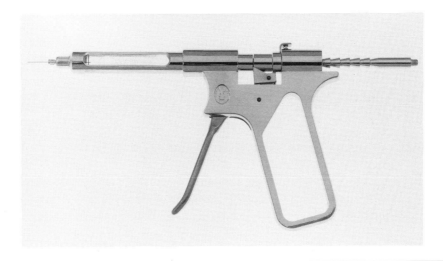

Figure 6–11.   Pistol-grip style of periodontal ligament injection syringe.

syringes has been enclosed in either a metal or plastic sheath to better support the anesthetic cartridge and protect the patient. The recent trend of plastic coating glass cartridges or the use of plastic cartridges has also largely overcome this problem. Because the pressure needed during periodontal ligament injections can be fatiguing for the clinician, several designs include a pistol grip mechanism, allowing more than one finger to be used in expressing the anesthetic (Fig. 6–11). Another design, relying on the principles of leverage, has a less-threatening appearance to the patient and also is easier to manipulate in the mouth (Fig. 6–12).

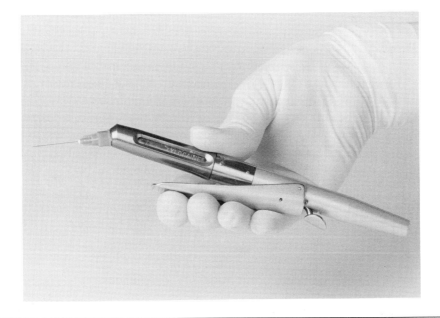

Figure 6–12.   Pen-grip style of periodontal ligament injection syringe.

STERILIZATION

The aspirating syringe is normally the only piece of equipment employed in regional anesthesia that is not designed for single patient use. Because it is usually not a disposable item, it must be properly cleaned, packaged, sterilized, and stored in a manner to ensure proper infection control. Sterilization is defined as any process that completely destroys all forms of microbial life. It is distinguished from terms such as disinfection, asepsis, antisepsis, sanitization, and bacteriostasis, which by definition do not include complete eradication of microorganisms. A chemical solution for sterilization of syringes is not normally recommended. Glutaraldehyde, which may be capable of producing sterilization, requires complete immersion for a minimum of 10 hours to destroy resistant pathogenic spores. The possibility of contaminating the syringe during rinsing (to remove the disinfectant), handling, and storage further rules against this method.

Proper preparation of the syringe before sterilization is essential. It should be washed, preferably in an ultrasonic cleaner, and rinsed. If the syringe is to be cleaned by hand, gloves should be worn to avoid unnecessary contact with blood or tissue debris. The syringe should be dried and packaged in a paper sterilization bag and sealed with a special autoclave indicator tape. Although use of the indicator tape does not guarantee sterility, it does change color or otherwise demonstrate that the item has been exposed to a sufficient temperature for a long enough time period that one can assume adequate sterilization.

The steam or chemical autoclave is the most common type of sterilizer used. These sterilizers are compact, lightweight, easy to use, and readily available. The dry heat sterilizer is also acceptable, although longer exposure is required to guarantee sterility. The ethylene oxide gas unit is a thoroughly acceptable, if expensive, alternative to the above. Ethylene oxide is fully capable of destroying all forms of microbial life, but its effectiveness depends on several factors: the concentration of gas, exposure time, temperature, and humidity. Because of these variables, it is a more difficult process to control than either pressurized steam, dry heat, or chemical vapor. In addition, nonmetallic supplies such as rubber goods or certain plastics must be ventilated to eliminate a residual toxic residue before use. Thus, for porous materials, the total sterilization and ventilation time can exceed 10 hours.

Anesthetic Cartridges

Commercial introduction of the disposable glass cartridge for administration of local anesthetics represented a major advance in oral regional anesthesia. This convenient dosage form provides for purity and sterility of the local anesthetic solution as well as easy observation of aspirated blood. Each cartridge consists of a tube with a rubber stopper on one end and a rubber diaphragm enclosed with a metal cap on the other (Fig. 6–13). In a recent modification of this format, the glass cartridge is replaced by plastic, which is consistent with the present trend of drugs being stored in plastic containers. The advantage is the reduced likelihood of breakage during transportation or use. This is of particular importance with periodontal ligament injections because of the increased pressure required. However, two main problems have arisen with the substitution of plastic for glass. The clarity of plastic is not equal to that of glass and gives anesthetic solutions a slight milky appearance. Also, in early production runs, the rubber stopper did not work as smoothly as in glass cartridges. Recently this situation has improved with a change of lubricant as well as altering the manufacturing process to ensure a uniform internal diameter. In North America, anesthetic cartridges generally consist of a barrel with a volume of 2.0 mL. However, when the rubber stopper is added, the net volume of fluid is 1.8 mL. Other cartridge sizes occasionally encountered include net volumes of 1.7, 2.0, and 2.2 mL, particularly in Europe, Asia, and Australia.

The contents of a cartridge are identified by labeling on the tube. The information provided includes the volume of solution and the trade and/or nonproprietary name of the anesthetic, along with its percentage concentration. Also included are the name and concentration of the vasocon-

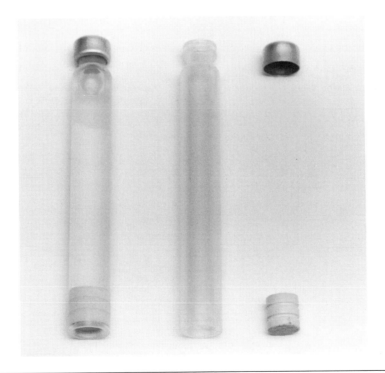

Figure 6–13. A plastic anesthetic cartridge disassembled into its constituent parts.

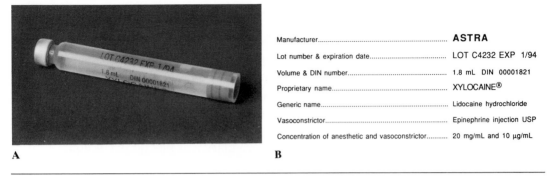

Manufacturer	**ASTRA**
Lot number & expiration date	LOT C4232 EXP 1/94
Volume & DIN number	1.8 mL DIN 00001821
Proprietary name	XYLOCAINE®
Generic name	Lidocaine hydrochloride
Vasoconstrictor	Epinephrine injection USP
Concentration of anesthetic and vasoconstrictor	20 mg/mL and 10 µg/mL

A   **B**

Figure 6–14.   Drug identification label. **A**. Label on a representative cartridge. **B**. Close-up of label information.

strictor, the name and address of the supplier, the manufacturer's lot number, and an expiration date. Finally, coded data are often included that identify the sterilization processes or batch number of the anesthetic (Fig. 6–14).

MANUFACTURING PROCESS

Each year millions of anesthetic cartridges are used whose sterility and purity of contents are taken for granted. The proven reliability of cartridges produced by major pharmaceutical companies is based on a complicated manufacturing process that involves many steps and quality control checks. As outlined in Figure 6–15, the process begins with water

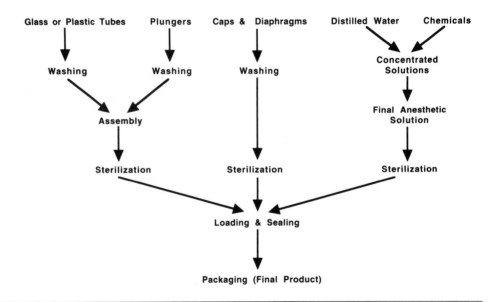

Figure 6–15.   Steps in the manufacture of local anesthetic cartridges.

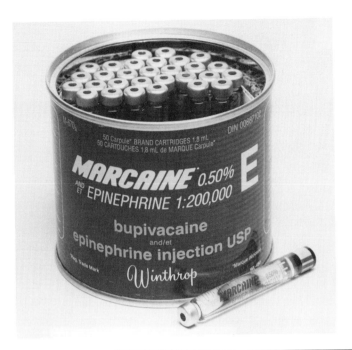

Figure 6–16.   Metal cannister of local anesthetic cartridges.

purification and the production of concentrated anesthetic solutions. These solutions are mixed in reduction chambers and held in sterile tanks until needed. After mixing and dilution, the anesthetic solution is placed into individual cartridges with rubber or silicon plungers in place and then sealed in place with aluminum caps enclosing a rubber diaphragm. All manufactured cartridges are inspected for flaws and then vacuum-packed in metal cans (Fig. 6–16) or blister packs (Fig. 6–17). Pharmaceutical companies routinely quarantine anesthetic agents for testing before shipment. Also, control samples of each production run are set aside for 6 months of continued evaluation. Should any problem subsequently develop, the U.S. Food and Drug Administration has the authority to recall selected anesthetic batches.

STORAGE AND DEFECTS

Most damage to cartridges occurs during shipment. Any cans that exhibit external damage such as corrosion, breakage, or major dents should not be accepted, even if the cartridges within appear normal (Fig. 6–18). When a container is opened, several cartridges should be randomly selected and inspected for imperfections. Examples of the various defects are described below.

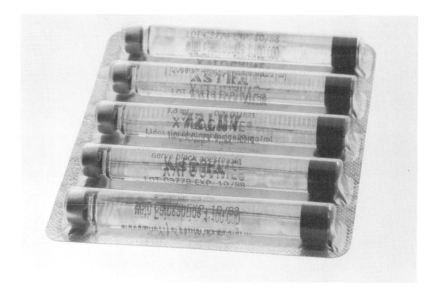

Figure 6–17. Blister pack of local anesthetic cartridges.

Breakage

When the cartridge is examined in adequate light, minute cracks or chips may become evident. These flaws will most often occur at either end of the cartridge where the glass barrel meets the aluminum cap or in the

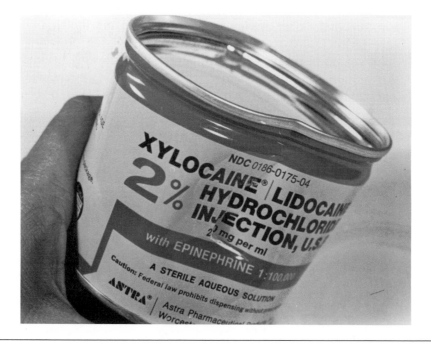

Figure 6–18. Storage cannister damaged in transport.

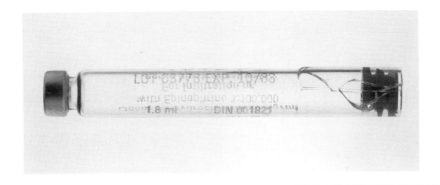

Figure 6–19. Example of a damaged glass cartridge.

region of the rubber stopper (Fig. 6–19). They are usually the result of rough handling during shipment. Use of cartridges with seemingly minor glass blemishes may result in breakage when seating the harpoon or during injection.

Bubbles

Small bubbles of nitrogen are normally present in cartridges as a result of the manufacturing process in order to remove oxygen, which would cause vasoconstrictor deterioration. Larger, "pea-sized" bubbles, however, indicate that the cartridge may have been frozen during shipment or storage (Fig. 6–20). Such cartridges should be returned to the supplier.

Extruded Plungers

When a plunger is noticeably extruded from the cartridge with an accompanying bubble of air, the cartridge has probably been exposed to temperatures that caused freezing of the solution. In this situation the solution cannot be relied on for sterility and should be returned to the supplier (Fig. 6–21). In rare cases, the plunger may extrude with no accompanying bubble as a result of other solutions diffusing into the cartridge and forcing the plunger out. This can occur when cartridges are stored in sterilizing solutions such as alcohol for long periods of time. Such cartridges should not be used, for reasons described below, and the practice of storing cartridges in alcohol solutions should be abandoned.

Altered Appearance of Anesthetic Solutions

The anesthetic solution should be crystal clear. Any evidence of color changes such as yellowing, cloudiness, or sedimentation may indicate a

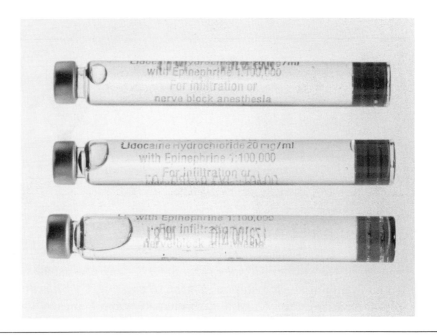

Figure 6–20.   Cartridges with bubbles. The top cartridge has a normal-sized nitrogen bubble. In the bottom two cartridges the nitrogen bubbles are enlarged, suggesting prior freezing of the solution.

breakdown of the chemical formulation of the solution (Fig. 6–22). If a cartridge shows any of these signs, the consignment of anesthetic should be sent back to the manufacturer for replacement. The most common reason for such discoloration is breakdown of the vasoconstrictor. This is accelerated by exposure of the solution to excess heat or light. Therefore, unopened containers of cartridges should be kept in a controlled

Figure 6–21.   Extrusion of rubber stoppers, suggesting diffusion of fluid into the cartridges.

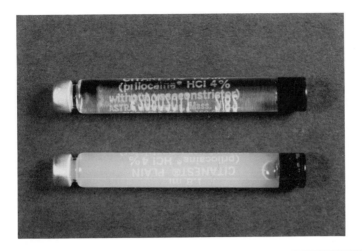

Figure 6–22.   Chemically altered anesthetic solution (*top*) compared with normal clear solution (*bottom*).

environment of 68° to 72° F (20° to 22° C). The storage of cartons in an unheated basement or attic is undesirable because of extremes in temperature. Anesthetic solutions contained in a cartridge have a shelf-life of 12 to 18 months, depending on the type of anesthetic and vasoconstrictor. The vasoconstrictor will degrade first. Expiration dates are clearly printed on each cartridge and on the metal container or blister pack. Any anesthetic that has passed the expiration date should not be used.

Corrosion

Corrosion of the aluminum cap is identifiable by a white powdery deposit that usually occurs when the cartridge is immersed in disinfecting solutions containing quaternary ammonium salts (e.g., benzalkonium chloride) or nitrate antirust materials. These salts react electrolytically with the aluminum, producing corrosion. This can be avoided by disinfecting cartridges with alternative solutions such as isopropyl or ethyl alcohol before use. Any sign of corrosion should prohibit the use of the cartridge (Fig. 6–23).

Leakage

Leakage of local anesthetic into a patient's mouth during injection usually indicates that the needle has perforated the rubber diaphragm at an angle rather than a central location. This produces an ovoid hole around the needle that is prone to leakage. This can be prevented by careful insertion of the needle into the cartridge.

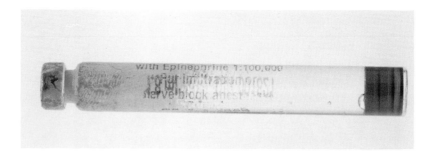

Figure 6–23.   Anesthetic cartridge demonstrating corrosion of the aluminum cap.

Sticky Plunger

At one time, paraffin was used as a sealant around the rubber stopper. However, when the paraffin hardened, the plunger was difficult to advance within the glass tubing. In recent years, this problem has been largely overcome with the use of silicon coating. However, occasionally a sticky plunger may still be encountered. To avoid such an occurrence, a few drops of local anesthetic should be extruded before injection is attempted.

DISINFECTION

Although the local anesthetic solution inside a cartridge is sterile (assuming no error in manufacture or damage to the cartridge has occurred), the external surface may not be. It is often desirable to sterilize cartridges before use, especially the rubber diaphragm through which the needle penetrates. Unfortunately, no entirely suitable method for this is available. Autoclaving, for example, causes the rubber stopper to be dislodged when the anesthetic solution expands. In addition, sympathomimetic amine vasoconstrictors are sensitive to high temperatures and are oxidized by brief exposure to steam heat. Thus, the only practical recourse for the clinician is to employ a disinfecting solution. It is a common practice to place cartridges in disinfectants such as alcohol. However, studies have shown that alcohol, phenol, and other disinfectants diffuse through the rubber diaphragm into the cartridge. This diffusion process will continue as long as the cartridge remains in the solution. Significant contamination of the anesthetic by a disinfectant results in pain, prolonged anesthesia, and possibly tissue injury. Because of the potential problems associated with submerging cartridges in disinfectants, a simple method of sanitizing the rubber diaphragm may be substituted. The diaphragm and metal cap should be wiped with gauze soaked in either 91% isopropyl or 70% ethyl alcohol, U.S.P., just before use. Some commercially available cartridge dispensers are designed to accept a gauze pad expressly for this purpose. Cartridge heaters have also been advocated to increase patient comfort during injection. However, since heat will accelerate breakdown of the vasoconstrictor and there is no evidence of benefit to the patients, the use of a cartridge heater is not recommended.

Needles

The hypodermic needle has undergone numerous changes since its invention in 1853. Over the years, research and manufacturing advances have resulted in needles that are strong yet flexible, sharp, sterile, and, most important, designed for single patient use. Since sterile disposable needles were first introduced, they have gained universal acceptance.[9] Disposable needles greatly reduce the risk of infection and, when properly used, eliminate the possibility of cross-contamination between patients. Patient discomfort is minimized by the sharpness of the point and cutting bevel, and needle breakage due to metal fatigue is extremely rare. Because of these advantages, the reusable needle is no longer recommended. Disposable needles are constructed of stainless steel. For patient comfort, the point of the needle, in addition to being very sharp, should have a bevel that offers little resistance to tissue.[10,11] Several tip configurations have been used, including a short bevel, a long bevel, and a multibevel (Fig. 6–24). The multibeveled point (lancet point) is de-

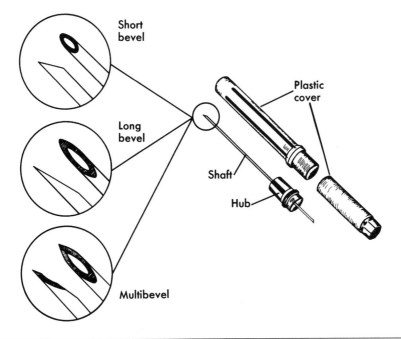

Figure 6–24. Types of bevels on disposable needles.

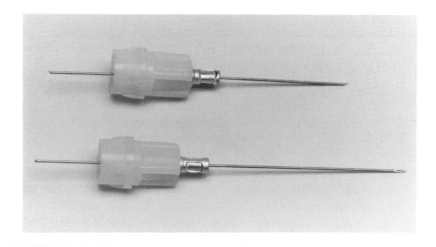

Figure 6–25.   Examples of short and long 27-gauge needles.

signed to produce the most efficient puncture with minimal trauma to the mucosa and subcutaneous tissues. The heel of a multibeveled tip is also specially ground to minimize coring and the creation of tissue tags. Most disposable needles are chemically treated with an antifriction substance to further ensure easy passage through oral tissues. Occasionally it is possible that the point of a needle may have been accidentally bent either during syringe preparation or during a previous injection where bony contact was made. This can produce a barb that would tear the tissues on removal following an injection. This defect may be unobservable by the human eye but can be checked for by drawing the needle backward over a sterile gauze swab. If a barb is present, it will pick up the threads of the gauze, indicating its presence.

Needles are generally categorized by length and diameter. Disposable cartridge needles are usually manufactured in two lengths, long and short (Fig. 6–25). Depending on the manufacturer, a "long" needle may be anywhere from 1⅛ to 1⅝ inches (28.9 to 41.5 mm) in length from hub to tip and a "short" needle from ¾ inch to 1 inch (19.4 to 25.5 mm). The external diameter of the needle shank is referred to as the gauge. The most commonly used gauges for intraoral anesthesia are 25, 27, and 30, with the higher numbers representing smaller diameters of the shank and lumen. Although most manufacturers adhere to the standard sizes (Table 6–1), some variation does exist.[12] Indeed, some specifications for the lumen diameter of the 30-gauge needle range from 0.003 to 0.015 inch.

NEEDLE SELECTION

The type of injection (infiltration versus block) and individual operator preference will determine whether a short or long needle is used. It is neither recommended nor routinely necessary for the entire needle shaft

Table 6–1. **COMMON NEEDLE GAUGES**

Gauge	Outside Diameter (mm)	Lumen Diameter (mm)
25	0.50	0.25
27	0.40	0.20
30	0.30	0.15

to be inserted into tissue. Breakage, although rare, normally occurs at the hub and is usually the result of lateral pressure exerted against the shank by improper insertion force or sudden movements of the syringe or patient. A sufficient length of the shaft must be visible in the oral cavity to permit retrieval of the terminal fragment in case of breakage. The current popularity of the fine-gauge needles (27 and 30 gauge) stems from the erroneous belief that ultra-fine needles cause less discomfort during insertion. Comparisons have shown, however, that a 25-gauge needle can be used as painlessly as a 30-gauge needle, and more safely.[13,14] Although it is possible to aspirate with the finer needles, their smaller lumens do significantly impede flow. Because the 25-gauge shaft is considerably stronger than its thinner counterparts, the possibility of breakage, however remote, is reduced.[15,16]

A major advantage of the 25-gauge needle is its relative nonpliance.[11,17] As demonstrated in Figure 6–26, for every increase in gauge number

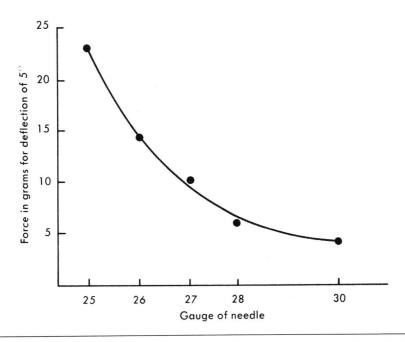

Figure 6–26. Relationship between needle gauge and force necessary to produce a 5-degree deflection at the tip. (Data from Smith, N: Aust. Dent. J., *13*:158–163, 1968.)

there is about a 1.5-fold decrease in force required to bend the needle. It is sometimes necessary with block injections, especially those of the inferior alveolar nerve, to redirect the needle after initial insertion. With highly flexible needles (i.e., 27 and 30 gauge), moving the syringe may appear to reorient the needle tip, when in reality the shank merely bends and the tip is marginally influenced. In such situations the local anesthetic may be deposited some distance from the intended target. Because the needle tip is asymmetric and located off the central axis of the shaft, there is even a tendency for the needle to deflect away from the bevel during straight insertion. Several factors determine the degree of deflection, the most important of which is needle diameter. The 30-gauge needle is the most susceptible to deflection and the 25-gauge needle is the least. Depending on the gauge, length, and bevel and the resistance of the tissue, a needle inserted 20 mm may deflect up to 5 mm. Therefore, while 27- and 30-gauge needles are acceptable for clinical use, their inherent flexibility can result in less accurate needle placement.

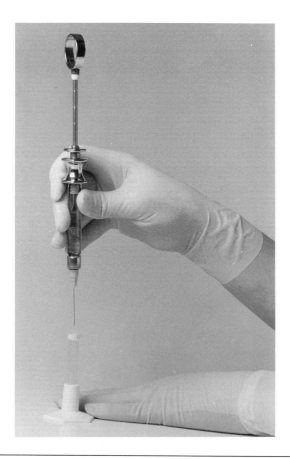

Figure 6–27.   Recapping device.

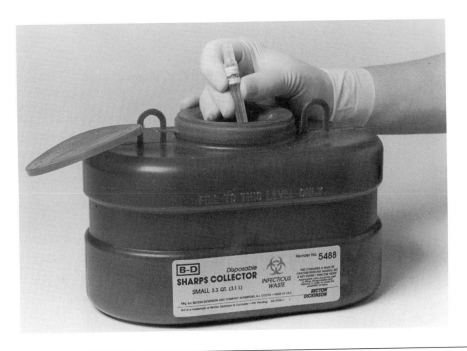

Figure 6–28.   Disposable needle collector.

HANDLING AND DISPOSAL OF CONTAMINATED NEEDLES

Accidental penetration of the clinician's hand when attempting to replace a protective cap is reportedly one of the most common accidents in hospitals and as a result has led to the development of needle guards.[18] Several companies have marketed devices that are designed to hold the needle cover during reinsertion, thus reducing the risk of accidentally stabbing one's fingers after injection (Fig. 6–27). Alternatively, recapping a contaminated needle is possible by inserting it into its cover positioned on a horizontal surface. In this manner, no hands are used to hold the cap until it is almost fully covering the needle.

A system must be established for the disposal of contaminated needles to minimize exposure for personnel who dispose of them. In this regard, contaminated material boxes are readily available from several manufacturers (Fig. 6–28).

References

1. Council on Dental Materials and Devices: New American National Standards Institute/American Dental Association Specification No. 34 for Dental Aspirating Syringes. J. Am. Dent. Assoc., 97:236–238, 1978.

2. Council on Dental Materials, Instruments, and Equipment: Addendum to American National Standards Institute/American Dental Association Specification No. 34 for Dental Aspirating Syringes. J. Am. Dent. Assoc., *104*:69–70, 1982.
3. Persson, G., Keskitalo, E., and Evers, H.: Clinical experiences in oral surgery using a new self-aspirating injection system. Int. J. Oral Surg., *3*:428–434, 1974.
4. Blair, G.S., and Meechan, J.G.: Local anaesthesia in dental practice: I. A clinical study of a self-aspirating system. Br. Dent. J., *159*:75–77, 1985.
5. Meechan, J.G., Blair, G.S., and McCabe, J.F.: Local anaesthesia in dental practice: II. A laboratory investigation of a self-aspirating system. Br. Dent. J., *159*:109–113, 1985.
6. Meechan, J.G.: A comparison of three different automatic aspirating dental cartridge syringes. J. Dent., *16*:40–43, 1988.
7. Meechan, J.G., and Blair, G.S.: Clinical experience in oral surgery with two different automatic aspirating syringes. Int. J. Oral Maxillofacial Surg., *18*:87–89, 1989.
8. Faulkner R.K.: The high-pressure periodontal ligament injection: A study involving undergraduate operators. Br. Dent. J., *154*:103–105, 1983.
9. Council on Dental Materials and Devices: Guide to Dental Materials and Devices, 8th ed. Chicago, American Dental Association, 1976.
10. Aldous, J.A.: Needle deflection: A factor in the administration of local anesthetics. J. Am. Dent. Assoc., *77*:602–604, 1968.
11. Jeske, A.H., and Boshart, B.F.: Deflection of conventional versus nondeflecting dental needles in vitro. Anesth. Prog., *32*:62–64, 1985.
12. Wittrock, J.W., and Fischer, W.E.: The aspiration of blood through small gauge needles. J. Am. Dent. Assoc., *76*:79–81, 1968.
13. Fuller, N.P., Menke, R.A., and Meyers, W.J.: Perception of pain to three different intraoral penetrations of needles. J. Am. Dent. Assoc., *99*:822–824, 1979.
14. Brownbill, J.W., Walker, P.O., Bourcy, B.D., and Keenan, K.M.: Comparison of inferior dental nerve block injections in child patients using 30-gauge and 25-gauge short needles. Anesth. Prog., *34*:215–219, 1987.
15. Marks, R.B., Carlton, D.M., and McDonald, S.: Management of a broken needle in the pterygomandibular space: Report of a case. J. Am. Dent. Assoc., *109*:263–264, 1984.
16. Burke, R.H.: Management of a broken anesthetic injection needle in the maxilla. J. Am. Dent. Assoc., *112*:209–210, 1986.
17. Smith, N.: An investigation of the influence of gauge on some physical properties of hypodermic needles. Aust. Dent. J., *13*:158–163, 1968.
18. Council on Dental Materials, Instruments and Equipment, Council on Dental Practice, and Council on Dental Therapeutics: Infection control recommendations for the dental office and the dental laboratory. J. Am. Dent. Assoc., *116*:241–248, 1988.

Chapter 7

Neuroanatomy of the Fifth Cranial Nerve

A ny discussion of anesthetic techniques of the oral cavity and face requires familiarity with the primary sensory nerve of that area, the fifth cranial nerve. The fifth or trigeminal nerve is the largest of the 12 cranial nerves that serve the muscles and the general and special sense organs of the head and neck region. It conveys the sensations of touch, pressure, pain, and temperature from the skin of the face and anterior scalp, the hard and soft tissues of the mouth, and the mucosal linings of most of the spaces of the head. The trigeminal nerve also carries the proprioceptive sensations of position, strain, and movement from the masticatory apparatus. A mixed nerve, it supplies motor stimulation to the muscles of mastication and to several other important muscles in the region. Finally, by means of communicating branches from the seventh and ninth cranial nerves and from the cervical sympathetic nerves, portions of the trigeminal nerve convey autonomic fibers (parasympathetic and sympathetic) that control secretory glands of the head and visual accommodation of the eye. Some of the special sense of taste is also transmitted along branches of the fifth nerve via its connections with the seventh.

Intracranial Structures

Besides an extensive peripheral distribution, the trigeminal system includes several distinct intracranial structures. These are the trigeminal ganglion, sensory and motor nuclei, and various tracts with interconnections to other cranial nerve nuclei and higher centers of the brain.

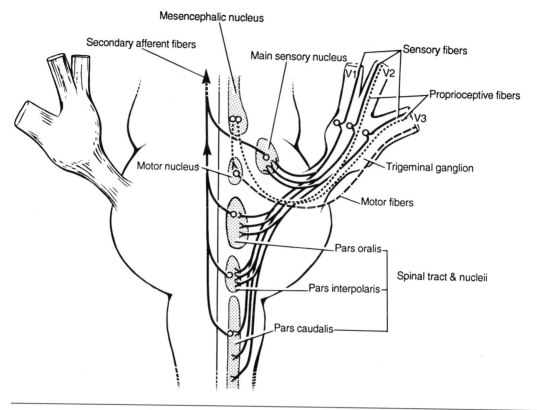

Figure 7–1.   Intracranial distribution of the trigeminal nerve.

TRIGEMINAL GANGLION

One of the easiest intracranial structures to identify is the large collection of sensory cell bodies variously called the trigeminal, semilunar, or gasserian ganglion. This sizable structure rests on the intracranial surface of the petrous bone in the middle cranial fossa. As the term *trigeminal* implies, the neurons of the ganglion give rise to peripheral processes that form three major divisions: the ophthalmic, the maxillary, and the mandibular. Each division leaves the cranial cavity through a separate opening. Centrally directed fibers from ganglion neurons collectively form a single sensory root. After entering the brainstem through the lateral surface of the pons, the sensory root courses to the pontine tegmentum (a collection of nerve fibers and cells in the dorsal pons), where it divides into short ascending and long descending arms (Fig. 7–1).

MAIN SENSORY NUCLEUS

Nerve fibers within the short ascending arm, most of which carry the sensation of touch, terminate at the main sensory nucleus of the fifth cranial nerve (CN V) located in the pontine tegmentum.

SPINAL V TRACT AND NUCLEUS

The long descending fibers of the sensory root become part of a descending spinal CN V tract, with terminal endings within the medially located spinal CN V nucleus (see Fig. 7–1). The trigeminal spinal tract and nucleus extend inferiorly through the medulla (a part of the brainstem just caudal to the pons) and into the upper two or three segments of the spinal cord, where the cells of the nucleus become continuous with those of the substantia gelatinosa of the cervical spinal cord. The substantia gelatinosa—"jelly-like substance"—is thought to be intimately related to modification of incoming pain and temperature sensations.

The spinal nucleus of CN V has been divided on the basis of cell structure into three distinct regions or parts. Superiorly (rostrally) to inferiorly (caudally), these are the pars oralis, pars interpolaris, and pars caudalis. The caudal portion of the nucleus is thought to receive predominantly pain and temperature sensations, whereas superior segments receive tactile information as well. The spinal nucleus also receives terminals from other cranial nerve tracts, specifically those of the seventh (facial), ninth (glossopharyngeal), and tenth (vagus) cranial nerves.

MOTOR NUCLEUS

The motor nucleus of the trigeminal nerve is a distinct collection of multipolar cells lying medial to the main sensory nucleus in the pontine tegmentum. Peripheral fibers leaving this area pass ventral to the trigeminal ganglion and become incorporated in the mandibular division of the trigeminal nerve before it leaves the middle cranial fossa. These fibers provide motor control to the muscles of mastication and to several other muscles of the head and neck.

MESENCEPHALIC NUCLEUS

The mesencephalic nucleus is a narrow column of cells originating in the pons lateral to the fourth ventricle and extending through the midbrain and lateral to the cerebral aqueduct. The peripheral processes of these cells (see Fig. 7–1) form the mesencephalic tract of CN V, which provides proprioception for the trigeminal system and sends collateral fibers to the motor nucleus, for reflex arc activity. Functionally this nucleus appears to relay proprioceptive information concerning the muscles of mastication, joint capsules, and periodontal ligaments to the motor nucleus for modulation of jaw position and movement.

SECONDARY PROJECTIONS

Cells of both the main sensory nucleus and the spinal nucleus of CN V give off extensive projections to higher neural levels, principally to various nuclei in the thalamus. Additionally, the mesencephalic nucleus appears to send fibers into the cerebellum. The exact functional organization and significance of some of these projections are currently the subject of active investigation.

Extracranial Distribution

Within the middle cranial fossa, as the fibers of the trigeminal nerve leave the ganglion, they separate into three major divisions: the ophthalmic (V_1), the maxillary (V_2), and the mandibular (V_3). The ophthalmic and maxillary divisions are entirely sensory (except for autonomic fibers that originate from other sources), whereas the mandibular division is a mixed sensory and motor nerve. Figure 7–2 illustrates the cutaneous innervation of these three major divisions. It should be noted that the ophthalmic and maxillary divisions give off very small branches intracranially that provide sensation to the dura mater. The mandibular division also contributes a similar branch but only after it leaves the cranium. This branch reenters the cranium accompanied by the middle meningeal artery via the foramen spinosum.

OPHTHALMIC DIVISION (V_1)

The ophthalmic division is the smallest of the three major divisions of the trigeminal nerve. At or just before its exit from the middle cranial fossa by way of the superior orbital fissure, the ophthalmic division separates into three branches: the lacrimal, frontal, and nasociliary nerves (Fig. 7–3). These nerves, via their terminal branches, provide exteroceptive sensation to the globe, conjunctiva, and corner of the eye, to the skin of

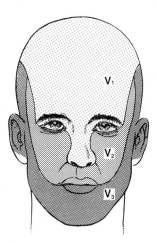

Figure 7–2.　　Front view of the cutaneous distribution of the trigeminal nerve.

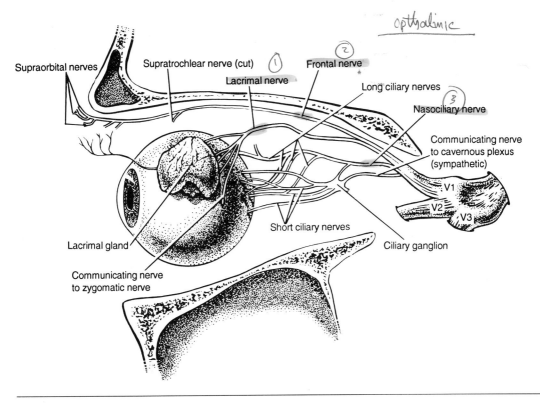

Figure 7–3.   Ophthalmic division (V₁).

the upper and part of the lower eyelid, to the forehead, anterior scalp, and part of the nose, and to the mucosa of the anterior nasal cavity and the frontal, ethmoidal, and sphenoidal air sinuses. Additionally, autonomic fibers provide for control of pupillary dilation and for lacrimal gland secretion. (See discussion under Autonomic Distribution.)

MAXILLARY DIVISION (V₂)

The maxillary division (Fig. 7–4) originates from the anteromedial portion of the trigeminal ganglion. It passes forward and exits from the middle cranial fossa via the round foramen (foramen rotundum) located in the greater wing of the sphenoid bone. As it passes through the foramen, the maxillary division immediately enters the pterygopalatine fossa, at which point it gives off the zygomatic nerve, two pterygopalatine trunks, the posterior superior alveolar nerve, and the infraorbital nerve. The last exits the fossa by passing anteriorly through the inferior orbital fissure. It then continues forward along the orbital floor, initially within a groove and subsequently through a canal. During its passage through the orbital floor, the infraorbital nerve gives off two branches: first the middle superior alveolar nerve (when present) and then the anterior superior

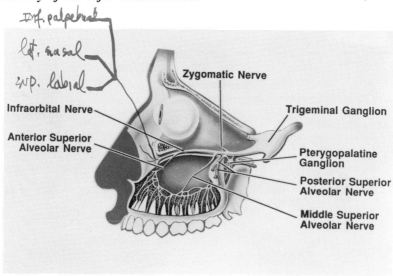

Figure 7–4. Maxillary division (V₂) and its major branches.

alveolar nerve. Finally, it emerges at the infraorbital foramen and divides shortly thereafter into several terminal branches: the inferior palpebral, external nasal, and superior labial nerves.

From the pterygopalatine fossa, the previously mentioned branches of the maxillary division follow independent courses. The zygomatic nerve exits anteriorly and laterally by passing through the inferior orbital fissure. In the orbit it gives off a communicating branch to the lacrimal nerve (V₁) and then enters a small foramen (zygomaticoorbital) in the zygomatic bone forming part of the lateral wall of the orbit. Within the substance of the zygomatic bone, it divides into the zygomaticofacial branch, which exits the zygoma via a small surface foramen (zygomaticofacial) to provide cutaneous sensation over the zygomatic prominence, and the zygomaticotemporal branch, which passes through the zygomaticotemporal foramen to innervate the skin overlying the anterior temporal region.

The short trunks of the pterygopalatine nerve (usually two are present) leave the main trunk of the maxillary nerve and descend vertically, merging with the pterygopalatine ganglion. This relationship is only one of proximity, however, because these sensory fibers pass through the area without synapsing.

Orbital branches leaving the pterygopalatine ganglion enter the orbit through the inferior orbital fissure to supply the ethmoidal and sphenoidal sinuses and the periosteum of the orbit. A pharyngeal branch also exits from the pterygopalatine ganglion posteriorly to serve portions of the sphenoidal sinus and the nasopharyngeal mucosa posterior to the auditory tube.

At the level of the ganglion, the posterior superior nasal branches are given off to enter the nasal cavity through the sphenopalatine foramen.

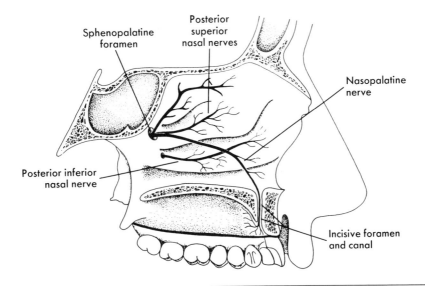

Figure 7–5.   Course of the nasopalatine nerve along the nasal septum and the posterior nasal nerves along the lateral wall of the nasal cavity.

Although these nerves, along with the posterior inferior nasal branches mentioned below, primarily provide sensation to the nasal mucosa, a long branch, the nasopalatine nerve, passes medially to the nasal septum (where it supplies the septal mucosa) and continues anteriorly and downward until it traverses the incisive canal and foramen to serve the soft tissue of the anterior palate (Figs. 7–5 and 7–6).

After leaving the ganglion, the pterygopalatine nerve descends within

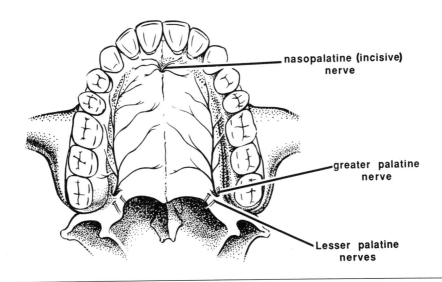

Figure 7–6.   Innervation of the hard palate by the nasopalatine and greater palatine nerves.

the pterygopalatine canal in the form of several distinct bundles. During its passage, the posterior inferior nasal branches are given off. The remaining nerves then leave the canal by two or three foramina located on the posterolateral aspect of the hard palate. The largest and most anterior of these branches is the greater palatine nerve, which emerges from the greater palatine foramen to supply general sensation to the soft tissues of the hard palate and adjacent soft palate and the gingiva up to the nerve's confluence in the vicinity of the canines with terminal fibers of the nasopalatine nerve (Fig. 7–6). The middle and posterior branches exit the canal through much smaller openings collectively known as the lesser palatine foramina and then turn posteriorly to supply general sensation to the tissues of the soft palate, uvula, and tonsillar area.

The posterior, middle, and anterior superior alveolar nerves constitute the primary sensory innervation of the maxillary bone, teeth, and periodontium, buccolabial gingiva, and maxillary antral mucosa (see Fig. 7–4). The anterior superior alveolar nerve also supplies a portion of the inferior meatus and floor of the nasal cavity. The posterior superior alveolar nerve separates from the main maxillary trunk and courses inferiorly from the pterygopalatine fossa, either as a single nerve or as two or three distinct branches. It enters the maxilla through one or more small foramina located at midheight on the infratemporal surface. Just before entering the foramina, small twigs supplying the gingiva and mucosa of the tuberosity and a variable part of the buccal mucosa are usually given off. The posterior superior alveolar nerve then descends anteriorly within the maxilla, along the posterior wall of the antrum, ultimately to join with fibers of the middle and anterior superior alveolar nerves in forming the superior dental plexus. Individual nerve strands issue from this plexus to innervate tooth pulps and adjacent tissues. The posterior superior alveolar nerve normally supplies the maxillary molar teeth (except for the mesiobuccal root of the first molar), their investing periodontium and adjacent buccal gingiva, and the posterior mucosa of the maxillary sinus. The middle superior alveolar nerve generally originates from the infraorbital nerve in the posterior segment of the infraorbital canal and runs downward along the lateral wall of the maxillary sinus to mingle with posterior superior alveolar nerve fibers. It usually provides sensation for the two premolar teeth and the mesiobuccal root of the first molar and for their surrounding periodontium, bone, buccal gingiva, and adjacent antral mucosa. Actually, this nerve is absent in over 50% of all individuals, in which case its fibers are incorporated into the posterior superior and anterior superior alveolar nerves.

The anterior superior alveolar nerve arises from the infraorbital nerve just before the latter emerges from the infraorbital foramen. The anterior superior alveolar nerve then descends through the anterior wall of the sinus to contribute to the superior dental plexus. Specifically, it provides sensation to the incisor and canine teeth, periodontium, and labial gingiva, to the anterior portion of the antral mucosa, and to the floor of the nasal cavity.

MANDIBULAR DIVISION (V₃)

The mandibular nerve is the largest of the three divisions of the trigeminal nerve and is the only one that carries both sensory and motor fibers (Fig. 7–7). It leaves the middle cranial fossa through the oval foramen (foramen ovale) to enter the infratemporal fossa, where it promptly divides into a smaller anterior and a larger posterior root. Before this division, however, a small sensory branch that accompanies the middle meningeal artery intracranially through the foramen spinosum is given off, as are several small nerves (in close proximity to the otic ganglion) that provide motor function to the medial pterygoid, tensor veli palatini, and tensor tympani muscles. The anterior root then courses forward and downward. In a position medial to the lateral pterygoid muscle, it ramifies to yield several motor nerves: the masseteric, deep temporal, and lateral pterygoid. Passing between the two heads of the lateral pterygoid muscle, the anterior trunk, now termed the buccal (long buccal) nerve, descends along the anteromedial aspect of the temporalis tendon until, at the level of the occlusal plane, it crosses the coronoid notch of the ramus in an anterolateral direction. Ultimately it divides into several branches, some of which supply the cheek as far forward as the angle of the mouth and others that penetrate the buccinator muscle to serve the buccal mucosa and gingiva adjacent to the mandibular molars. The exact area of innervation varies somewhat. Occasionally the buccal nerve serves the mucosa and gingiva up to the canine or the premolars, but in other instances it innervates a much smaller area, excluding even the posterior molar region. Some variation also exists at its junction with fibers of the gingival branch of the posterior superior alveolar nerve, at times permitting the buccal nerve to convey sensation from the gingivae of the maxillary third molar region.

The posterior root of the mandibular nerve is predominantly sensory; however, it does provide motor innervation for the mylohyoid and digastric (anterior belly only) muscles. As the posterior root descends, it separates into three branches. The first of these, the auriculotemporal nerve, runs posteriorly and then laterally behind the neck of the mandibular condyle, turns superiorly, and emerges from the parotid gland. The remainder of the auriculotemporal nerve finally divides into several superficial temporal branches as it crosses the root of the zygoma. These peripheral branches supply the skin of the temporal region of the head.

The lingual nerve originates deep to the lateral pterygoid muscle and courses downward within the anterior portion of the pterygomandibular space. During this descent, it receives a communicating branch from the facial nerve 1 to 2 cm below the oval foramen. This branch, the chorda

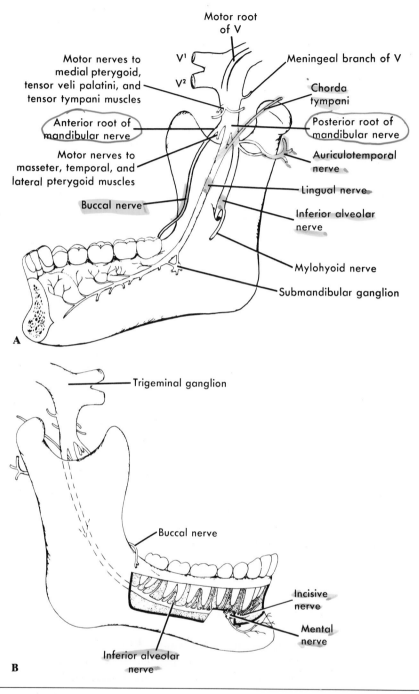

Motor root of V

Motor nerves to medial pterygoid, tensor veli palatini, and tensor tympani muscles

V¹

V²

Meningeal branch of V

Chorda tympani

Anterior root of mandibular nerve

Posterior root of mandibular nerve

Motor nerves to masseter, temporal, and lateral pterygoid muscles

Auriculotemporal nerve

Lingual nerve

Buccal nerve

Inferior alveolar nerve

Mylohyoid nerve

Submandibular ganglion

A

Trigeminal ganglion

Buccal nerve

Incisive nerve

Mental nerve

Inferior alveolar nerve

B

Figure 7–7. Mandibular division (V₃) and its major branches. **A**. Medial view of mandible. **B**. Lateral view of mandible.

tympani, adds parasympathetic and taste fibers to the lingual nerve. The lingual nerve then passes between the medial pterygoid muscle and the medial aspect of the mandibular ramus and courses downward into the floor of the mouth, where it continues anteriorly above the mylohyoid muscle toward the tongue. In the floor of the mouth, it communicates with the submandibular ganglion. Terminal filaments of the lingual nerve provide general sensation for all of the lingual gingiva, the mucosa of the floor of the mouth, and the anterior two-thirds of the tongue.

The inferior alveolar nerve, the third branch of the posterior root of the mandibular nerve, passes inferior to the lateral pterygoid muscle and runs in a somewhat lateral direction within the pterygomandibular space posterior to the lingual nerve. From 5 to 25 mm before the inferior alveolar nerve enters the mandibular canal on the medial surface of the ramus, the mylohyoid nerve branches off. This nerve continues inferiorly and anteriorly along the mylohyoid groove. Passing superficial (ventral) to the mylohyoid muscle, it provides motor function to that muscle as well as to the anterior belly of the digastric muscle. Terminal fibers of the mylohyoid nerve have a sensory component that serves the skin over the lower chin and occasionally contributes to the innervation of the mandibular incisor teeth.

The inferior alveolar nerve provides sensation to all mandibular teeth up to the midline. In a manner analogous to that of the superior alveolar nerves, the inferior alveolar nerve sends nerve fibers that innervate tooth pulps and periodontium and pierce adjacent alveolar bone to provide sensation to nearby gingival tissues (e.g., interdental papillae). The nerve has two terminal branches: the mental and the incisive. The mental nerve exits the mandible through the mental foramen, usually located several millimeters inferior to the apex of the second premolar or slightly anterior or posterior (but still inferior) to it. This nerve provides sensation to the labial gingiva and alveolar mucosa from the premolar region to the midline, and to the mucosa and skin of the lower lip and chin. The incisive branches supply the incisors and canines, their investing alveolar bone, periodontium, and labial gingiva.

Autonomic Distribution

The discussion to this point has dealt largely with the somatosensory and motor distribution of the fifth cranial nerve, with only cursory mention of the parallel but separate distribution of the autonomic nervous system. Composed of two major subdivisions, the parasympathetic and the sympathetic, the autonomic nervous system is primarily concerned with visceral functions and homeostasis. Although the motor nucleus of the trigeminal system itself does not give rise to autonomic fibers, a portion of the parasympathetic and sympathetic innervation of the head is carried by branches of the fifth nerve.

Parasympathetic pathways utilizing the trigeminal system regulate pupillary diameter and lacrimal, mucous membrane, and salivary gland secretion. Presynaptic fibers originating in certain motor nuclei of the third, seventh, and ninth cranial nerves course from the central nervous system (CNS) to synapse on postganglionic neurons in the parasympathetic ganglia (ciliary, pterygopalatine, otic, and submandibular) that lie adjacent to, or in the path of, major branches of the fifth nerve. Postganglionic fibers arising from these ganglia then communicate with nearby trigeminal branches to reach their respective target organs.

Sympathetic postganglionic axons that are conveyed by the trigeminal nerve arise from the superior cervical ganglion and ascend as a plexus in close association with the internal and external carotid arteries. These axons eventually pass through the aforementioned ganglia, without synapsing, to travel with their parasympathetic counterparts. Sympathetic fibers associated with the trigeminal system provide for pupillary dilation and influence glandular secretion and local blood flow in the areas innervated.

The various autonomic tracts that accompany branches of the trigeminal nerve will be considered briefly in relation to the parasympathetic ganglia that are involved.

CILIARY GANGLION

The ciliary ganglion receives its preganglionic parasympathetic innervation from the oculomotor (third cranial) nerve. Postganglionic fibers leave this ganglion in the short ciliary nerves. When stimulated, these fibers cause constriction of the pupil (miosis) and contraction of the ciliary muscle of the iris (for lens accommodation). Sympathetic fibers traversing this ganglion also exit via the short ciliary nerves. Stimulation of these fibers causes dilation of the pupil (mydriasis). In this case, the actions of the parasympathetic and sympathetic nerves are opposed, with a balance between them maintaining proper pupillary diameter.

PTERYGOPALATINE GANGLION

Secretomotor function to the lacrimal glands and to the mucous glands of the nose, hard and soft palate, upper part of the nasopharynx, and mucosa of the upper lip and cheek is transmitted through the pterygopalatine ganglion (Fig. 7–8). The parasympathetic preganglionic fibers derive from the seventh cranial nerve, leaving it as the greater superficial petrosal branch. A group of sympathetic fibers collectively known as the deep petrosal nerve leave the sympathetic nervous plexus surrounding the internal carotid artery to join the greater superficial petrosal nerve just before it disappears into the pterygoid (Vidian) canal within the sphenoid

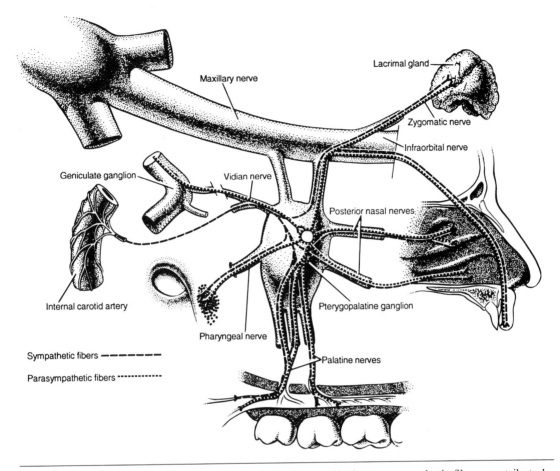

Figure 7–8.   Nerves of the pterygopalatine fossa. Preganglionic parasympathetic fibers contributed by the seventh cranial nerve (via the geniculate ganglion) synapse in the pterygopalatine ganglion. Postganglionic parasympathetic fibers then follow branches of the maxillary division of the trigeminal nerve to supply the secretory glands as shown. Postganglionic sympathetic fibers from the superior cervical ganglion (via the internal carotid artery) are similarly distributed.

bone. Appropriately termed the nerve of the pterygoid canal (or vidian nerve), the collected autonomic fibers enter the pterygopalatine fossa by emerging from the pterygoid canal just posterior to the pterygopalatine ganglion. After synapsing in the ganglion, parasympathetic postganglionic fibers are routed to the lacrimal gland via a pathway involving the maxillary, zygomatic, and lacrimal nerves. They are also carried to various mucus-secreting glands by way of the infraorbital, posterior nasal, pharyngeal, and palatine branches of the maxillary nerve. Accompanying sympathetic fibers are similarly distributed. Here, the two subdivisions of the autonomic nervous system exert relatively independent actions, with the parasympathetic outflow primarily controlling glandular secretion and the sympathetic distribution regulating vascular resistance and local blood flow.

OTIC GANGLION

The otic ganglion receives parasympathetic preganglionic fibers from the lesser superficial petrosal nerve, a branch of the glossopharyngeal nerve. Parasympathetic postganglionic axons providing secretomotor innervation to the parotid gland leave the ganglion, along with accompanying sympathetic fibers, by associating with branches of the auriculotemporal nerve.

SUBMANDIBULAR GANGLION

The submandibular ganglion receives its preganglionic parasympathetic fibers from the chorda tympani, a branch of the facial nerve that joins the lingual nerve (Fig. 7–9). After traveling with the lingual nerve, the parasympathetic fibers leave it to enter the submandibular ganglion, where they synapse. Postganglionic fibers then leave the ganglion, along with their associated sympathetic fibers, to provide secretomotor control of the sublingual, submandibular, and adjacent minor salivary glands. In regard to salivation, the parasympathetic and sympathetic systems have complementary functions, with the former stimulating copious secretion of a serous saliva and the latter stimulating secretion of a mucous saliva rich in organic material.

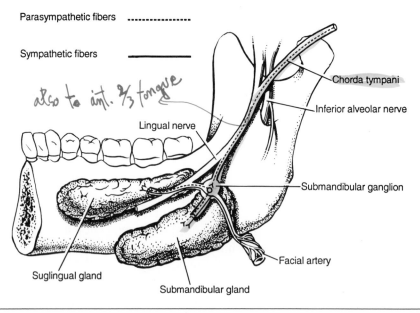

Figure 7–9.   Submandibular ganglion. After synapsing in the ganglion, parasympathetic fibers are distributed to the submandibular and sublingual salivary glands. Sympathetic fibers pass through the ganglion without synapsing to travel with the parasympathetic fibers.

Taste Pathways

As with autonomic fibers, neurons of the facial nerve that subserve the special sense of taste travel in part with branches of the trigeminal system. Some of the cell bodies in the geniculate ganglion extend their peripheral processes via the chorda tympani to join the lingual nerve and thus provide the sense of taste for the anterior two thirds of the tongue. Additionally, some fibers accompany the greater superficial petrosal nerve passing through the pterygopalatine ganglion and then with the lesser palatine nerves to supply taste buds in the soft palate. It should be noted that the posterior third of the tongue receives its special and general sensory innervation from the glossopharyngeal nerve and that a few taste buds about the epiglottis are served by the vagus nerve. In neither case are trigeminal branches used to route these sensory fibers to their destination.

Bibliography

1. Bossy, J.: Atlas of Neuroanatomy and Special Sense Organs. Philadelphia, W.B. Saunders Co., 1970.
2. Carpenter, M.B.: Human Neuroanatomy, 7th ed. Baltimore, Williams & Wilkins Co., 1976.
3. DuBrul, E.L.: Sicher and DuBrul's Oral Anatomy, 8th ed. St. Louis, Ishiyaku EuroAmerica, Inc., 1988.
4. Ferner, H., ed.: Eduard Pernkopf Atlas of Topographical and Applied Human Anatomy, 2nd ed. Vol. 1. Head and Neck (transl. by H. Monsen). Baltimore, Urban & Schwarzenberg, Inc., 1980.
5. Warfel, J.H.: The Head, Neck and Trunk, 4th ed. Philadelphia, Lea & Febiger, 1973.
6. Williams, P.L., ed.: Gray's Anatomy, 37th ed. New York, Churchill Livingstone, 1989.
7. Williams, P.L., and Warwick, R.: Functional Neuroanatomy of Man. Philadelphia, W.B. Saunders Co., 1975.

Basic Principles of Injection Technique

Successful delivery of local anesthesia often depends on a variety of factors, including proper preparation of the injection site, appropriate selection of the local anesthetic technique for the procedure to be performed, and competent patient management. This chapter defines the different anesthetic techniques in common usage and discusses the various factors that go into successful administration of a local anesthetic.

Classification of Administration Techniques

Local anesthetics are administered in a variety of ways to obtain anesthesia of oral structures. One method of classifying these techniques of administration is to consider the portion of peripheral nerve that is affected (Fig. 8–1).

Nerve block anesthesia is the term given to the injection of a local anesthetic solution close to a nerve trunk. This approach has the advantage of blocking sensations from a large portion of the anatomy (as defined by the peripheral distribution of the nerve) with a single injection and is used extensively in the oral cavity. A potential disadvantage is that major blood vessels frequently accompany nerve trunks, and the possibility of accidentally piercing an artery or vein is significantly enhanced. Another limitation to block anesthesia is that some nerve trunks are not readily accessible by conventional methods of injection.

Field block anesthesia is a form of regional anesthesia commonly employed in the maxillary arch. As with the nerve block, areas distal to the

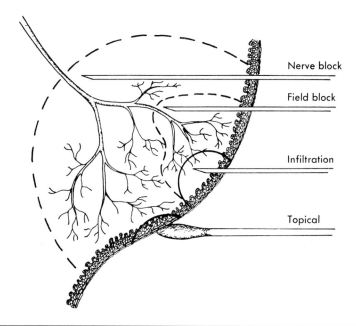

Figure 8–1.   Administration techniques used for anesthesia. Dashed lines and solid lines represent
the areas of anesthesia produced by regional (nerve block, field block) and local (infiltration, topical application) anesthetic techniques, respectively.

site of injection are rendered insensitive to noxious stimuli. Because
the target of a field block injection is the smaller distributing branches of
the nerve, however, the area of anesthesia is usually more restricted in
scope.

Infiltration anesthesia provides pain relief solely in the area bathed by
the drug solution. By definition, only terminal nerve endings are affected
by infiltration, and the region of anesthesia does not extend beyond the
diffusion boundary of the local anesthetic. Infiltration is commonly employed for soft tissue anesthesia and, in gingival surgery, for the hemostasis afforded by the vasoconstrictor.

Topical anesthesia refers to the surface application of a local anesthetic to block free nerve endings supplying the mucosal surfaces. The
technique is useful for a variety of procedures and conditions (e.g., taking radiographs, palliation of aphthous ulcers) in which only superficial
anesthesia is required. Topical anesthesia is also used in obtunding the
pain of needle insertion.

General Procedures for Injection

The patient's opinion of the clinician is strongly governed by his or her
experiences during the administration of local anesthesia. To provide
anesthesia safely, effectively, and atraumatically, the clinician must fol-

low certain steps in managing the patient, preparing the tissue for injection, and making the injection.

PATIENT MANAGEMENT

Most patients dislike injections, and some are overtly fearful. Such feelings are particularly intense regarding injections within the oral cavity. Not only is the mouth richly supplied with sensory nerves, resulting in enhanced sensitivity to painful stimuli, it is also a major expressive part of the face and a primary route of visceral gratification. Thus, the oral cavity is of great psychologic importance to the patient. In one sense, intraoral anesthesia can be interpreted as a form of physical assault on a physiologically sensitive and psychologically important region. Obviously, most patients are not conscious of this association, but its existence is verified by the large number of patients who willingly accept injections in other parts of the body but who become a moving target for the dentist's needle.

Although there is no technique or approach that eliminate all fears in all patients, much can be done to minimize the perceived trauma of oral injection. Patient comfort, for instance, is very important. A semisupine position is far more comfortable to the patient than an upright posture, particularly in the modern contour chair. Anesthesia can be easily administered to the reclining patient (Fig. 8–2); as an added benefit, the possibility of syncope in the acutely anxious individual is greatly reduced.

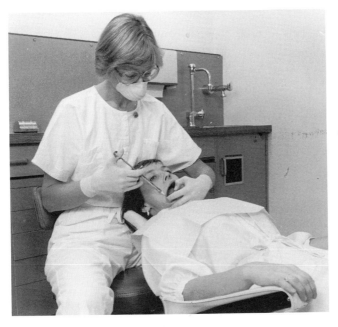

Figure 8–2.   Administration of local anesthesia to a patient in a comfortable reclining position.

Gentleness of manner, speech, and injection technique is vitally important. A patient who is very fearful will nevertheless often fully cooperate with a clinician who is perceived as being concerned and careful. In fact, the one major criterion of clinical excellence that patients are most cognizant of is gentleness of the operator, especially during administration of anesthesia.

The anesthetic syringe and needle assembly is a forbidding device. The syringe should be loaded and tested for anesthetic flow prior to the arrival of the patient and kept out of the patient's field of vision, particularly when the needle cover has been removed (Fig. 8–3).

The wise clinician avoids use of such psychologically charged words as "needle" or "shot" in conversations with patients. For example, "pain" can be described as discomfort.

In many instances, the use of conscious sedation is helpful in decreasing patient anxiety, and, with some methods, it can provide additional pain control over that afforded by local anesthesia alone. One of the simplest and safest techniques is nitrous oxide and oxygen inhalation sedation. This form of pain and anxiety control is rapidly induced and readily reversed, and it usually does not impose any dietary or functional restrictions on the patient (Fig. 8–4). Also useful is intravenous sedation, particularly with a benzodiazepine, such as diazepam or midazolam, which frequently permits difficult patients to be managed effectively with regional anesthesia. These drugs normally produce a period of amnesia during which the injections are not remembered. Oral sedation is also popular among clinicians and avoids the use of complex equipment or

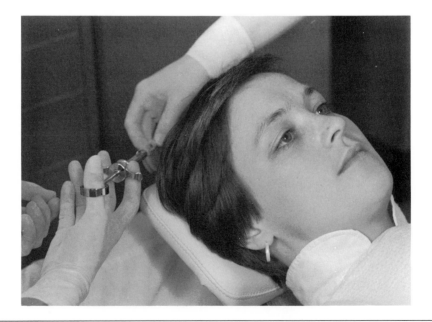

Figure 8–3.   Syringe transfer and needle exposure performed out of the patient's view.

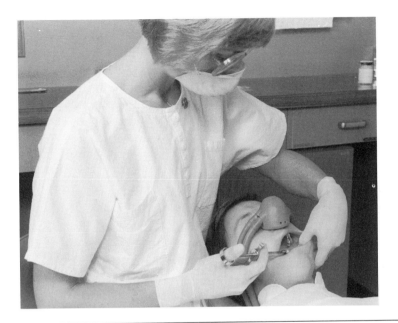

Figure 8–4. Local anesthetic injection with inhalation sedation for pain and anxiety control.

techniques. Drugs frequently administered for oral sedation include the benzodiazepines, chloral hydrate, various barbiturates, and sedative antihistamines.

TISSUE PREPARATION

Preparing the tissue for an intraoral injection includes application of a topical anesthetic, physical debridement, and manipulation of tissue about the site of administration. Topical anesthesia has a definite role in regional anesthesia (Fig. 8–5). When a topical anesthetic is applied to oral mucosa, good surface anesthesia can often be achieved, and the patient may be rendered insensitive to the penetration of the needle. Topical anesthesia of attached gingival tissue is less reliable, however, and it may be of no benefit when given before a palatal injection because of its poor penetration of cornified epithelium. However, one major reason why topical anesthetics sometimes fail is that insufficient time is allowed for the drug to take effect. Onset of anesthesia may vary from 30 seconds for some concentrated benzocaine preparations to several minutes for lidocaine ointments and gels.

Although topical anesthetics are generally recommended, even in areas where their effectiveness is equivocal, opinion is divided over the need for topical antiseptics. The mouth harbors a dense microbial flora that precludes effective disinfection of any mucosal injection site. All that can be gained by application of an antiseptic solution is some reduction in the number of bacteria that are introduced into the submucosal

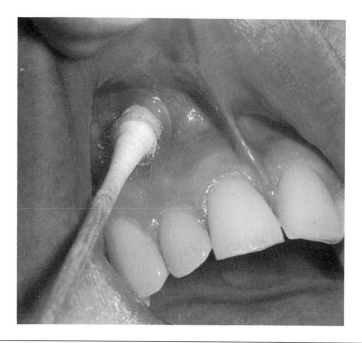

Figure 8–5.   Topical anesthetic placement in the maxilla.

tissues during needle insertion. Because of the small surface area of the needle and the antibacterial action of the topical anesthetic (described in Chapter 2), this number is already low and generally of little consequence in the healthy patient. Moreover, some topical antiseptics are irritating to mucosa, and most have a somewhat unpleasant taste. Thus, no real benefit may be realized. However, a liberal attitude toward the use or nonuse of an intraoral antiseptic solution must not breed laxity concerning the absolute necessity for sterile needles and anesthetic solutions. Although a needle or cartridge may be employed for several injections in the same individual, it bears reiteration that a needle or cartridge should never be used on more than one patient. Also, insertion of a needle into an acute abscess is undesirable.

Just before insertion, the site of administration should be wiped with sterile gauze to remove any surface debris, saliva, and remaining topical anesthetic (Fig. 8–6). The tissue should be made taut with the free hand and the patient's head stabilized securely yet comfortably (Fig. 8–7).

SYRINGE STABILIZATION

Anesthetic solutions must be deposited accurately to be consistently effective, which normally requires insertion of the needle and deposition of solution in a specific anatomic region. In this regard, a metal syringe containing a full cartridge of local anesthetic solution and an attached needle can be a surprisingly cumbersome device unless a sensible han-

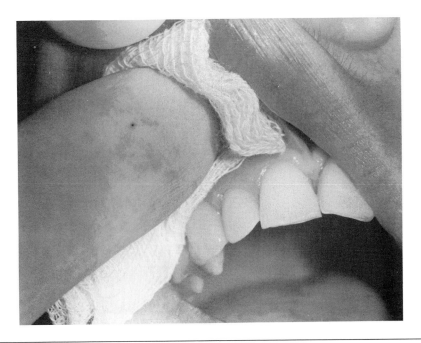

Figure 8–6.   Sterile gauze is used to remove saliva, debris, and excess topical anesthetic prior to needle insertion.

dling technique is adopted. Figure 8–8 demonstrates the recommended "palms-up" handling technique.

Note that the palms-up method permits easy use of finger rests on either the syringe barrel or patient, thus eliminating excessive needle movement prior to tissue insertion. It is very important to avoid uncontrolled syringe movement, as the patient will invariably detect such instability and interpret it as careless technique, inexperience, or poor training and will lose confidence in the operator.

OPERATOR POSITION

The position of the operator in relation to the patient is a matter of considerable importance. The clinician in most instances will be providing patient care for many years. An uncomfortable or unstable body position leads to fatigue, bad technique, and poor-quality dentistry. In some instances, acute or chronic musculoskeletal strain or injury may be caused. A comfortable, well-supported sitting position is therefore essential (Fig. 8–9). To maintain this optimal position, the patient's head can be turned to assist vision and the dental chair adjusted to further enhance the operator's access to the patient's mouth (Fig. 8–10).

It is usually unnecessary for the operator to rest an arm on the patient's chest or shoulder during the injection. Indeed, doing so may result in the operator's hand being jolted unexpectedly during the injection, with the

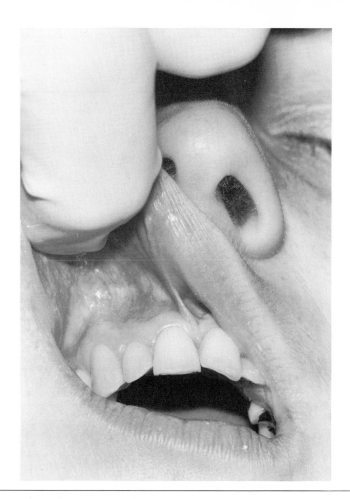

Figure 8–7.   Tissue is retracted before a maxillary supraperiosteal injection is performed.

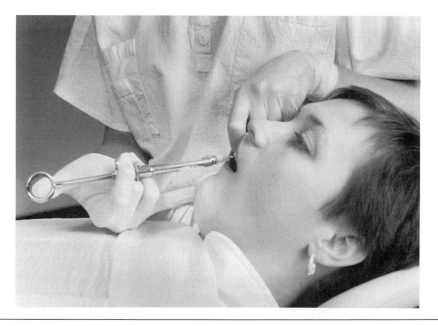

Figure 8–8.   The correct palms-up syringe technique with a finger rest on the patient's face.

192

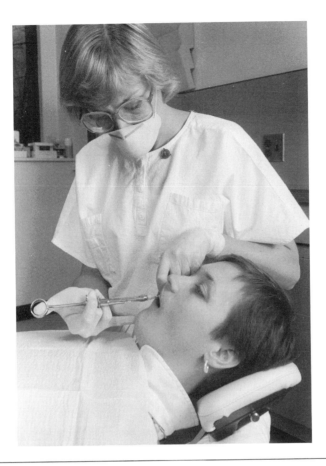

Figure 8–9.   A straight sitting posture during the administration of a maxillary injection.

possible loss of needle position, tearing of mucosa, failure of anesthesia, and, in rare instances, needle breakage. Also, using the patient's chest as an armrest has led to accusations of unprofessional behavior of male dentists treating female patients. At the very least, leaning or resting against the patient can be uncomfortable to that individual.

THE INJECTION

The injection technique is summarized in Table 8–1. For needle insertion to be as accurate and as painless as possible, the syringe should be properly oriented before the mucosa is punctured. If the needle must be redirected after insertion, as sometimes occurs during the inferior alveolar nerve block, it should be nearly withdrawn and then reinserted along a corrected pathway. Attempting to "torque" the needle during a deep block injection often does little but bend the needle or unnecessarily tear connective tissues.

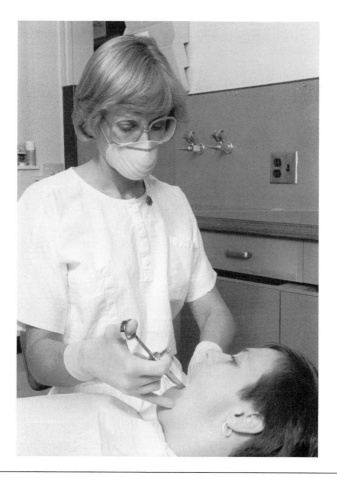

Figure 8–10. Operator position during the administration of a mandibular (inferior alveolar) injection. The clinician is in front of the subject with the patient's head turned and the patient's chair lowered to permit better vision and access to the mouth.

Penetration of alveolar mucosa can be made relatively pain free by employing distraction, such as vibrating the cheek. Once the needle tip has been inserted through the mucosa, a few drops of anesthetic can be given as the needle is slowly advanced to the intended target.

Before the anesthetic solution is injected, aspiration should be carried out to ensure that a blood vessel has not been entered. Several seconds may be required for blood to appear in the cartridge if small-diameter needles are used. If a positive aspirate is obtained but the amount of blood that enters the cartridge is small, the needle can be moved a few millimeters and aspiration reattempted. When a negative result is obtained, the drug may then be administered (Fig. 8–11). When injecting, especially near vascular areas such as the pterygoid venous plexus, it is often prudent to perform several aspirations during the injection.

Even though aspiration prior to injecting anesthetic solution is a universally recommended precaution, it is not an infallible indicator of intra-

Table 8–1. **SUMMARY OF CORRECT INJECTION TECHNIQUE**

1. Seat the patient in a comfortable reclining position.
2. Position yourself correctly and adjust the patient's position to optimize access and vision (e.g., raise or lower the chair, turn the patient's head).
3. Apply topical anesthetic when appropriate, allowing sufficient time for the anesthetic to take effect.
4. Retract the mucosa in order to enhance vision and minimize needle insertion trauma.
5. Dry the injection site with a sterile gauze.
6. Penetrate the mucosa using distraction (e.g., vibration of lip) to minimize the pain of insertion.
7. Insert the needle gently and slowly to its intended position. Use a palms-up technique with finger rests. Do not rely on the patient's upper body for arm support.
8. Aspirate prior to injection. If positive, reposition the needle gently until a negative aspirate is obtained.
9. Inject solution at a rate of 2 mL/min or slower.
10. Remove the needle slowly along the path of insertion.

vascular needle placement. Thin needles (e.g., 25, 27, and 30 gauge) commonly used for intraoral anesthesia can enter a blood vessel and during the aspiration maneuver can be blocked by the vessel wall (Fig. 8–12). For this reason, *any* blood in the cartridge is considered a positive aspirate, and appropriate repositioning of the needle should be carried out.

The rate of injection should not normally exceed 2 mL/min. At this rate, if the needle tip is unexpectedly in a blood vessel, the contents of the cartridge will be dispersed throughout the vascular system, and a high transient concentration of drug will be avoided. To minimize local complications, even slower rates of administration (e.g., 0.5 mL/min) are

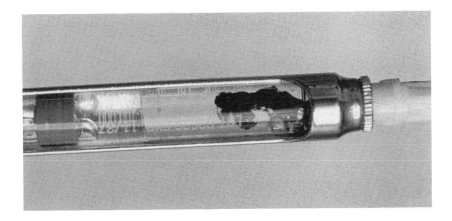

Figure 8–11. A positive aspiration.

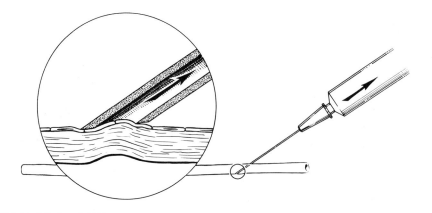

Figure 8–12.   Intimal obstruction of a needle lumen during aspiration.

used during injection into dense connective tissue, such as in the palate. A slow injection also allows distribution of anesthetic solution without painful tissue distention.

Once the injection has been completed, the needle should be removed slowly along the path of insertion. Depending on the particular injection and anesthetic solution employed, anesthesia may take anywhere from a few seconds to 10 minutes to develop. In most instances, however, anesthesia is complete within 5 minutes.

Intraoral Anesthesia and the Child

Children are not small adults. Psychologically, the child requires an approach somewhat different from that used with adults. Anatomically, there are also some important differences in both size and proportion that need to be considered when anesthesia is administered.

BEHAVIORAL AND MANAGEMENT CONSIDERATIONS

Children often have an unreasonable fear of needles and injections. The intensity of this problem varies with the child's age and emotional maturity, family background, basic intelligence, and prior experience with medical and dental treatment.

If a child is well-behaved and expresses fear in a relatively mature manner appropriate for his or her age, the clinician is often able to teach the child about "numbing" the tooth or "putting it to sleep."

Patience and a gentle manner are even more important with children than with adults. Although an occasional adult with a pathologic fear of intraoral injections can become uncooperative, this is much more likely to happen with the young child, particularly if the clinician is rough,

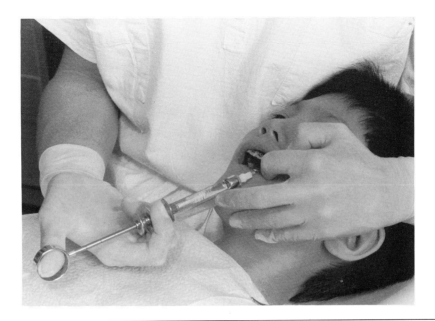

Figure 8–13. Example of a young child receiving an injection of a local anesthetic. The child's head is held gently but firmly against the operator's body to minimize sudden undesirable movement.

uncaring, and impatient or fails to observe critical aspects of patient management. These simple rules are offered for effectively managing the young patient:

1. Never lie about pain, but don't overemphasize it either.
2. Tell the child what to expect in a simple, direct manner at his or her level of understanding. For instance, nonthreatening terms such as a "pinch" can be used to describe the injection.
3. Manage delaying tactics (e.g., repeated questions) with a gentle but inexorable progression through the planned procedure.
4. Use topical anesthetics that have a pleasing taste.
5. Avoid showing the needle to the child.
6. Insert the needle with care and inject the solution very slowly.
7. Support the child's head. Assume that young patients will move during injection (Fig. 8–13).
8. If possible, avoid giving palatal injections, because they are poorly tolerated by young children. The use of jet injection in this instance is a useful alternative.

This approach will succeed with most but not all young patients. A child who gives indications of being unduly frightened or uncooperative may be much more easily managed by using oral, parenteral, or inhalation sedation.

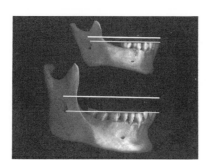

Figure 8–14.   Comparison of the mandible of an adult and young child. The lingula in the child mandible is lower and more anterior.

ANATOMIC AND PHYSIOLOGIC CONSIDERATIONS

Because of their proportionately smaller size, children require less local anesthetic solution for an equivalent anesthetic effect. For example, if an adult requires 1.8 mL for a combined inferior alveolar and lingual nerve block, a small child can be successfully anesthetized with 1.0 mL of the same agent. Contributing to a decreased volume requirement for supraperiosteal injections is the fact that juvenile bone is thinner, more porous, and thus more permeable to anesthetics than is adult bone. Indeed, a supraperiosteal administration in young children is often effective in eliciting anesthesia of mandibular posterior teeth.

Besides the obvious disparity in size, certain anatomic relationships are also different in the child. The location of the lingula (and mandibular foramen) on the medial surface of the ramus is of particular significance. Although individual variations exist and children of the same age can exhibit enormous differences in physical size and maturity, between the ages of 2 and 5 years the mandibular lingula lies approximately at the level of the occlusal plane. As the child develops, the location of the lingula moves upward and backward in relation to the occlusal plane. Finally, in the teenager the lingula is situated at the level of the deepest concavity of the coronoid notch at about 1 cm above the occlusal plane. The varying location of the lingula must be taken into account when an inferior alveolar nerve block is performed (Fig. 8–14).

The decreased size of the ramus in smaller children makes it possible to safely administer an inferior alveolar block using a short needle. Penetration is generally 15 mm, and this is less than the typical length of a short needle (20 to 25 mm). Although the choice of a short versus long needle is unimportant in regard to the production of pain, children psychologically often equate long needles with increased discomfort, and should they see the needle, they are more apt to accept an injection if a short needle is used.

Maxillary Anesthesia

Anesthesia of the maxillary arch involves blocking one or more of the peripheral nerves of the maxillary division of the fifth cranial (trigeminal) nerve. When pain control for the maxillary teeth, attendant alveolar bone, and facial gingiva is necessary, the superior alveolar nerves must be anesthetized (Fig. 9–1). When restorative or surgical procedures involving the palatal mucoperiosteum are contemplated, additional injections to block the nasopalatine and greater palatine nerves become necessary.

A commonly used method for securing anesthesia of individual maxillary teeth and supporting periodontium is the supraperiosteal injection, in which the anesthetic solution is placed adjacent to the periosteum of the alveolar bone overlying the apex of the tooth (Fig. 9–2). Because the maxilla is relatively porous and has a thin cortical plate, the anesthetic is able to penetrate the bone and anesthetize terminal fibers of the superior dental plexus. The supraperiosteal injection is often referred to as an infiltration, but this terminology is somewhat misleading. The injection is more appropriately classified as a field block, because some structures (e.g., interdental papilla, tooth pulp) may become anesthetized without ever having been exposed to a pharmacologically effective concentration of the administered agent. It is most frequently used for anesthesia of the more anterior teeth, being somewhat less employed in the maxillary molar region, where the posterior superior alveolar nerve block may be administered. Although individual supraperiosteal injections can be given for each tooth to be treated, it is usually propitious to anesthetize the anterior or middle superior alveolar nerves when a wide area of coverage is needed, thus avoiding multiple injections to achieve adequate pain control. Alternatively, the second division, or maxillary, nerve block can be used to anesthetize the entire hemimaxilla with a single injection.

Injection of local anesthetics into palatal tissue is considered the most uncomfortable of all intraoral anesthetic techniques. For this reason, and

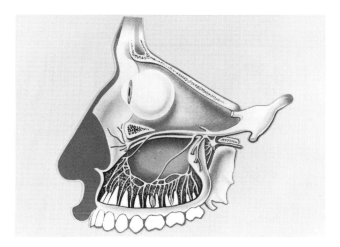

Figure 9–1.   Innervation of the maxillary teeth by the superior alveolar nerves.

because the anesthesia obtained is essentially limited to the palatal mucosa, periosteum, and underlying bone, the use of palatal injections is normally restricted, particularly in children, to situations when direct manipulation of these structures is performed. Indications for palatal injections include the extraction of teeth, palatal surgery, and the extensive stimulation of palatal nerves during crown preparation, gingival retraction, or subgingival scaling and curettage.

The supraperiosteal and nerve block injections most commonly employed for regional anesthesia of the maxilla are described in this chap-

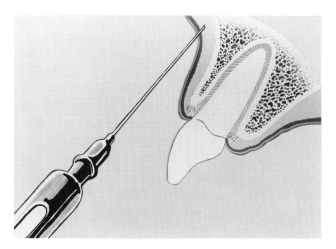

Figure 9–2.   Supraperiosteal injection. The anesthetic solution is administered submucosally but supraperiosteally adjacent to the apex of the tooth. The solution then spreads through the alveolar bone to anesthetize nerve fibers supplying the tooth pulp and adjacent periodontium.

ter. Other techniques, such as the periodontal ligament and intraosseous injections, are described in Chapter 11.

Supraperiosteal Injection—Single Tooth

The supraperiosteal injection is ideally suited for anesthesia of a single tooth or circumscribed portion of the maxilla. The discussion that follows applies to all the maxillary teeth; modifications of the standard technique that are useful for individual teeth are also provided.

ANATOMIC CONSIDERATIONS

The objective of all supraperiosteal injections is to insert the needle under the mucosa so that it lies adjacent to the bone without impinging on the richly innervated periosteum (Fig. 9–3). For maximum effect, the needle tip should overlie the apex of the tooth being anesthetized. Inasmuch as the maxillary teeth have different root lengths, insertion endpoints will vary among teeth and, for that matter, among patients. Table 9–1 lists the average root lengths of selected maxillary teeth.[1]

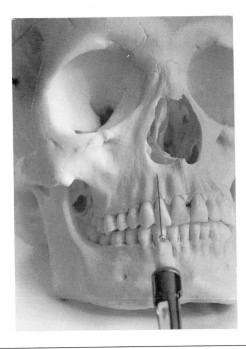

Figure 9–3.   Supraperiosteal injection of the maxillary lateral incisor. The needle is nominally aligned along the long axis of the tooth, with the tip overlying the apex of the root.

Table 9–1. **AVERAGE SIZE AND ROOT LENGTH OF SELECTED MAXILLARY TEETH**

Tooth	Total Length (mm)	Root Length (mm)
Central incisor	24.0	12.4
Lateral incisor	22.5	13.5
Canine	27.0	17.0
First premolar	22.5	13.8
Second premolar	21.5	13.0
First molar	20.5	12.8
Second molar	19.5	12.0

Data from DuBrul.[1]

TECHNIQUE

The patient's cheek or lip is retracted with the operator's free hand sufficiently to expose the tooth and area to be anesthetized and to stretch the vestibular mucosa. After applying topical anesthesia and drying the mucosa, the operator inserts the needle at or near the greatest concavity of the mucobuccal fold and directs it toward the apex of the tooth (Fig. 9–4). The depth of insertion varies but is usually 3 or 4 mm. If bone is contacted, the needle should be withdrawn slightly to avoid injection under the periosteum. The local anesthetic solution is slowly injected after a negative aspirate is obtained. The amount of solution needed will vary from 0.5 to 1.5 mL, depending on the tooth to be anesthetized, the procedure that is planned, the patient's size, and the density of bone.

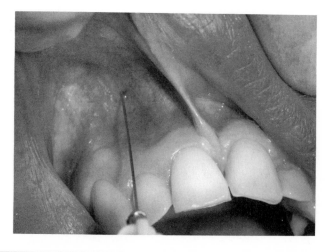

Figure 9–4.   Supraperiosteal injection of the maxillary lateral incisor. The lip is retracted and the vestibular mucosa made taut with the operator's free hand.

Smaller amounts are usually adequate for anterior teeth, whereas larger volumes are often necessary for multirooted posterior teeth.

Normally, as shown in Figure 9–4 of a lateral incisor injection, the puncture point is over the root of the tooth. However, in the case of the maxillary central incisor, the anterior nasal spine, with its exquisitely sensitive periosteum, often encroaches on the apex. Here a much more comfortable technique for the patient is to insert the needle from a distal position, as shown in Figure 9–5.

A supraperiosteal injection directly over the roots of the maxillary first molar may be ineffective because of the overlying zygomatic process, whose bulk and density can preclude adequate penetration by the anesthetic. In such instances, anesthesia is often best accomplished by two injections, one over the apex of the second premolar and the second over the roots of the second molar.

AREA AND SIGNS OF ANESTHESIA

The area of anesthesia for a single-tooth supraperiosteal injection includes the pulp and labial/buccal tissues adjacent to the tooth. Figure 9–6 illustrates the limited area of anesthesia that can be obtained when a minimal amount (0.5 mL) of anesthetic is injected over the apex of the lateral incisor. It should be noted that adjacent teeth, periodontal tissues, and facial structures (e.g., lateral aspect of the nose) may be affected, depending on the spread of the local anesthetic. It is also important to note that palatal tissues are not affected by supraperiosteal injections on the facial side of the alveolar process.

Patients are quite responsive to the altered sensorium of the labial tissues after anterior supraperiosteal injections. They are less cognizant

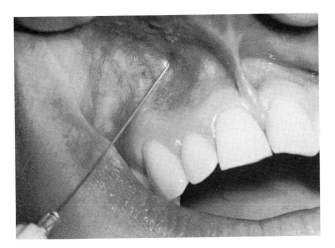

Figure 9–5.   Supraperiosteal injection of the maxillary central incisor. The distal insertion of the needle is used to avoid the anterior nasal spine.

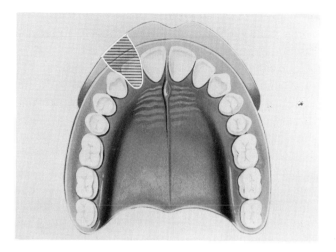

Figure 9–6.   Approximate area of anesthesia after a supraperiosteal injection of the lateral incisor.

of the effects of posterior injections, and the depth of anesthesia is best gauged with an explorer or by judiciously beginning treatment.

Anterior Superior Alveolar Nerve Injection   ASA

The anterior superior alveolar nerve injection normally provides anesthesia for the three anterior teeth and their associated periodontal ligaments, alveolar bone, and labial gingiva. However, because of presumed cross-innervation from the contralateral nerve, anesthesia of the central incisor and/or overlying mucosa may be incomplete without a supplemental injection near the midline over the apex of that tooth. A nasopalatine nerve block may on rare occasions also be required to provide full anesthesia for the central incisors.

ANATOMIC CONSIDERATIONS

The needle should be inserted such that the tip opposes the periosteum adjacent to the apex of the maxillary canine (Fig. 9–7). The anterior superior alveolar nerve usually divides within the maxillary bone at that point, providing branches that innervate all three anterior maxillary teeth (see Fig. 9–1).

TECHNIQUE

As during the single-tooth supraperiosteal injection, the operator's free hand retracts the lip, thereby placing tension on the vestibular mucosa and affording direct access to the injection site. After applying topical

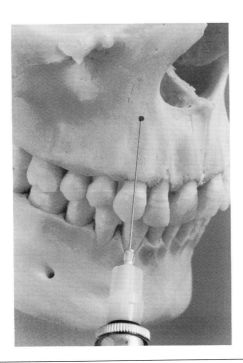

Figure 9–7. Anterior superior alveolar nerve injection. The needle parallels the long axis of the canine, and the tip approximates the root apex.

anesthetic, waiting an appropriate time, and drying the mucosa, the operator inserts the needle at the height of the vestibular fold and advances it until the tip is just above the periosteum adjacent to the apex of the canine (Fig. 9–8). After a negative aspiration, the anesthetic solution is injected slowly until 1 to 1.5 mL has been deposited. The needle is then slowly withdrawn.

AREA AND SIGNS OF ANESTHESIA

Figure 9–9 provides an approximate outline of the structures anesthetized with an anterior superior alveolar nerve injection. Anesthesia excludes the palatal tissues and may be incomplete near the midline because of the accessory innervation previously described. Although the extent of anesthesia shown is restricted to the three anterior teeth, the anterior superior alveolar nerve often provides innervation posteriorly; thus, anesthesia can variably include the first and second premolars in some patients. The close proximity of the apex of the canine to the infraobital foramen usually results in some anesthesia of the distal branches of the infraorbital nerve.

Patients reliably detect loss of sensation of the teeth, adjacent soft tissues, and upper lip. However, depending on the volume injected and the diffusion of the anesthetic solution, lip anesthesia may be incomplete.

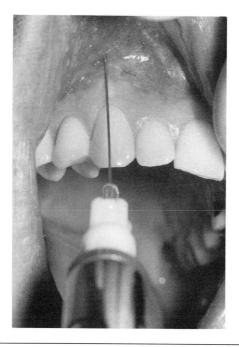

Figure 9–8.   Anterior superior alveolar nerve injection. Lip retraction provides access to the maxillary canine area.

If a surgical procedure is to be performed on the upper lip, an infraorbital block is often a more reliable anesthetic technique.

Middle Superior Alveolar Nerve Injection   MSA

The middle superior alveolar nerve injection is primarily indicated for anesthesia of the premolars, mesiobuccal root of the maxillary first mo-

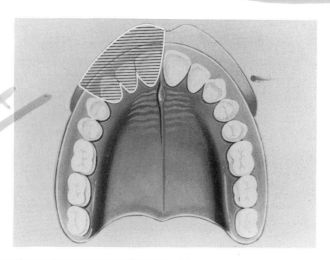

Figure 9–9.   Approximate area of anesthesia after an anterior superior alveolar nerve injection.

lar, and the adjacent bone, periodontal ligaments, and soft tissues. Actually, the middle superior alveolar nerve as a discrete entity is absent in approximately 60% of patients. Its function is then provided by the anterior and/or posterior superior alveolar nerves. Nevertheless, it is still possible to obtain reliable anesthesia by placing anesthetic solution in the area adjacent to the presumed location of the middle superior alveolar nerve.

ANATOMIC CONSIDERATIONS

Ideally, the solution is placed supraperiosteally at or slightly above the apex of the maxillary second premolar (Fig. 9–10). If one of the premolars is missing (as frequently happens in orthodontically treated patients), the remaining premolar serves as the principal landmark. This injection (similar to the anterior superior alveolar injection) depends on local spread of the anesthetic, and minor differences in root position are usually unimportant.

TECHNIQUE

The operator's free hand retracts the corner of the mouth and the buccal mucosa adjacent to the premolars. This maneuver affords visual access to the injection site and places tension on the vestibular mucosa, permitting a more pain-free needle insertion. After providing topical anesthesia and drying the mucosa, the operator inserts the needle at or near the height of the mucobuccal fold adjacent to the second premolar. The needle is slowly advanced until the tip is estimated to be at or just above the root apex (Fig. 9–11). After negative aspiration, 1.0 to 1.5 mL of

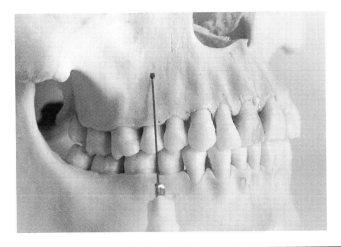

Figure 9–10.   Middle superior alveolar nerve injection. The needle is placed adjacent to the root apex of the second premolar.

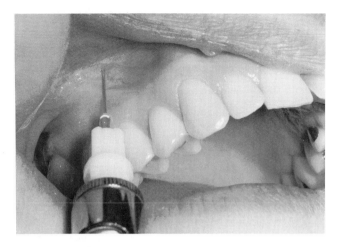

Figure 9–11. Middle superior alveolar nerve injection. The needle is inserted near the height of the vestibule, with access obtained by retracting the lip with the operator's free hand.

anesthetic is injected slowly, and the needle is withdrawn in a similarly deliberate manner.

AREA AND SIGNS OF ANESTHESIA

Patients are usually able to discern the loss of sensation over the corner of the upper lip, adjacent buccal mucosa, and premolar teeth (Fig. 9–12). This injection normally permits conservative treatment of both premolars and, when combined with an appropriate palatal injection, their surgical removal. The middle superior alveolar nerve injection is also used as a

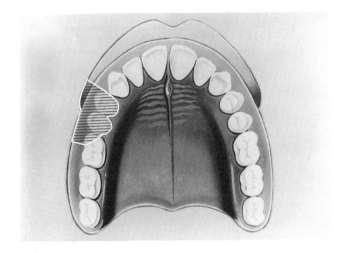

MSA

Figure 9–12. Approximate area of anesthesia after a middle superior alveolar injection.

supplemental injection with the posterior superior alveolar nerve block in the treatment of the first maxillary molar.

Posterior Superior Alveolar Nerve Block PSA

Unlike anesthesia of the anterior maxilla, anesthesia of the maxillary molar region is most readily accomplished by a block injection of the posterior superior alveolar nerve. This nerve courses laterally and inferiorly from the pterygopalatine fossa to enter the maxilla through one or more small foramina located at midheight on its posterior wall above the tuberosity. Once within the bone, the posterior superior alveolar nerve contributes to the superior dental plexus. Ultimately it provides sensation to the maxillary molars (with the possible exception of the mesiobuccal route of the first molar) and their adjacent bone, periodontal ligaments, and buccal gingiva. In addition, small branches of the nerve innervate buccal soft tissues and mucosa and gingiva around the tuberosity, but the extent of this distribution varies considerably.

ANATOMIC CONSIDERATIONS

The site of the injection lies on the posterolateral aspect of the maxilla about 1 cm above and behind the apices of the last molar (Fig. 9–13). The

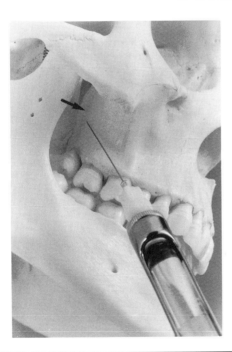

Figure 9–13.   Posterior superior alveolar nerve block. The tip of the needle approximates the posterior superior alveolar nerve foramina (arrow). Access is achieved through the superiorly inclined angle of the needle and the position of its hub beneath the zygomatic process.

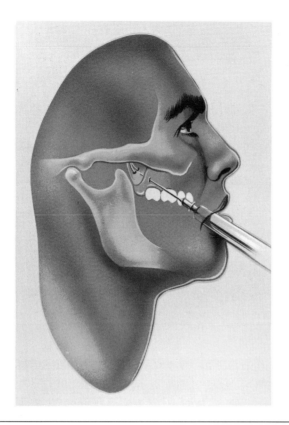

Figure 9–14.   Relative position of the needle and syringe to the posterior superior alveolar nerve. Partially closing the mouth and shifting the mandible to the side of injection permits the proper orientation of the syringe.

PSA

maxilla in this area is convex and access is limited; thus, the needle must be directed inward, upward, and backward. A major anatomic landmark is the zygomatic process of the maxilla, which lies in front of the target area and is easily palpated buccal to the first molar. Figure 9–14 shows the needle position with the tip adjacent to the entry point of the posterior superior alveolar nerve into the maxilla and the hub of the needle below the zygomatic process.

TECHNIQUE

To determine correctly the proper insertion point for this injection, the distal boundary of the zygomatic process should be palpated with the thumb or forefinger. The puncture point is in the height of the vestibule immediately posterior to the process. Normally it will lie somewhere between the distobuccal root of the second molar and the mesiobuccal root of the third molar. Because of the inward curvature of the posterior surface of the maxilla, the needle will have to be directed medially as well as posteriorly and superiorly. A good rule of thumb is that the needle axis

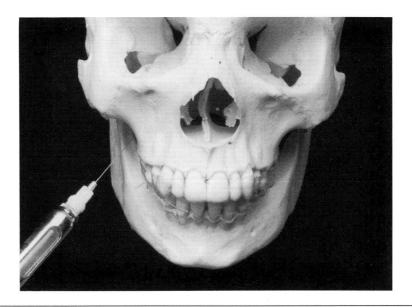

Figure 9–15. Normal orientation of the needle for the posterior superior alveolar nerve block.

should be at an angle of 45 degrees to the patient's occlusal and midsaggital planes (Fig. 9–15). However, individual patients may have structural variations that require a slightly different orientation of the needle.

For easy access, the patient's mouth should be nearly closed and the mandible shifted toward the side to be injected. This maneuver relaxes the cheek and moves the coronoid process of the ascending ramus of the mandible away from the maxillary tuberosity. After securing topical anesthesia (Fig. 9–16) and drying the mucosa, the operator retracts the

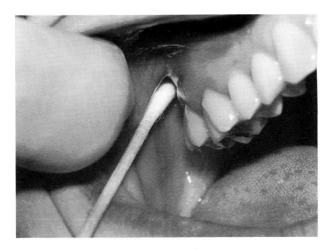

Figure 9–16. Placement of topical anesthetic behind the zygomatic process. The cotton swab is oriented in the same direction as the subsequent needle insertion for a posterior superior alveolar nerve block.

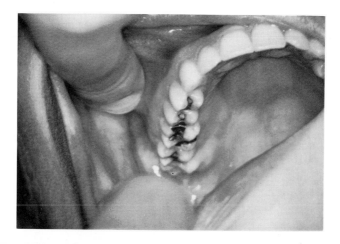

Figure 9–17.   Palpation of the zygomatic process. The point of needle insertion lies within the mucosal pocket posterior to the palpating finger.

cheek and palpates the zygomatic process (Fig. 9–17). The needle is then inserted through the mucosa and underlying buccinator muscle to a depth of about 1.5 cm (Fig. 9–18). A total of 1.0 to 1.8 mL of anesthetic solution is slowly deposited after negative aspiration, and the needle is withdrawn along its insertion path.

If the needle is inserted too far laterally, as commonly occurs with beginners unused to contending with the pressure of the cheek on the syringe, penetration of the pterygoid venous plexus may occur. Besides the possibility of minor hematoma formation, anesthesia may be incomplete. If the needle is inserted too far anteriorly or too close to the maxilla (i.e., not in the depth of the vestibule), bone may be encountered prema-

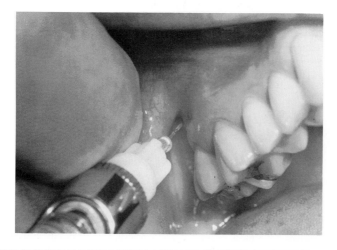

Figure 9–18.   Needle insertion for the posterior superior alveolar nerve block.

turely. In these situations, care should be taken to withdraw the needle almost completely before repositioning it. Failure to heed this admonition may cause laceration of the posterior superior alveolar artery, which is rather tortuous and held rather tightly to the posterior maxilla by inelastic connective tissues. A hematoma in this case develops quickly and may assume substantial proportions.

Because the posterior superior alveolar artery is in close proximity to the nerve and cannot always be avoided even with proper technique, a supraperiosteal injection instead of a posterior superior alveolar nerve block is sometimes advocated.[2] The approach is identical to that described above except that the needle is inserted to a depth of no more than 1.0 cm. Should the needle not penetrate the buccinator muscle, anesthesia will depend on diffusion of the anesthetic through the buccal plate of the maxillary alveolar bone. Although this method of injection may prevent an occasional hematoma from occurring, it is also less likely to produce profound anesthesia. In fact, many successful "supraperiosteal" injections are probably unintentional posterior superior alveolar nerve blocks.

AREA AND SIGNS OF ANESTHESIA

The posterior superior alveolar nerve block provides pain control for procedures performed on the maxillary molars and adjacent buccal soft tissues, periodontal ligaments, and bone, as diagramed in Figure 9–19. A separate injection is often necessary, however, to block the mesiobuccal root of the first molar. Patients can rarely determine the extent of anesthesia without being subjected to the actual dental treatment itself.

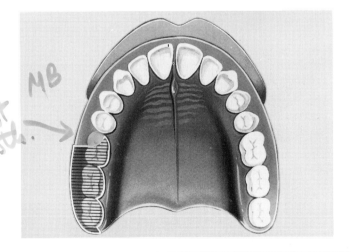

Figure 9–19.   Approximate area of anesthesia after a posterior superior alveolar nerve block. In this case, the absence of anesthesia of the mesiobuccal root of the first molar indicates the presence of the middle superior alveolar nerve.

Infraorbital Nerve Block

The infraorbital nerve block anesthetizes the anterior superior alveolar nerve, the middle superior alveolar nerve (when present and in an anterior location), and all peripheral branches of the infraorbital nerve: the inferior palpebrals, lateral nasals, and superior labials. Although the infraorbital injection is rarely used for routine restorative procedures, it should be considered when multiple procedures are planned for maxillary anterior teeth, since it obviates the need for multiple injections. The infraorbital block is especially helpful when supraperiosteal administration is contraindicated (as would be the case with periapical inflammation) or proves ineffective.

There are three basic techniques for achieving an infraorbital nerve block. Two are intraoral injection techniques and are described in detail; the third is an extraoral technique performed by direct puncture of overlying skin. This last approach has no particular advantage over the intraoral methods and has several liabilities, including the requirement for skin disinfection, lack of effective topical anesthesia, and possibly increased patient fear of needle insertion visibly close to the eye.

ANATOMIC CONSIDERATIONS

The site of injection is the infraorbital foramen. Although the needle may actually penetrate into the foramen, it is not a requirement for successful anesthesia. In fact, overinsertion will cause unnecessary discomfort and increase the possibility of direct injury to the nerve. Penetration of the orbital floor and damage to the eye may occur if the needle is inserted too deeply and posteriorly, but this is highly unlikely to occur with either of the techniques described below.

Deposition of the anesthetic solution just over the infraorbital foramen or just within its aperture will usually permit posterior flow down the infraorbital canal sufficient to reach the anterior superior alveolar nerve before it descends within the anterior wall of the maxillary sinus. Anesthesia of the middle superior alveolar nerve may also occur when it is a separate entity but located in a relatively anterior position within the maxillary sinus.

Several extraoral landmarks exist that are helpful in identifying the location of the infraorbital foramen. Figure 9–20 illustrates the linear relationship between the pupil of the eye (with the patient gazing straight ahead), the zygomaticomaxillary suture (infraorbital notch), the infraorbital foramen, and the corner of the mouth. Figure 9–21 shows the needle end-point using either the vertical approach along the axis of the second premolar or the midline approach over the incisors. In either case, the needle tip is barely within the foramen, and no attempt is made to penetrate into the canal.

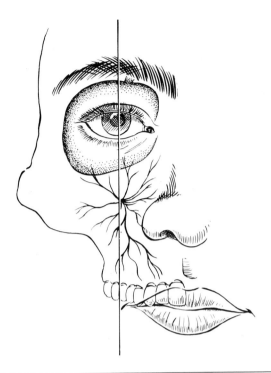

Figure 9–20. Linear relationship between the pupil of the eye, zygomaticomaxillary suture, infraorbital foramen, and corner of the mouth.

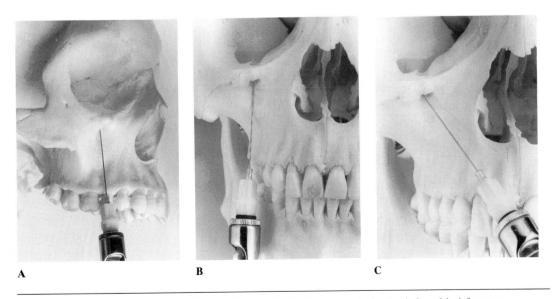

A B C

Figure 9–21. Infraorbital nerve block. The needle tip lies just within the infraorbital foramen. **A.** Vertical approach, lateral view. **B.** Vertical approach, frontal view. **C.** Midline approach.

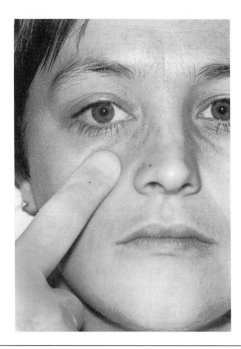

Figure 9–22.   Palpation of the infraorbital depression (foramen area) just below the infraorbital rim. The tip of the finger is in a line between the pupil and the corner of the mouth.

TECHNIQUE

Before injection, the location of the infraorbital foramen should be confirmed. An easy method of locating the foramen is to palpate, with the index finger, a notch or roughness on the infraorbital rim. This irregularity corresponds to the zygomaticomaxillary suture. Sliding the finger inferiorly 5 to 10 mm will bring it to rest in a depression that contains the infraorbital foramen (Fig. 9–22).

Vertical Approach

While the finger is kept in place over the foramen, the patient's upper lip is retracted by the operator's thumb. After application of topical anesthesia and drying the mucosa with a sterile gauze, the operator makes a puncture in the taut vestibular mucosa about 5 mm lateral to the second premolar and parallel to the long axis of its crown (Fig. 9–23). The orientation of the needle as seen from the front of the patient should mirror a vertical line defined by the medial aspect of the pupil and the infraorbital foramen. The needle is slowly advanced over the canine fossa (and through the levator anguli oris muscle) until the tip arrives at the foramen. The average depth of insertion is about 1.5 cm, which may

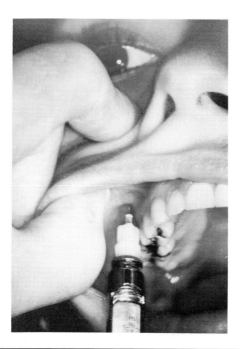

Figure 9–23. Infraorbital nerve block, vertical approach. The index finger is firmly palpating the infraorbital depression while the thumb is retracting the lip. The needle parallels the axis of the second maxillary premolar.

appear excessive when first attempted and give rise to fears of penetrating the orbit. However, the eye is protected from needle puncture by the bony infraorbital rim just above the target area.

Although the needle need not actually enter the foramen, it must closely approximate the opening to permit the anesthetic solution to pass easily into the infraorbital canal. After negative aspiration, injection of 1.0 mL of local anesthetic solution is carried out slowly, with the palpating finger firmly pressed over the infraorbital depression to help direct the flow of anesthetic into the canal.

Midline Approach

For the alternative midline approach, palpation of the infraorbital foramen and reflection of the lip are the same as previously discussed. The needle pathway to the foramen, though, is defined by a line running from the incisal edge of the central incisor to the foramen (Fig. 9–24). Puncture of the mucosa usually occurs in the depth of the vestibule opposite the lateral incisor. This injection technique may avoid penetration of facial musculature; on the other hand, it is a longer, less direct route to the foramen.

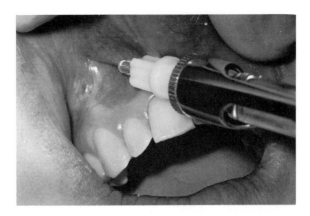

Figure 9–24.   Infraorbital nerve block, midline approach. The retraction of the lip and palpation of the infraorbital depression are similar to that of the vertical approach, but the needle is inserted in the vestibule adjacent to the lateral incisor, with the barrel of the syringe over the central incisors.

AREA AND SIGNS OF ANESTHESIA

When performed correctly, the infraorbital block will anesthetize the incisor and canine teeth, their supporting labial periodontium, and the upper lip, anterior cheek, lower eyelid, and lateral aspect of the nose. Anesthesia may also include the premolar region and extend as far back as the mesiobuccal root of the first molar (Fig. 9–25).

Inadequate anesthesia of the incisors may result from accessory innervation. A supplemental supraperiosteal injection over the central incisor

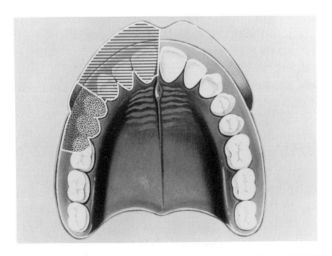

Figure 9–25.   Approximate area of anesthesia after an infraorbital nerve block. The primary area of anesthesia is associated with blockade of the infraorbital and anterior superior alveolar nerves. The secondary extension of anesthesia (darker shading) may result from blockade of the middle superior alveolar nerve.

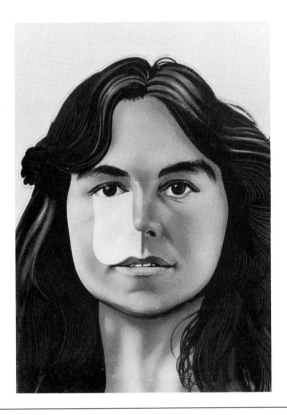

Figure 9–26.   Facial view of the distribution of cutaneous anesthesia after an infraorbital nerve block.

(or its contralateral mate) will block any fibers crossing over from the opposite anterior superior alveolar nerve. The same injection should also block labially directed fibers contributed by the nasopalatine nerve; however, a separate injection of that nerve occasionally may be necessary.

The patient readily detects anesthesia of the infraorbital nerve. The upper lip on the side of injection is profoundly numb, and surgical anesthesia usually includes the lower eyelid and skin overlying the anterior maxilla inferiorly to the midline of the upper lip (Fig. 9–26). The depth of pulpal anesthesia, particularly in the more posterior teeth, is not as easily determined by the patient before the procedure is attempted.

Nasopalatine (Incisive Canal) Nerve Block

The nasopalatine nerve block is indicated for surgical procedures involving the mucoperiosteum of the anterior palate, for restorative procedures in which the palatal gingiva must be retracted or is likely to be injured, and occasionally for supplementary anesthesia of the incisor teeth.

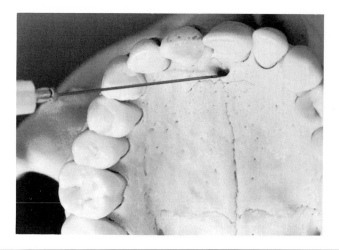

Figure 9–27.   Nasopalatine nerve block. The tip of the needle is just within the incisive foramen.

ANATOMIC CONSIDERATIONS

The bilateral nasopalatine nerves descend along the nasal septum, enter the incisive canals, and exit the incisive foramen in the anterior palate. The foramen is usually located midway on a line drawn between the canines, or about 5 mm behind the lingual border of the central incisors. The needle need not penetrate the foramen deeply (Fig. 9–27), but the tip must be inserted sufficiently to pass under the thick palatal mucosa.

TECHNIQUE

The patient's mouth ideally should be opened widely and the head tipped back to assist in visualizing the incisive papilla, which overlies the foramen. Topical anesthesia may be applied, but evidence is lacking as to its effectiveness in this area. After the mucosa is dried, the needle is inserted from a lateral direction, through the mucosa at the edge of the papilla, and 3 to 5 mm until bone is gently contacted or the needle tip is well beneath the mucosa (Fig. 9–28). After negative aspiration, 0.2 to 0.3 mL is slowly injected. Typically, there will be considerable resistance to the injection, and the incisive papilla will noticeably blanch.

A variety of techniques have been used to minimize the pain of needle insertion. As with all injections, deposition of several drops of local anesthetic as soon as the mucosa is punctured will quickly anesthetize tissues immediately ahead of the advancing needle, and avoidance of needless overinsertion will be appreciated by the patient. Some loss of sensation can also be obtained by applying pressure to the papilla with a cotton-tipped applicator or other blunt instrument, beginning 20 to 30 seconds before the injection and continuing until the needle is fully inserted and deposition of anesthetic has begun (Fig. 9–29). If a supra-

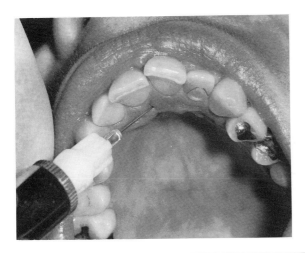

Figure 9–28.   Nasopalatine nerve block. The needle is inserted at the lateral edge of the incisive papilla and directed superiorly and medially.

periosteal injection of the central incisor has been performed, the needle can be advanced through the anesthetized interdental papilla between the central incisors and an infiltration given close to the incisive canal. Properly performed, this approach may enable the nasopalatine block to be administered without discomfort.

AREA AND SIGNS OF ANESTHESIA

The field of anesthesia produced by a nasopalatine block includes the palatal gingiva of the six anterior teeth and the mucoperiosteum of the anterior third of the hard palate (Fig. 9–30). Because communicating

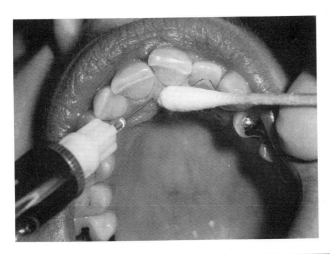

Figure 9–29.   Pressure anesthesia with a sterile cotton swab during needle insertion at the incisive foramen.

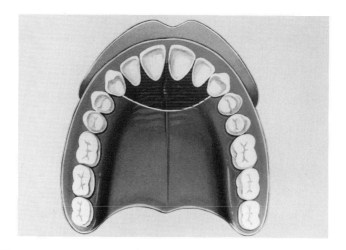

Figure 9–30.   Approximate area of anesthesia after a nasopalatine nerve block.

fibers from the greater palatine nerve also supply the canine region, a supplementary injection to block these fibers is necessary for full anesthesia of that area. Patients can usually detect the loss of sensation in the anterior palate by rubbing the tongue over the affected area.

Greater (Anterior) Palatine Nerve Block

The greater palatine nerve block anesthetizes the mucoperiosteum of the posterior two-thirds of the hard palate. It is generally reserved for situations in which palatal soft tissue in the region of the molars and premolars is involved. When coupled with a nasopalatine block, it will also provide anesthesia of the palatal mucosa adjacent to the canine.

ANATOMIC CONSIDERATIONS

The greater palatine nerve emerges onto the hard palate via the greater palatine foramen. This foramen is situated on the lateral aspect of the hard palate, generally opposite the second or third molar. The nerve runs forward in the angle formed by the horizontal process of the palate and the vertical wall of the alveolar process, giving off terminal branches to the mucoperiosteum as it progresses anteriorly. Injection of a local anesthetic anywhere along the course of the nerve will anesthetize the tissues forward of the administration site. Figure 9–31 illustrates the bony architecture of the hard palate with the greater palatine foramen (and lesser palatine foramina) located medially to the molar teeth. The needle is ideally placed just anterior to the foramen. As one moves forward from this point, the submucosal thickness along the lateral palate diminishes considerably, making needle insertion more difficult to accomplish and

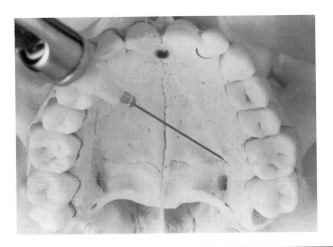

Figure 9–31.   Greater palatine nerve block. The needle tip in this example is opposite the second molar and several millimeters anterior to the greater palatine foramen.

for the patient to tolerate. Posteriorly, injection directly over the greater palatine foramen will often result in anesthesia of the lesser palatine nerves innervating the soft palate.

TECHNIQUE

The patient's mouth should be opened widely and the head hyperextended to permit direct vision of the injection site. The greater palatine foramen lies underneath a depression or fovea located about 3 or 4 mm anterior to the vibrating line at the junction of the horizontal and vertical plates of bone. A cotton-tipped applicator applied to the area is often useful in locating the foramen tactually. The insertion point is normally approximately halfway between the midline and the gingival margin and several millimeters anterior to the foramen.

As with the nasopalatine nerve block, topical anesthesia may be used but is of limited efficacy. Instead, a cotton-tipped applicator is held with considerable pressure over the injection site while the needle is inserted gently from the opposite side of the mouth and through the mucosa for 5 mm or until bone is gently contacted (Fig. 9–32). A total of 0.25 to 0.5 mL of solution is slowly deposited after a negative aspiration. During injection, care should be taken to ensure that the needle is not withdrawn prematurely (causing anesthetic to leak into the oral cavity) or forced against the palatal periosteum accidentally (causing unnecessary discomfort).

AREA AND SIGNS OF ANESTHESIA

Patients can invariably detect a sensation of anesthesia from the midline to the gingival margin of the posterior teeth (Fig. 9–33). The anterior limit

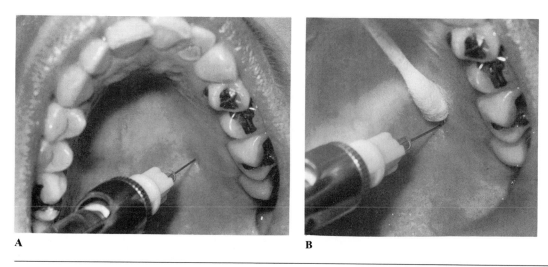

A   B

Figure 9–32.   Greater palatine nerve block. **A**. The needle approaches from the opposite side of the mouth and is inserted adjacent to the second molar at the junction of the horizontal and vertical aspects of the hard palate. **B**. The use of a cotton swab to apply pressure minimizes pain of insertion.

of anesthesia is the soft tissue adjacent to the maxillary canine. If a large amount of anesthetic is used (or its placement is more posterior than usual) and the lesser palatine nerves are blocked, anesthesia of the soft palate, uvula, and tonsilar area will result. In this situation, some patients may misinterpret the loss of sensation in the soft palate as an inability to swallow. Should a patient be concerned about the unanticipated loss of sensation, reassurance of its temporary nature and of the retained ability to swallow will usually suffice to allay apprehension.

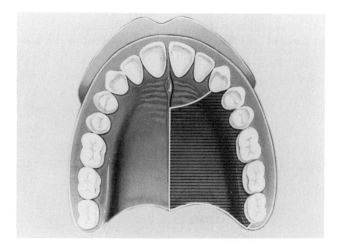

Figure 9–33.   Approximate area of anesthesia after a greater palatine nerve block.

Maxillary (Second Division) Nerve Block

The maxillary, or second division, nerve block anesthetizes the entire hemimaxilla. It is rarely employed for restorative dentistry but is useful when extensive maxillary surgery is planned, when infection necessitates a more centrally placed injection, and in the differential diagnosis of oral and maxillofacial pain syndromes. The target of the block is the maxillary nerve as it passes through the pterygopalatine fossa. Three approaches are possible: up the pterygopalatine canal, a lateral or "high tuberosity" approach, and an extraoral technique. The extraoral method of second division block is rarely used and will not be covered in depth. It involves percutaneous insertion of the needle medially under the zygomatic arch, between the coronoid process and the condyle, and into the pterygopalatine fossa.[3] It requires careful antisepsis and, because of the depth of insertion required (4 to 5 cm), cannot be performed with the conventional cartridge syringe and needle.

The most widely used method for anesthetizing the maxillary nerve is the pterygopalatine canal approach. The alternative high tuberosity approach is perhaps a more comfortable injection and is sometimes required when the pterygopalatine canal cannot be easily negotiated with the needle. On the other hand, it is a less reliable technique and requires more anesthetic volume to be injected.

ANATOMIC CONSIDERATIONS

The anesthetic solution is ideally deposited within the pterygomaxillary fossa. This fossa contains the main trunk of the maxillary nerve as it gives off its major sensory branches, including the infraorbital nerve, posterior superior alveolar nerve, and the pterygopalatine nerve roots (through which course fibers that ultimately make up the palatine and nasal nerves). In the pterygopalatine canal approach, the needle must be inserted through the greater palatine foramen and advanced approximately 2.5 to 3.0 cm for the tip to reach the pterygopalatine fossa (Fig. 9–34). With the high tuberosity approach, the needle is advanced upward and behind the maxilla 2.5 to 3.0 cm and through the pterygomaxillary fissure to enter the fossa (Fig. 9–35). In either case, the needle tip lies about 1 cm below the main trunk of the maxillary nerve.[4]

The position of the greater palatine foramen and the orientation of the pterygopalatine canal vary between patients. In 90% of patients the foramen is located anteroposteriorly within the distal half of the second molar and the mesial half of the third molar; in the remainder it generally lies adjacent to the distal half of the third molar (Fig. 9–36). Table 9–2 details the variation in the angle formed in the saggital plane by the pterygopalatine canal and the palatal bone. As shown, 75% of patients fall within a relatively narrow range of 35 to 55 degrees but the complete distribution may range from 20 to 70 degrees.[5]

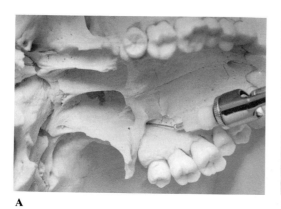
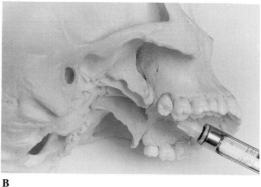

A   **B**

Figure 9–34.   Maxillary nerve block, pterygopalatine canal approach. The needle is bent 30 degrees near the hub to facilitate insertion. **A.** View of the needle inserted up the greater palatine foramen. **B.** View of needle tip within the pterygopalatine fossa.

TECHNIQUE

Pterygopalatine Canal Approach

The patient's head should be hyperextended and the mouth opened as widely as possible to allow direct vision of the injection site. To minimize discomfort with this injection, the greater palatine foramen should be located and a greater palatine block performed, as described in the previous section, but with a minimal volume (0.1 to 0.2 mL) of anesthetic. In this instance, the insertion should be made directly over the foramen,

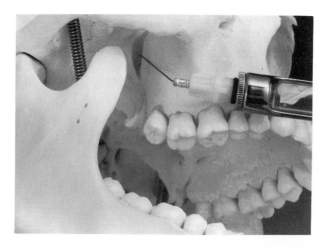

Figure 9–35.   Maxillary nerve block, high tuberosity approach. Lateral view of the needle gaining access to the pterygopalatine fossa via the pterygomaxillary fissure. The needle is bent 30 degrees near the hub to facilitate insertion.

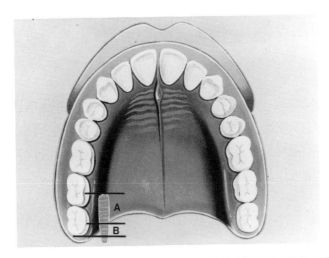

Figure 9–36.   Location of the greater palatine foramen in relation to the posterior maxillary molars. **A** indicates the region including the distal half of the second molar and the mesial half of the third molar; **B** indicates the region inclusive of the distal half of the third molar.

because the lesser palatine nerves will not be spared by the maxillary block to follow and anesthesia of the pterygopalatine canal tissues will be enhanced. After 2 or 3 minutes, the needle is then gently inserted into the greater palatine canal and slowly advanced up the pterygopalatine canal in a superior and posterior direction.

Although it may be theoretically desirable to insert the needle up the pterygopalatine canal without altering the angle of the needle with re-

Table 9–2.   **ANGLE FORMED IN THE SAGITTAL PLANE BY THE GREATER PALATINE CANAL AND THE HORIZONTAL SURFACE OF THE HARD PALATE***

Angle (degrees)	Number (%)
<35	24 (12.1)
35–42.5	53 (26.6)
45–47.5	34 (17.1)
50–57.5	63 (31.6)
>57.5	25 (12.6)

* *Measurements of 199 adult skulls were taken to the nearest 2.5 degrees.*
Data from Malamed et al.[5]

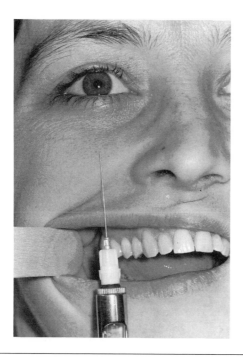

Figure 9–37.   Use of the gingival margin–infraorbital rim distance to estimate the insertion depth of the maxillary nerve block.

spect to the syringe axis, most patients will be unable to open widely enough to permit it comfortably, and in some cases (e.g., patients with small mouths) it is an impossibility. Ergo, to facilitate insertion the needle is bent at a 30-degree angle near the hub before the injection is begun. It may be necessary to probe gently for the foramen entrance, and a midcourse redirection is sometimes required, since the canal may have small bony obstructions or a tortuous path. On rare occasions it is impossible to pass the needle through the canal at all, and an alternative technique must be used. The needle should never be forced up the canal as this can lead to needle breakage, perforation of the thin medial wall of the pterygopalatine canal, or deflection of the needle into the infratemporal fossa.

A useful method for determining the correct depth of insertion in a given patient is to measure the distance between the infraorbital rim and the alveolar crest in the premolar region. This measurement roughly corresponds to the distance between the gingival margin in the posterior molar area and the target site in the pterygopalatine fossa (Fig. 9–37). At maximal insertion (normally 2.5 to 3.0 cm), the entire content of the anesthetic cartridge is slowly deposited after having obtained a negative aspiration (Fig. 9–38).

If, during aspiration, air is drawn back into the syringe, it is probable that the needle has entered the nasopharynx. In this case injection of the

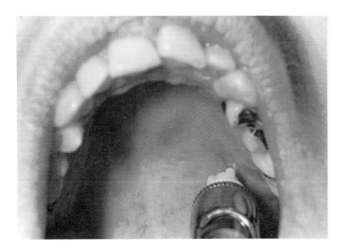

Figure 9–38.   Maxillary nerve block, pterygopalatine canal approach. Maximal insertion up the pterygopalatine canal is facilitated by having the syringe on the injection side of the mouth (in contrast to the greater palatine block).

anesthetic will usually cause the patient to comment that the solution is running down the throat. Alternatively, if significant resistance is noted during the injection, it is likely that the needle has not been advanced far enough to be outside of the confines of the canal and into the pterygomaxillary fossa. Attempting to force anesthetic up the canal will likely not result in satisfactory anesthesia and may cause damage to the palatine nerves. In rare patients (usually children or small adults), full advancement of the needle to 3 cm will place the needle high enough in the pterygomaxillary fossa where diffusion of anesthetic can cause transient anesthesia of the optic nerve and/or cranial nerves controlling the extraocular muscles.

High Tuberosity Approach

The lateral or high tuberosity approach is similar to the posterior superior alveolar nerve block except that the needle is advanced much deeper (2.5 to 3.0 cm) to enter the pterygopalatine fossa by way of the pterygomaxillary fissure. As with the pterygopalatine method, the depth of insertion can be estimated by the infraorbital ridge–gingival margin distance. Also, the needle is generally bent close to the hub to help direct it medially during insertion.

At least one full cartridge of anesthetic solution is required, and frequently a second cartridge is needed. Especially in larger adults, the needle may not penetrate into the fossa but reach only to the pterygomaxillary fissure; the extra anesthetic is then necessary for effective spread of the anesthetic solution to the maxillary nerve. Figure 9–39 illustrates the similarity of this block to a deep posterior superior alveolar block.

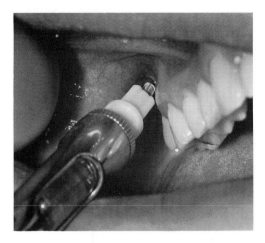

Figure 9–39.   Maxillary nerve block, high tuberosity approach. The injection is similar to a posterior superior alveolar nerve block in which the depth of insertion is doubled.

AREA AND SIGNS OF ANESTHESIA

Because the maxillary nerve and its major branches are blocked, the extent of anesthesia intraorally includes the entire maxilla on the side of the injection (Fig. 9–40). A possible exception is in the maxillary central incisor region, where crossing fibers from the contralateral maxillary nerve (specifically its anterior superior alveolar and nasopalatine branches) may provide some innervation. To block such fibers, supplemental injections (supraperiosteal or nasopalatine, as necessary) may be given with minimum discomfort on the side already anesthetized.

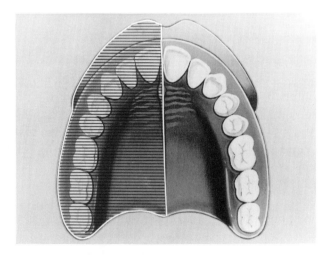

Figure 9–40.   Approximate area of anesthesia after a maxillary nerve block. The entire hemimaxilla is affected.

The patient will experience profound "numbness" of the middle face, including the skin overlying the upper lip and cheek, infraorbital region, and zygomatic process. Patients may also complain of a perceived difficulty in swallowing and, because of autonomic blockade, nasal stuffiness and inhibition of lacrimal gland secretion.

References

1. DuBrul, E.L.: Sicher and DuBrul's Oral Anatomy, 8th ed. St. Louis, Ishiyaku EuroAmerica, Inc., 1988.
2. Malamed, S.F.: Handbook of Local Anesthesia, 3rd ed. St. Louis, Mosby-Year Book, Inc., 1991.
3. Roberts, D.H., and Sowray, J.H.: Local Analgesia in Dentistry, 2nd ed. Bristol, England, John Wright & Sons Ltd., 1979.
4. Mercuri, L.G.: Intraoral second division nerve block. Oral Surg. Oral Med. Oral Pathol., *47*:109–113, 1979.
5. Malamed, S.F., and Trieger, N.: Intraoral maxillary nerve block: An anatomical and clinical study. Anesth. Prog., *30*:44–48, 1983.

Chapter 10

Mandibular Anesthesia

The vast majority of injections used for anesthesia of mandibular structures are nerve blocks of branches of the third division of the trigeminal nerve: the inferior alveolar (and its mylohyoid, incisive, and mental branches), the buccal (or its branches serving the oral mucous membranes), and the lingual (Fig. 10–1). Two reasons account for the popularity of nerve block techniques in the mandible. First, the nerves supplying the mandible are readily accessible. Second, the comparatively dense cortical plate of bone normally precludes effective anesthesia from supraperiosteal injections in all areas except perhaps the incisor region. This chapter reviews the injection techniques commonly used for mandibular anesthesia; supplemental methods of administration that may be used in the mandible are covered in Chapter 11.

Supraperiosteal Injection

The supraperiosteal injection is of limited use for pulpal anesthesia in the adult mandible. It is most effective in young children and in the anterior region of older children and young adults with a small stature and light bone structure. In large adults, particularly older men, the dense cortical bone may effectively prevent the anesthetic from reaching the nerve fibers supplying the teeth.

When successful, the supraperiosteal administration of a local anesthetic in the incisor region will anesthetize fibers from the incisive and mental branches of the inferior alveolar nerve supplying the teeth, periodontium, and labial gingiva. Although the supraperiosteal injection is sufficient for most restorative needs, a separate injection to block the lingual nerve is necessary for tooth extraction or surgery involving the lingual gingiva. On the other hand, even if another injection (e.g., mental or inferior alveolar block) is used to provide anesthesia of the incisor

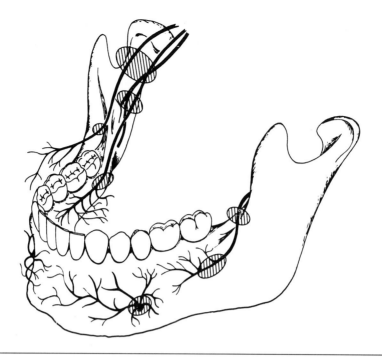

Figure 10–1. Diagram of the sensory innervation of the mandible. *Hatched areas* represent locations of local anesthetic deposition.

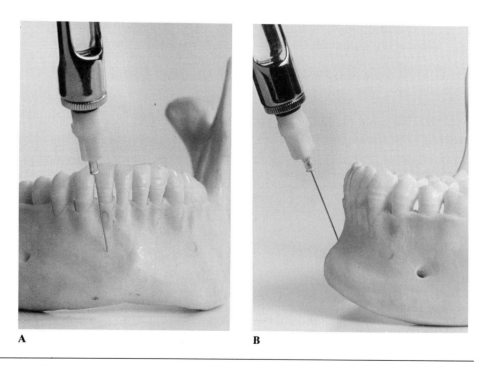

A   B

Figure 10–2. Needle placement for a mandibular supraperiosteal injection of the lateral incisor. **A.** Anterior view. **B.** Lateral view.

teeth, a supraperiosteal administration near the midline to block fibers crossing from the contralateral side is often necessary for profound anesthesia of the area.

ANATOMIC CONSIDERATIONS

The needle tip is placed adjacent to the mandibular periosteum overlying the root tip of the tooth to be anesthetized (Fig. 10–2). Alternatively, placement between the apices of the incisors may be used when anesthesia of both teeth is desired.

TECHNIQUE

The lower lip is retracted with the operator's thumb and forefinger to provide good vision and a taut mucosal surface (Fig. 10–3). After the topical anesthetic is applied, the mucosa is dried and the needle inserted in the depth of the vestibule. The needle is advanced slowly to the target (Fig. 10–4). The depth of penetration is only a few millimeters; care

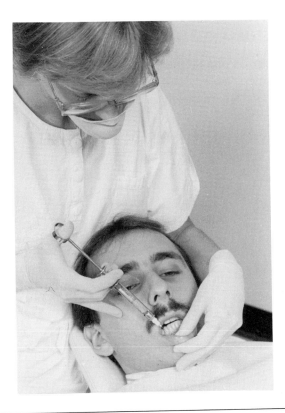

Figure 10–3.   Clinical view of a mandibular supraperiosteal injection.

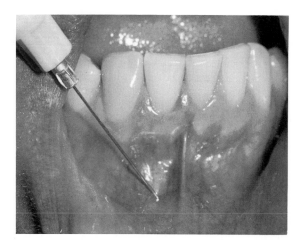

Figure 10–4.   Intraoral view of a mandibular supraperiosteal injection. Here the needle end-point is adjacent to the central incisor.

should be taken not to overinsert, since deposition of the anesthetic in the mentalis muscle may result in incomplete anesthesia. Approximately 1 mL of solution is slowly injected after a negative aspiration.

AREA AND SIGNS OF ANESTHESIA

The anatomic distribution of a single discrete mandibular supraperiosteal injection is quite limited. Soft tissue anesthesia will include the gingiva and adjacent labial mucosa, including a small portion of the lower lip. If

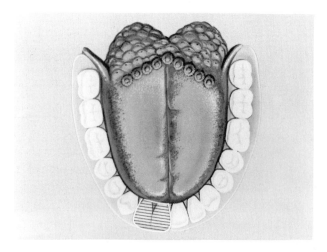

Figure 10–5.   Approximate area of anesthesia after a supraperiosteal injection adjacent to the mandibular central and lateral incisors.

extensive surgery is to be performed on the lower lip, a different technique providing full anesthesia of the mental nerve will be required. Figure 10–5 illustrates the area of anesthesia achieved by a supraperiosteal injection between the roots of the mandibular right central and lateral incisors.

Mental (Incisive) Nerve Block

The mental nerve is a superficial terminal branch of the inferior alveolar nerve that leaves the inferior alveolar canal via the mental foramen. The other terminal branch of the inferior alveolar nerve is the incisive nerve, which courses anteriorly within the mandible. Whereas the mental nerve provides sensation for the labial mucosa, gingiva, and lower lip adjacent to the incisors, canine, and, to a variable degree, the premolars, the incisive nerve innervates the tooth pulps, periodontal ligaments, and investing bone of these teeth.

Profound anesthesia of the mental nerve is relatively easy to achieve; anesthesia of the incisive nerve is more technique sensitive. The incisive nerve is located some distance from the mental foramen aperture, through which the anesthetic agent must pass to reach its site of action. Unfortunately, the mental foramen is often quite small and difficult to enter, and thus the majority of anesthetic solution is typically deposited outside of the canal. In that case, diffusion of the anesthetic is hampered by the heavy and dense cortical plate of the mandible, and the net result, particularly in the larger or older adult, may be inconsistent pulpal anesthesia.

ANATOMIC CONSIDERATIONS

The target for the injection is the mental foramen, which is situated immediately below the apex of the mandibular second premolar or just anterior or posterior to it. Because the usual intention of this injection is to anesthetize the incisive nerve within the body of the mandible, the needle must enter the foramen or at least overlie it so that the anesthetic solution will flow into it.

The mental foramen opens superiorly and posteriorly. It can sometimes be palpated, and its location can be estimated from a radiograph. Figure 10–6 illustrates, from a lateral view, the correct placement of the needle. It is often difficult, and generally not recommended, to insert the needle more than 1 to 2 mm into the canal.

TECHNIQUE

This injection is best accomplished with the clinician positioned behind the patient (Fig. 10–7A). The lip is retracted between the thumb and the

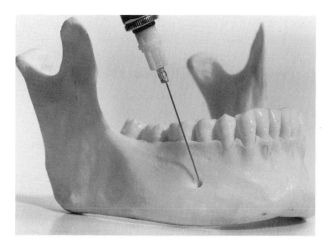

Figure 10–6.   Needle placement for a mental (incisive) nerve block.

forefinger. After applying topical anesthetic and drying the mucosa, the operator inserts the needle into the vestibule approximately 1 cm lateral to the buccal surfaces of the teeth and somewhat distal to the foramen (Fig. 10–7B). A small amount of solution (0.25 mL) is infiltrated to provide local anesthesia of the area. After 20 to 30 seconds, the needle is advanced about 1 cm inferiorly and medially to contact the buccal plate of bone. The entrance to the canal is found by gentle probing. It may be useful to orient the bevel of the needle toward the bone while probing; doing so helps the needle glance off the mandible until a firm positive stop is obtained when the needle tip impinges on the inferior border of the mental foramen.

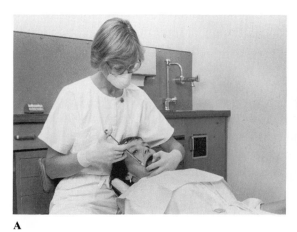

A

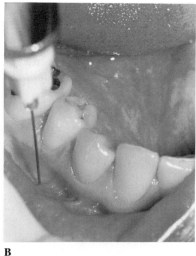

B

Figure 10–7.   Mental (incisive) nerve block. **A.** Operator position. **B.** Intraoral view.

After a negative aspiration, 1.0 mL of anesthetic solution is slowly injected, and the needle is then slowly removed. A supraperiosteal injection in the central incisor region may be necessary to provide complete anesthesia of that area because of possible cross-innervation from the contralateral incisive nerve.

AREA AND SIGNS OF ANESTHESIA

A satisfactory mental-incisive nerve block will provide pulpal anesthesia of the mandibular incisors, canine, and variably the first and second premolars and their investing bone and periodontal ligaments. Soft tissue anesthesia includes the facial gingiva and mucosa of these teeth and the lower lip to the midline (Fig. 10–8). The full extent of anesthesia of the anterior cheek depends on the relative contributions to the area by the buccal and mental nerves.

Buccal Nerve Block

Anesthesia of the cheek and posterior buccal mucous membranes is accomplished by blocking the buccal nerve (sometimes referred to as the long buccal nerve). The injection is often reserved for those situations in which the buccal gingiva and mucosa are directly manipulated. However, many clinicians routinely block the nerve to reduce discomfort associated with conservative dental treatment (e.g., gingival irritation from a rubber dam clamp or retraction cord placement) and to anesthetize any fibers providing accessory innervation to the posterior teeth. The success rate of this injection is very high, regardless of the exact technique selected to achieve anesthesia. If carefully administered, it is also a relatively painless injection.

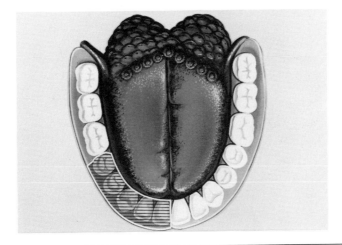

Figure 10–8.   Approximate area of anesthesia after a mental (incisive) nerve block.

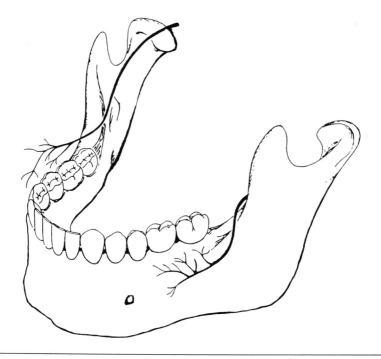

Figure 10–9.   Diagram of the buccal nerve as it crosses the coronoid notch anteriorly.

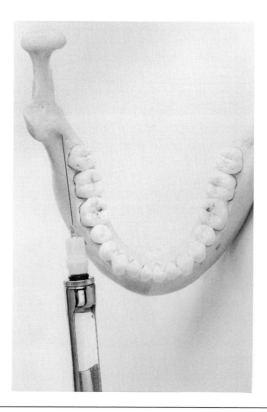

Figure 10–10.   Needle placement for a buccal nerve block at the coronoid notch.

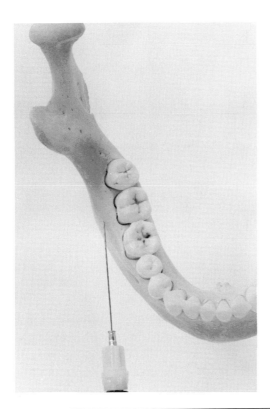

Figure 10–11.   Needle placement for a buccal nerve block in the vestibule area.

ANATOMIC CONSIDERATIONS

The buccal nerve crosses the deep tendon of the temporalis, retromolar triangle, and oblique line (external oblique ridge) at about the level of the occlusal plane. After emerging onto the external surface of the buccinator from underneath the masseter muscle, the nerve ramifies to supply the cheek and to send branches medially through the buccinator to innervate the vestibule and buccal alveolar mucosa in the molar region.

Figure 10–9 demonstrates the usual pathway taken by the buccal nerve. It is obvious that depositing anesthetic solution anywhere along the course of the nerve will block impulses originating distal to the blockade. Hence, the nerve can be injected as it crosses the anterior border of the ramus (Fig. 10–10), submucosally in the cheek 1 cm below the parotid duct, or in the buccal vestibule (Fig. 10–11).

TECHNIQUE

Two of the several methods for anesthetizing the buccal nerve or its peripheral branches will be detailed. The first approach blocks the nerve just medially to the oblique line of the ramus (Fig. 10–12). The buccal fat

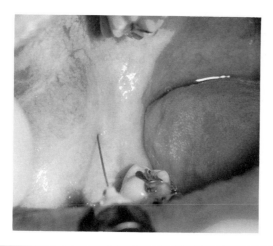

Figure 10–12. Intraoral view of a buccal nerve block at the coronoid notch.

pad and cheek are retracted by the operator's thumb or forefinger. Topical anesthesia is applied and the area is dried with sterile gauze. Needle puncture is made lateral and generally distal to the last mandibular molar at the level of the occlusal plane. The insertion depth is limited to 2 to 3 mm by the anterior border of the ramus. After a negative aspiration, about 0.5 mL of solution is slowly injected. The needle is then removed slowly.

The second method of providing buccal anesthesia is to inject the anesthetic solution submucosally in the depth of the vestibule at or just distal to the tooth of interest (Fig. 10–13). In this case, terminal branches of the buccal nerve are blocked, and the area of anesthesia is more limited. After preparing the tissues as before, the cheek is reflected later-

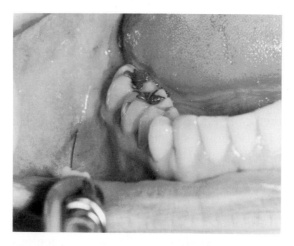

Figure 10–13. Intraoral view of a buccal nerve block in the mandibular vestibule.

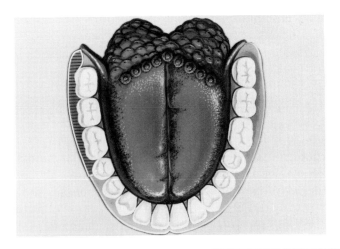

Figure 10–14. Approximate area of anesthesia after a buccal nerve block.

ally with the thumb and forefinger, and the needle is inserted just under the mucosa.

AREA AND SIGNS OF ANESTHESIA

The area of anesthesia produced by a complete buccal block is indicated in Figure 10–14. The anterior and posterior extent of anesthesia is variable, depending on the distributions of the mental nerve and gingival branch of the posterior superior alveolar nerve. Because some accessory innervation to the mandible may be blocked when the injection is made in the retromolar area, a decreased responsiveness to noxious stimuli may be noted, especially during the treatment of mandibular third molars (see Chapter 11). The more limited area of anesthesia obtained with vestibular injections often excludes much of the cheek, and accessory nerve fibers to the mandibular teeth are less likely to be affected.

Because the buccal nerve provides sensation to a restricted area, patients do not often perceive numbness. Indeed, buccal nerves permanently injured during surgery or trauma rarely cause noticeable symptoms for patients, most of whom are largely unaware of the loss of sensation. Ergo, the only consistent finding of anesthesia after a buccal block is the lack of pain during physical manipulation of buccal tissues.

Mandibular Nerve Block Anesthesia

Blockade of the inferior alveolar nerve is the single most commonly desired goal of mandibular anesthesia. It is also one of the most difficult to achieve. A variety of different intraoral injection techniques have been developed, but in all cases the target site for the inferior alveolar block is within the pterygomandibular space. A thorough understanding of this space and its contents is helpful in performing nerve block successfully and is indispensable in comprehending the possible causes for failure of anesthesia.[1]

THE PTERYGOMANDIBULAR SPACE

The pterygomandibular space (Fig. 10–15) is bounded medially by the medial pterygoid muscle, laterally by the mandibular ramus, superiorly by the lateral pterygoid muscle, and posteriorly by the parotid gland (which fills the retromandibular space and encompasses the external carotid artery, retromandibular vein, and facial nerve). Anteriorly, it is separated from the mouth by the oral mucosa, submucosal connective tissue, and a rather thin sheet of buccinator muscle. Within the pterygomandibular space are found the inferior alveolar and lingual nerves, the inferior alveolar artery and vein, and the sphenomandibular ligament. The remainder of the space is primarily filled with loose connective tissue and fat.

After separating from each other, the inferior alveolar and lingual nerves enter the pterygomandibular space by passing through a narrow cleft between the medial and lateral pterygoid muscles. The lingual nerve lies anterior and medial to the inferior alveolar nerve and follows a downward and lateral course through the space until it reaches the most anterior and inferior corner, where it exits forward into the floor of the

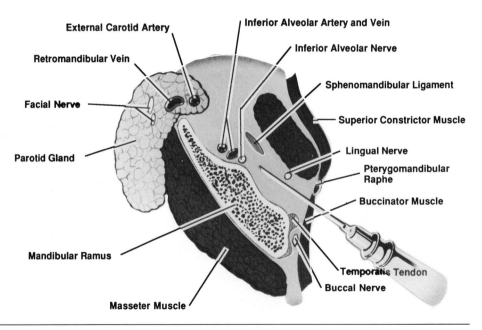

Figure 10–15. Transverse section of the pterygomandibular space and surrounding structures approximately 1 cm above the occlusal plane.

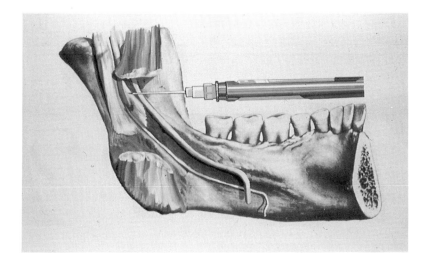

Figure 10–16. Medial view of the pterygomandibular space and mandible. A portion of the medial pterygoid muscle has been cut away to show the sphenomandibular ligament and the inferior alveolar, lingual, and mylohyoid nerves. The mandibular foramen and portions of the inferior alveolar and mylohyoid nerves normally covered by the sphenomandibular ligament are represented in shadow. The buccal nerve and the inferior alveolar blood vessels are not shown.

mouth. The inferior alveolar nerve passes laterally and downward in a slight S-shaped configuration until it reaches the ramus just behind and below the lingula, a bony projection in front of and superior to the mandibular foramen. The lingula serves as the attachment for the sphenomandibular ligament, which originates from the angular spine of the sphenoid bone. The lateral and downward convergence of the inferior alveolar nerve is approximated by a similar orientation of the medial pterygoid muscle and the sphenomandibular ligament, both of which lie medial to the nerve (Fig. 10–16).

Somewhat posterior and lateral to the inferior alveolar nerve are the accompanying artery and vein, all of which enter the ramus via the mandibular foramen. Before disappearing within the ramus, the inferior alveolar nerve gives off the mylohyoid nerve. This nerve penetrates the attachment of the sphenomandibular ligament inferiorly and courses downward and forward within the mylohyoid groove on the medial surface of the mandible.

OVERVIEW OF INJECTION TECHNIQUES

Several distinct approaches are possible for providing mandibular nerve blockade. With the so-called standard or orthodox approach, the most frequent description for this technique is "inferior alveolar nerve block." However, this terminology implies that only a single nerve (the inferior alveolar) is affected by the anesthetic. In fact, it is standard protocol for

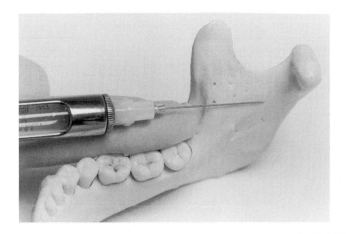

Figure 10-17.   Needle placement for a Clarke and Holmes high mandibular nerve block.

the lingual nerve to be anesthetized at the same time. Additionally, the buccal nerve is often injected during the administration of most inferior alveolar blocks, but by a separate and discrete injection of its own (see previous discussion under Buccal Nerve Block).

To further complicate this looseness of terminology, various "high" nerve block techniques have been described. These high blocks, although differing in approach from each other, anesthetize both the inferior alveolar and lingual nerve simultaneously and, in certain circumstances, also the buccal nerve without a separate injection. For example, Clarke and Holmes advocated a two-step injection technique in which the needle is advanced just medially to the ramus to end up just below the origin of the condylar neck and approximately 2 cm above the lingula and mandibular sulcus (Fig. 10–17).[2] Subsequently, George Gow-Gates described a "new" technique for mandibular conduction anesthesia.[3] The claim was made that this method was more reliable, less painful, and had the advantage of anesthetizing both lingual and inferior alveolar nerves simultaneously. Similarly, Vazirani in 1960[4] and Akinosi in 1977[5] each described the same "new" technique in which the mouth was kept closed during the injection, thus permitting mandibular nerve block anesthesia in patients who are unable to open their mouths (e.g., those with trismus from infection, hematoma, or tumor).

Three mandibular nerve block techniques are described separately below. Chapter 12 discusses the reported benefits of these differing techniques and suggestions for their selective use.

Standard Inferior Alveolar (Lingual) Nerve Block

This injection technique provides pain control for dental procedures on the mandible from the retromolar region to the midline. When accompa-

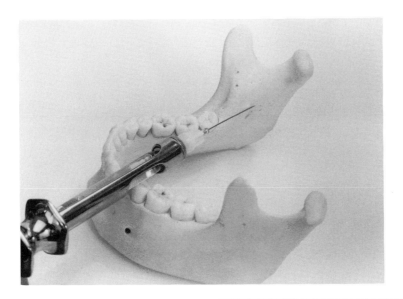

Figure 10–18.   Needle placement for a standard inferior alveolar (lingual) nerve block.

nied by a separate buccal nerve block, pain control encompasses the posterior buccal tissues, anterior labial region, and lingual areas to the midline with a single anesthetic procedure.

ANATOMIC CONSIDERATIONS

The needle end-point is the mandibular sulcus just behind the lingula. Within this depression, and partly covered by the lingula, is the mandibular foramen through which the inferior alveolar nerve, artery, and vein pass (Figs. 10–18 and 10–19).

Unlike the inferior alveolar nerve, the lingual nerve lies somewhat anterior to the lingula and does not enter the mandibular bone but instead courses downward and into the floor of the mouth. Thus, after depositing anesthetic solution adjacent to the mandibular foramen to anesthetize the inferior alveolar nerve, the operator withdraws the needle half-way, so that the tip lies about 1 cm anterior to the lingula, where the lingual nerve resides at this height within the pterygomandibular space.

TECHNIQUE

Although several variations on the standard technique have been described, the one that is most commonly employed is the direct approach in which the needle is advanced along a straight line to a point where the tip lies just over the mandibular foramen. Landmarks that need to be identified or palpated within the oral cavity include the deep tendon of the temporalis muscle located on the temporal crest of the ramus and,

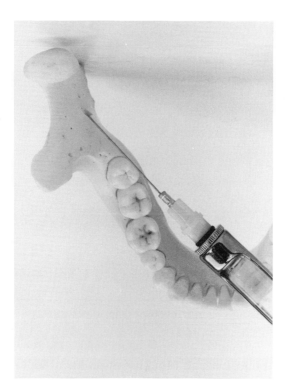

Figure 10–19. Superior view of the inferior alveolar (lingual) nerve block. The needle-syringe axis approaches the mandibular sulcus from the contralateral premolars.

just lateral to it, the coronoid notch of the ramus. Also visualized should be the pterygomandibular raphe (Fig. 10–20). Although challenged as not being a truly distinct entity, this roll of soft tissue running from just behind the mandibular third molar superiorly and medially to blend with

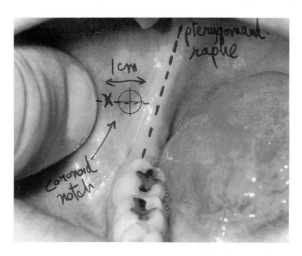

Figure 10–20. The insertion point for a standard inferior alveolar (lingual) nerve block just lateral to the pterygomandibular raphe. The clinician's thumb is retracting the mucosa laterally.

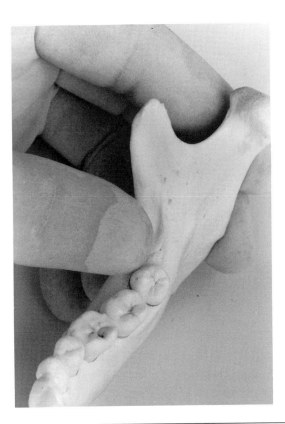

Figure 10–21. Hand position for a standard inferior alveolar (lingual) nerve block demonstrated on a mandible. The thumb is positioned over the coronoid notch, and the fingers are behind the ramus.

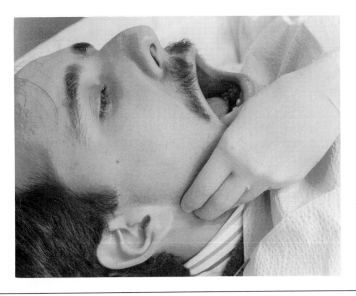

Figure 10–22. Extraoral view of the hand position during a standard inferior alveolar (lingual) nerve block.

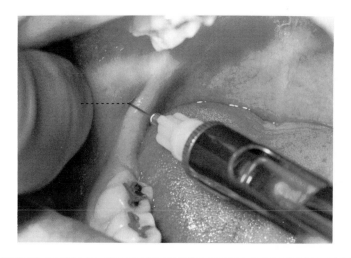

Figure 10–23.   Intraoral view of a standard inferior alveolar (lingual) nerve block. The height of insertion is determined by an imaginary line bisecting the thumb placed in the deepest concavity of the coronoid notch.

the soft palate is a convenient structure for delineating the medial border of the pterygomandibular space. In preparation for the injection, the posterior ramus is grasped by the operator's free hand and the thumb placed in the mouth to retract laterally the cheek and the underlying loose connective tissue and fat pad. The thumb then lies directly over the coronoid notch; just medially to it is the retromolar fossa, and medially to that the raphe (Figs. 10–20 through 10–22). Properly positioned, the thumb is parallel to mandibular occlusal plane and in the greatest concavity of the coronoid notch.

After placement of topical anesthetic and drying the area with gauze, the needle is inserted at a height approximating an imaginary line running through the bisected thumbnail (Fig. 10–23). This usually places the needle at least 1 cm above the mandibular occlusal plane. With the syringe and needle axis oriented from the opposing lower premolars, the needle is advanced gently through mucosa, buccinator muscle, and areolar tissue within the pterygomandibular space until it contacts bone at a depth of 2 to 2.5 cm. Then the needle is withdrawn slightly, aspiration performed and if negative, 1.0 to 1.5 mL of anesthetic solution injected at the rate of 2 mL/min or less. In some instances, owing to variations in ramus divergence with the mandibular body, ramus bone will not be contacted. Nevertheless, it usually is not necessary to insert the needle more than 2.5 cm, as it will still be adjacent to the mandibular foramen. Deeper needle placement will occasionally result in penetration of the parotid capsule and transient anesthesia of the seventh cranial (facial) nerve (see Chapter 13 for a discussion of facial paralysis). In contrast, inserting the needle in a too lateral approach will cause it to strike the temporal crest

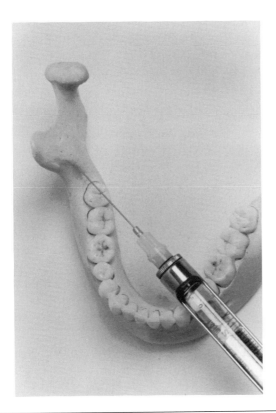

Figure 10–24. Standard inferior alveolar (lingual) nerve block: excessively lateral needle axis with the tip striking the anterior ramus.

of the ramus before sufficient depth is achieved (Fig. 10–24). If this occurs, partial withdrawal and reinsertion in a slightly more medial direction will permit the needle to bypass this structure and reach a terminal position just adjacent to the mandibular foramen.

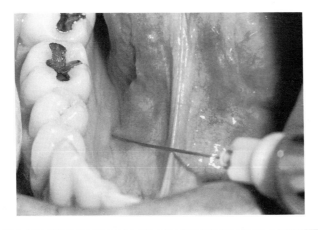

Figure 10–25. Clinical view of a partial lingual nerve block.

Although the lingual nerve is often simultaneously anesthetized when solution is injected at the mandibular foramen area, it is usual practice to inject additional anesthetic (0.3 to 0.5 mL) when the needle has been withdrawn half-way (and after a second aspiration attempt). Alternatively, the lingual nerve can be anesthetized just as it enters the floor of the mouth by injecting 0.3 to 0.5 mL of solution under the posterior lingual mucosa (Fig. 10–25). However, this injection technique is typically used only when the inferior alveolar nerve is not anesthetized and only lingual soft-tissue anesthesia is required.

AREA AND SIGNS OF ANESTHESIA

A satisfactory inferior alveolar (and lingual) nerve block provides bony, periodontal, and pulpal anesthesia of all mandibular molars, premolars, cuspid, and incisors on the side of the injection to midline. It also provides anesthesia of buccal/labial soft tissues served by the mental nerve and, with a lingual nerve blockade, the anterior two thirds of the tongue, floor of the mouth, and lingual gingiva (Figs. 10–26 and 10–27). However, supplementary anesthesia may be occasionally necessary in two instances. Mandibular central incisors occasionally receive cross-innervation from the contralateral side, requiring a supraperiosteal injection near the midline. Similarly, procedures performed on the mandibular second and third molars often require supplemental anesthesia of the buccal nerve or the initial use of a high mandibular block owing to inferior alveolar nerve branches originating in separate paths and not a part of the main nerve trunk (see Chapter 12).

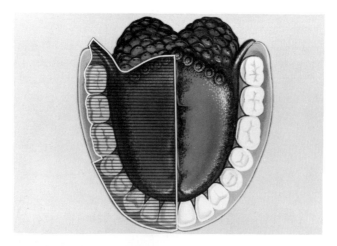

Figure 10–26. Approximate intraoral area of anesthesia after a standard inferior alveolar (lingual) nerve block.

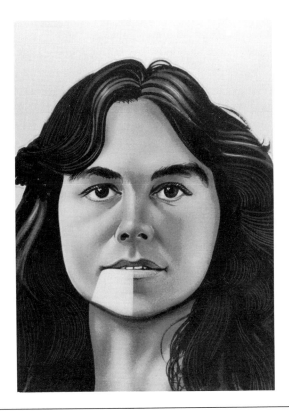

Figure 10–27. Facial view of lip anesthesia after an inferior alveolar nerve block.

Gow-Gates Mandibular Nerve Block

This technique is considered a high mandibular block, with needle placement considerably above that used for the standard inferior alveolar nerve block. The Gow-Gates injection has been reported to be more reliable and less uncomfortable for the patient. Its main disadvantages are difficulty in learning the technique and the possible requirement for more anesthetic solution for large patients than is contained in a 1.8-mL anesthetic cartridge. (Dr. Gow-Gates, an Australian, used an anesthetic cartridge containing 2.2 mL of anesthetic solution that is marketed in that country.)

ANATOMIC CONSIDERATIONS

The needle end-point is within the upper portion of the pterygomandibular space at the neck of the mandibular condyle just below the insertion of the external pterygoid muscle (Fig. 10–28). Although this end-point is at least 1 cm from the trunks of the inferior alveolar, lingual, and buccal nerves, the lack of restricting fascia within the pterygomandibular space at that height permits easy distribution of the anesthetic in a downward, forward, and medial direction. In this regard, the pterygomandibular

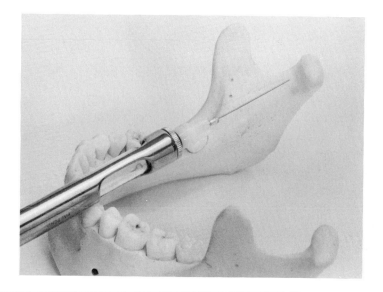

Figure 10–28. Needle placement for a Gow-Gates mandibular nerve block.

space has been estimated to contain a volume of about 2 mL.[6] Therefore 1.8 mL of anesthetic solution would mostly fill this space in an average-sized individual and anesthetize all the nerves within the area. Also, the condylar neck used as a target in this technique provides a definitive landmark absent in the alternative approaches. The patient is asked to open his or her mouth as widely as possible. The intertragic notch and the corners of the mouth then define a plane in which the needle will be aligned.

TECHNIQUE

A useful aid is to palpate the anterior border of the ramus with the thumb and to place the index finger on the intertragic notch. The tip of the finger then provides a tactile as well as a visual target for the needle. In fact, when this technique is used, the index finger usually lies directly over the lateral pole of the condyle (Figs. 10–29 and 10–30). After placement of topical anesthetic and drying the mucosa with gauze, the needle puncture is made medial to the deep tendon of the temporalis but considerably superior and lateral to the point used for the standard inferior alveolar nerve block. Normally, the insertion point is slightly distal to the maxillary second molar at the level of its mesiolingual cusp. Its exact location, however, is established by extraoral landmarks.

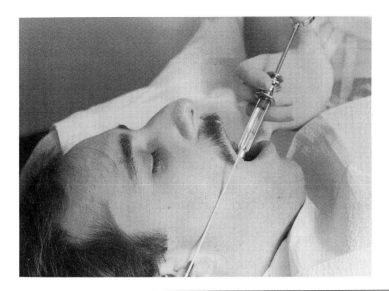

Figure 10–29. Gow-Gates mandibular nerve block. The needle-syringe axis is aligned to a line connecting the corner of the mouth and intertragic notch of the ear when the patient's mouth is open widely.

With the syringe oriented toward the intertragic notch (or the "target" finger) in the plane formed by the notch and the angles of the mouth wide open, the needle is slowly advanced until the neck of the condyle is reached, at a depth of insertion of about 2.5 cm. Then the needle is

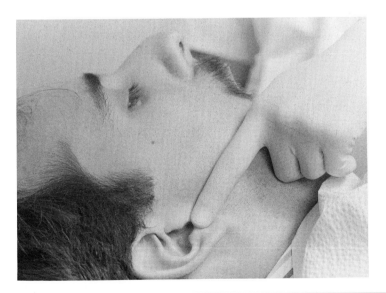

Figure 10–30. Extraoral hand position for the Gow-Gates mandibular nerve block.

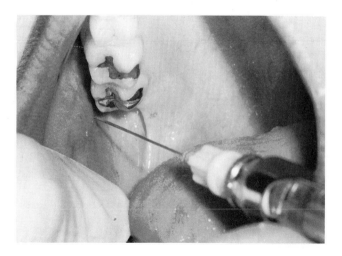

Figure 10–31.   Intraoral view of a Gow-Gates mandibular nerve block.

withdrawn slightly, and after a negative aspiration, the full cartridge is injected. Figure 10–31 illustrates the needle insertion 1 to 2 cm superior to that of a standard inferior alveolar block and just below the maxillary second molar. When using the Gow-Gates block, the clinician must estimate the divergence of the mandibular ramus from the body of the mandible. Gow-Gates and Watson[6] have stipulated that this angulation is paralleled by the orientation of the patient's tragus of the ear. Thus a flat tragus (and ramus) would require a needle axis originating over the contralateral mandibular canine (Fig. 10-32A), and a widely divergent tragus (and ramus) would require a more acute angle, achieved by placing the

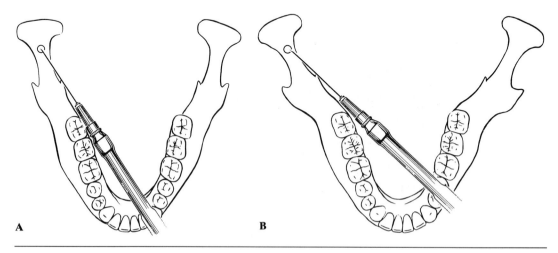

A   B

Figure 10–32.   Lateral angulation for the Gow-Gates mandibular nerve block. **A.** Needle orientation for a mandibular ramus (and tragus) with a relatively shallow divergence. **B.** Needle orientation for a mandibular ramus (and tragus) with a wide divergence.

syringe barrel over the contralateral premolars or even the first molar (Fig. 10–32B). In fact, the novice often has difficulty with this aspect of the technique and should consider that the needle axis may be either too shallow or too great if bone is not contacted. In such instances, repositioning of the needle axis is required.

To facilitate flow of the anesthetic around the nerves, the patient's mouth should be kept open for 30 seconds after injection. Because of the proximity of the maxillary artery, its accessory and middle meningeal branches, and the pterygoid plexus of veins, it is of paramount importance that careful aspiration be performed before administration of the local anesthetic.

AREA AND SIGNS OF ANESTHESIA

Although not a complete third division nerve block, this technique will often affect all three nerves providing sensation to mandibular structures of dental interest. It also has the advantage of anesthetic solution deposition high enough in the pterygomandibular space that unusual or aberrant sensory paths may be anesthetized. Figure 10–33 illustrates the cutane-

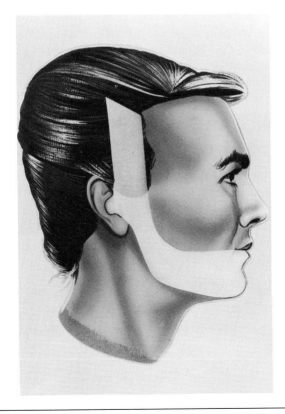

Figure 10–33. Approximate cutaneous distribution of anesthesia after a Gow-Gates mandibular nerve block.

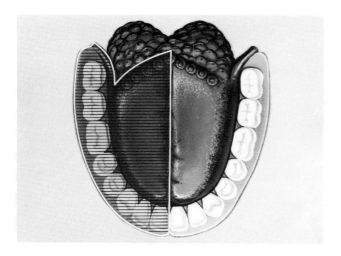

Figure 10–34.   Approximate intraoral area of anesthesia after a Gow-Gates mandibular block.

ous distribution, and Figure 10–34 the intraoral distribution, of a typical Gow-Gates mandibular block. The patient experiences a sensation of numbness from the midline laterally, which includes all teeth, periodontium, (usually) buccal and lingual soft tissue. The peripheral distributions of the mental and often the buccal and auriculotemporal nerves are also anesthetized. In some instances, especially with large individuals, anesthesia of the buccal nerve may be incomplete, and supplemental anesthesia may be necessary.

The Closed-Mouth Mandibular Nerve Block (Vazirani-Akinosi Technique)

The closed-mouth mandibular nerve block permits mandibular anesthesia to be achieved in patients who have difficulty opening their mouths (e.g., those with trismus) or who will not cooperate (young children). Although this technique is convenient and satisfactory for routine use, most clinicians tend to rely on it during specific instances of limited mouth opening.

ANATOMIC CONSIDERATIONS

The end-point of the needle lies within the superior portion of the pterygomandibular space. In this respect it is more medial and slightly inferior to the end-point of the Gow-Gates injection (condylar neck). However, the needle position is probably closer to the nerve trunks than with the Gow-Gates technique. Figures 10–35 and 10–36 illustrate the needle position within the pterygomandibular space and relative to the mandible and maxilla. There is normally no point of bony contact during this injection.

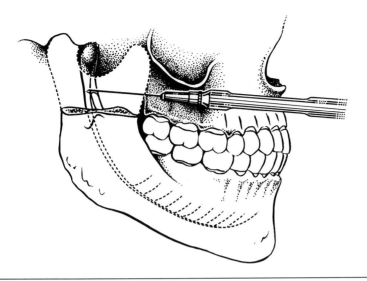

Figure 10–35. Diagram of the mandibular ramus showing the needle end-point during a closed-mouth mandibular nerve block. The buccal and mylohyoid nerves are not shown.

TECHNIQUE

The patient's teeth should be gently in occlusion, or, if the patient is edentulous, the jaw should be in a comfortable, closed resting position. Once topical anesthesia has taken effect and the mucosa is wiped with sterile gauze, the lip is retracted with the index finger of the operator's free hand, and the needle and syringe are then advanced into the maxil-

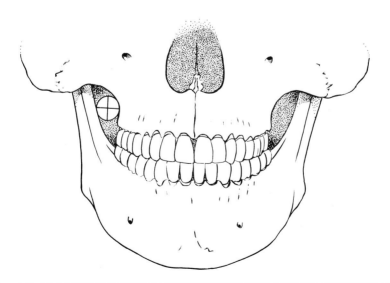

Figure 10–36. Anterior view of the target zone for needle insertion during a closed-mouth mandibular nerve block injection.

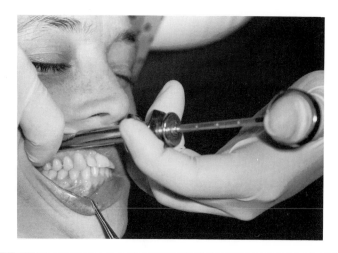

Figure 10-37.   Clinical view of a closed-mouth mandibular nerve block injection.

lary vestibule with the syringe axis parallel to the occlusal plane at the height of the mucogingival junction. The needle passes just under the zygomatic buttress adjacent to the first and second maxillary molars (it should not touch this structure) and penetrates the retromolar mucosa above the injection site for a standard inferior alveolar nerve block (Fig. 10-37). The needle is advanced until the tip is estimated to be halfway between the anterior and posterior borders of the ramus, or approximately 2.5 cm. Because it is difficult to see the needle insertion, the depth can be estimated by the hub of the needle being adjacent (and above) the maxillary second molar.

After injection of 1.8 mL of solution, the syringe is slowly removed. Onset of anesthesia usually occurs within 5 minutes. Technically, this injection, although difficult to visualize, is easier to perform than either the conventional or Gow-Gates technique.

AREA AND SIGNS OF ANESTHESIA

The pattern of sensory nerve anesthesia is similar to that of the Gow-Gates mandibular block (see Fig. 10-34). Both the inferior alveolar and lingual nerves are reliably blocked, and the buccal nerves are reportedly anesthetized in a majority of patients. The auriculotemporal nerve, however, may not be reliably blocked, but it is unimportant for intraoral procedures.

References

1. DuBrul, E.L.: Sicher and DuBrul's Oral Anatomy, 8th ed. St. Louis, Ishiyaku EuroAmerica, Inc., 1988.

2. Clarke, J., and Holmes, G.: Local anesthesia of the mandibular molar teeth: A new technique. Dent Pract., *10*(2):36–38, 1959.
3. Gow-Gates, G.A.E.: Mandibular conduction anesthesia: A new technique using extraoral landmarks. Oral Surg., Oral Med., Oral Pathol., *36*:321–330, 1973.
4. Vazirani, S.J.: Closed mouth mandibular nerve block: A new technique. Dent. Dig. *66*:10–13, 1960.
5. Akinosi, J.O.: A new approach to the mandibular nerve block. Br. J. Oral Surg., *15*:83–87, 1977.
6. Gow-Gates, G.A.E., and Watson, J.E.: The Gow-Gates mandibular block: Further understanding. Anesth. Prog., *24*:183–189, 1977.

Supplemental Injection Techniques

Several methods of providing local anesthesia for selected teeth or in special circumstances are available. These include the periodontal ligament (PDL) or intraligamentary injection, the intraseptal injection, intraosseous anesthesia, and the intrapulpal technique. The PDL and intraseptal injection techniques, although using distinct approaches, are fundamentally intraosseous injections. In both instances a small amount of anesthetic solution is deposited adjacent to the tooth to be anesthetized, and considerable diffusion of the anesthetic solution occurs within alveolar bone, which provides pulpal anesthesia of one or more adjacent teeth and surrounding periodontium. The use of a PDL, intraseptal, or introsseous injection technique is especially helpful when standard supraperiosteal or block anesthesia has failed to provide adequate anesthesia or when it is desirable to avoid the standard techniques (Table 11–1). In addition, a great advantage of these injections is their ability to achieve nearly instantaneous anesthesia of one or two teeth in the mandibular arch without use of the mandibular block technique.

Because supraperiosteal (infiltration) injection techniques are usually unreliable for providing pulpal anesthesia in the mandible (except in young children and in the anterior region of older children and adults), the only realistic alternative has been to administer a mandibular nerve block, which many patients find uncomfortable and inconvenient because of the extensive area of anesthesia. The use of a PDL, intraseptal, or intraosseous injection technique avoids discomfort and provides usable anesthesia when treating a limited area of the mandible. The use of these techniques in the maxillary arch is also possible but less frequent, except in the incisor area, where supraperiosteal injections can be painful. Intrapulpal injections, on the other hand, are almost exclusively used for

Table 11–1. INDICATIONS FOR AND ADVANTAGES OF THE PERIODONTAL LIGAMENT (PDL) INJECTION

1. Reducing patient anxiety about intraoral injections.
2. Only a small quantity of local anesthesia is required, and therefore the technique is useful in the medically compromised patient.
3. Provides a limited area of anesthesia.
4. A substitute for nerve block anesthesia in patients with hemorrhagic disorders (hemophilia).
5. An effective supplement to standard nerve block and supraperiosteal techniques.
6. Useful in children to limit lip anesthesia, which can lead to self-mutilation.

endodontic procedures when supplementary anesthesia is required during pulp canal instrumentation. Intrapulpal injection of anesthetic has no place in routine restorative dentistry on teeth not undergoing endodontic treatment. Although occasional concerns are voiced, PDL injections appear to have few real problems other than their essential limitations of scope. Mild transient postanesthetic sensitivity limited to the tooth or teeth injected may be expected. Pulpal blood flow has been noted to decrease to less than one-half of normal (Table 11–2) when intraseptal injection techniques are used. This is especially true with mandibular molar teeth, where less than 10% of blood flow may result when anesthetics containing a vasoconstrictor are used.[1] However, the clinical significance of these data is not yet clear, as no consistent long-term deleterious effect has been documented to date. Indeed, nearby bone resorption or direct PDL damage from needle insertion and injection can be best described as transient and minimal.

Successful use of either the PDL or intraseptal injection techniques depends on generating a considerable amount of pressure during the injection. In fact, the absence of resistance to the injection with both the PDL and intraseptal techniques is a hallmark of inadequate technique and probable anesthetic failure. Special syringes have been manufactured and marketed for these injections (Ligmaject, Peripress, etc.). They all possess the advantages of a measured (e.g., 0.2 mL) delivery of solution

Table 11–2. COMPARATIVE PULPAL BLOOD FLOW (mL/min-kg) AFTER INJECTION OF 2% LIDOCAINE + 1/100,000 EPINEPHRINE

	Canines		Molars	
	Control	Experimental (% Control)	Control	Experimental (% Control)
Supraperiosteal injection	333	77 (28%)	—	— —
Inferior alveolar nerve block	281	99 (33%)	263	120 (47%)
Intraseptal injection	274	82 (30%)	200	18 (9%)

Data from Kim et al.[1]

with each trigger pull, and a protective shield around the anesthetic cartridge to protect against accidental glass breakage. However:

1. They may appear imposing to the patient, since some resemble a small pistol.
2. They are generally expensive.
3. They generate very high pressure, which may be detrimental to a periodontally compromised tooth.

In this regard, a standard cartridge syringe has been reported to produce a pressure of up to 600 psi during PDL injection.[2] Recently, one manufacturer claimed 25 times the force of a standard syringe, or conceivably as much as 15,000 psi. Excessive injection force or speed of injection can cause unnecessary postoperative pain or undesirable damage to bony structures around the injected tooth. Therefore, such excessive force is best avoided. Despite the considerable pressure necessary, most clinicians have little difficulty achieving a satisfactory PDL or intraseptal injection using a standard cartridge syringe with a 27-gauge short needle. As to the cartridge breakage problem, manufacturers have recently begun coating individual anesthetic cartridges with a plastic laminate that effectively protects against accidental breakage.

One potential hazard with any intraosseous-type injection must be considered. Recent data have convincingly demonstrated that anesthetic solutions given in this manner penetrate the vascular system very rapidly.[2,3] Indeed, local anesthetics containing epinephrine have essentially the same effect pharmacologically as intravenous administration (Fig. 11–1),[4,5] and in spite of the small amount of drug used are clinically important. Thus, patients in whom vasoconstrictor-induced tachycardia or dysrhythmias would constitute a significant risk should not be subjected to an intraosseous-type injection, or, if these injections are absolutely necessary, they should be performed with great care. Intrapulpal injections do not seem to have this same liability.

Finally, concern has been expressed regarding use of the PDL injection where periodontal disease is present. The increase in periodontal pressure apically and the use of a vasoconstrictor may well allow extension of the disease.

Periodontal Ligament Injection

A 27-gauge short or 30-gauge ultrashort needle is placed on either the mesial or distal aspect of a single-rooted tooth and gently wedged between the root and alveolar bone. A total of 0.2 mL of solution is injected (Fig. 11–2). For multirooted teeth, a separate injection is required for each root. Considerable resistance should be encountered when injecting the anesthetic, and blanching normally will occur in the mucosa. Anesthesia is essentially immediate.

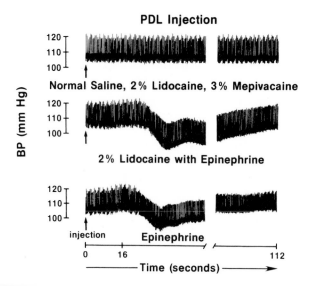

Figure 11–1.   Comparative blood pressure (BP) recordings in dogs given periodontal ligament (PDL) injections of normal saline, 2% lidocaine with and without 1 : 100,000 epinephrine, 3% mepivacaine, and 1 : 100,000 epinephrine alone. Blood pressure changes are solely due to the epinephrine. (Courtesy of Smith, G.N., and Pashley, D.H.: Oral Surg. Oral Med. Oral Pathol., *56*:571–574, 1983.)

AREA AND SIGNS OF ANESTHESIA

The area of anesthesia from a PDL injection is usually restricted to the tooth or teeth adjacent to the injection site. Although the injection of anesthetic with this technique produces surprisingly distant migration, anesthetically usable concentrations are achieved only in the immediate

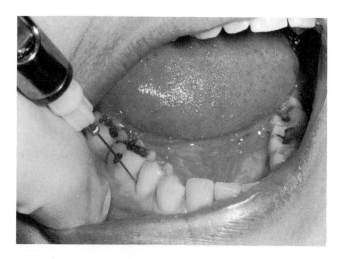

Figure 11–2.   Clinical view of a periodontal ligament injection of the mandibular premolar.

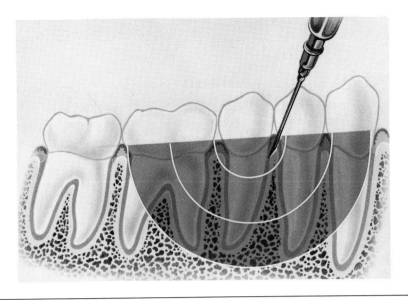

Figure 11–3. Approximate distribution of anesthesia after a single periodontal ligament injection.

area of the injection, including the pulp of the adjacent tooth (teeth), surrounding alveolar bone, gingiva, and periodontium (Fig. 11–3).

Unlike supraperiosteal (infiltration) or block anesthetic techniques, there is little or no sensation of soft-tissue anesthesia of the nearby mucosa, lip, chin, and so forth. However, what soft-tissue anesthesia does occur (periodontal ligament and gingiva) will considerably outlast tooth pulp anesthesia, much as occurs with a supraperiosteal or block anesthetic technique.

Intraseptal Injection

Although essentially producing the same anesthetic result as a PDL injection, the intraseptal technique is slightly different. A puncture is made at about 90 degrees to the intraseptal gingiva between the teeth to be anesthetized and 2 to 4 mm below the gingival crest (Figs. 11–4 through 11–6). The actual site of the injection depends on the underlying crestal bone, which may vary considerably because of periodontal disease. Preoperative periapical or bitewing radiographs may be helpful in determining the intraseptal bone height. A 27-gauge short needle is most conveniently used. The needle is advanced slowly while a small amount of anesthetic solution is injected within the soft tissue of the papilla. After bone is contacted, the needle is pushed 1 or 2 mm into the intraseptal bone. Then, 0.2 to 0.4 mL of anesthetic is slowly injected. If no resis-

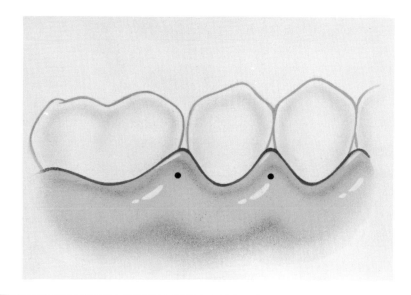

Figure 11–4.   Buccal view showing needle insertion points for an intraseptal injection.

tance to injection is encountered, the needle is unlikely to be within bone and should be repositioned or inserted more deeply. This injection is likely to be less detrimental to periodontally involved teeth than the PDL injection.

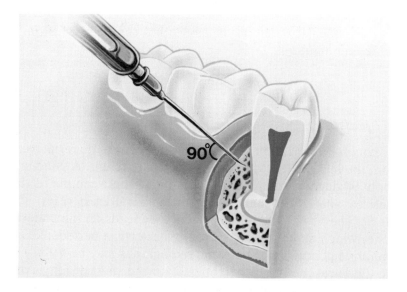

Figure 11–5.   Diagram of needle position during an intraseptal injection. The needle is inserted at a 90-degree angle to the gingival surface.

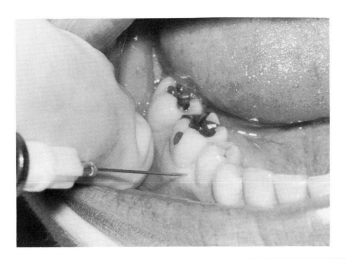

Figure 11-6.   Clinical view of an intraseptal injection.

AREA AND SIGNS OF ANESTHESIA

The intraseptal technique produces an onset and area of anesthesia essentially identical to that of the PDL injection technique (see Fig. 11–3). Also similar to that injection, little soft-tissue anesthesia is perceived by the patient.

Intraosseous Injection

The original method of intraosseous anesthesia used a small round bur to drill a hole through surgically exposed cortical bone. Recently, a new technique has been developed that is less invasive and solves many of the problems previously associated with intraosseous anesthesia. It employs an introducer device to make the hole in the cortical bone and an ultra-short needle to facilitate injection of the anesthetic (Fig. 11-7). The introducer (perforator) is a 27-gauge solid core needle mounted on a plastic shank that fits into a standard slow-speed, contraangle handpiece. The needle portion is approximately 8 mm in length and is supplied capped and sterile from the manufacturer. The injection needle is the same length and diameter as the perforating needle.

The injection site should be next to the tooth of interest, equidistant between it and the adjacent tooth. All injections are initiated 2 mm below a line connecting the gingival margins of the teeth bracketing the injection site. If anesthesia of the soft tissue has not been achieved previously, a small amount of local anesthetic is injected into the gingiva at the injection site. Prior application of a topical anesthetic may minimize discomfort with the injection.

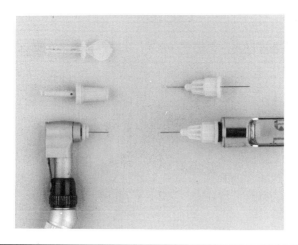

Figure 11–7.   Intraosseous injection system. *Left,* introducer devices. *Right,* intraosseous needles.

Two perforation methods have been described. For one approach, the introducer tip is held perpendicular to the surface at the injection site and is pushed through the gingiva, periosteum, and buccal plate by a short series of brief, sharp bursts of the handpiece. Perforation is complete when there is a sudden loss of resistance, indicating that the cancellous bone has been reached. With the second approach, the introducer is angled such that the needle tip will achieve a more apical position. An angle of 35 degrees to the alveolus is used for all maxillary injections. In the mandible, a very acute angle (10 degrees) is used in the incisor region, shifting incrementally to a 60-degree angle in the posterior molar region where the cortical plate is particularly dense. Once the proper angulation is achieved, the penetrator needle is introduced through the soft tissues and bone with light pressure and a slow revolution rate. Penetration continues until the collar of the introducer abuts the gingiva (Fig. 11-8A). After the perforation is made, the penetrator is removed, and the anesthetic needle is inserted into the hole along the same pathway as the penetrator needle using a pen grasp. The anesthetic is then injected slowly (Fig. 11-8B).

Certain areas of the mouth do not lend themselves to this technique. Intraosseous penetration is not recommended in the midline, near the location of the mental foramen, in the maxillary sinus area where penetration of the sinus is likely, and wherever adjacent teeth are so close that penetration of the periodontal ligament space becomes hard to avoid.

AREA AND SIGNS OF ANESTHESIA

The area of anesthesia after an intraosseous injection is determined in part by the volume of solution administered. A quarter to a third of a cartridge is sufficient for anesthesia of a single tooth or two adjacent

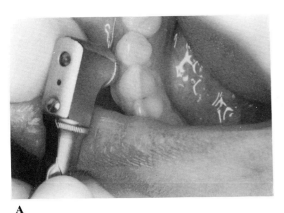 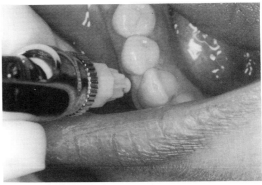

A   **B**

Figure 11–8.   Intraosseous injection. **A.** The introducer is used to penetrate the cortical bone. **B.** The needle is inserted in the hole for injection of the anesthetic.

teeth. A single injection of up to one cartridge can also be effective for multiple tooth anesthesia (up to eight in a maxillary quadrant). Multiple injections are required to anesthetize teeth in more than one quadrant. For instance, bilateral mandibular injections between the canine and first premolar can anesthetize the six anterior teeth and the first premolars.

Intrapulpal Injection

Intrapulpal injection of local anesthetic solution is helpful in endodontic patients to facilitate pain control during instrumentation of the tooth pulp. The needle can be placed in a natural (carious) pulp exposure, but technically the injection is better when a small pinpoint opening is made into the pulp chamber. The smaller the opening into the pulp chamber the better, for it allows pressure to build up within the pulp chamber. Larger openings allow the anesthetic solution to escape. The needle is gently inserted through the hole and wedged against the pulp canal walls. A small amount of anesthetic solution is injected under considerable pressure. In fact, it may be the pressure effect more than the anesthetic effect that produces pulpal anesthesia, as endodontists have had good success with this technique using a saline solution instead of an anesthetic. There may be a brief period of pain with the initiation of the injection, but this can be diminished to some extent by applying a cotton pledget soaked in local anesthetic to the exposure site. After injection, one can immediately proceed with the endodontic procedure (Fig. 11–9).

AREA AND SIGNS OF ANESTHESIA

Because the amount of anesthetic injected is quite small and because an intrapulpal injection technique is always used as a supplement to other

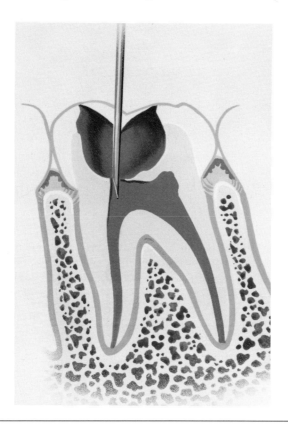

Figure 11–9.   Needle placement in the pulp canal of a mandibular molar. The small hole into the pulp is just large enough to permit the needle to pass through it.

(preceding) injections, the area of anesthesia is only definable by the patient having less or no pain during actual pulpal instrumentation. It is doubtful that a significant amount of anesthetic exits the pulp apex and contributes to the anesthesia of surrounding tissues.

Intrapapillary Infiltration

This is a simple technique in which the interdental papilla is injected with a small amount of anesthetic containing a vasoconstrictor until the papilla visually blanches. This technique is particularly useful with periodontal procedures in which profound hemostasis is desired. It is commonly used after supraperiosteal or nerve block anesthesia has been achieved (for pain control). All interdental papillae in the area to be treated are injected separately. It may also be used before application of a rubber dam clamp if the soft tissues involved are not already anesthetized.

Jet Injection

Although theoretically available to dentists since the late 1950s, the jet injection technique has never achieved much popularity because of cost and significant limitations to its use. Although pushing a small quantity (0.05 mL) of anesthetic under high pressure through very tiny holes will permit its passage through mucosa without the use of a needle, the only real use of this technique is for infiltration anesthesia of a limited area. The technique tends to be more successful in children than in adults, probably owing to the greater porosity of bone in children. Because the typical supraperiosteal injection can be administered painlessly, especially with prior use of a topical anesthetic, and because it has much more capability and flexibility than a jet technique, the use of a jet injector is uncommon. It is particularly useful, however, for palatal injections, rendering them almost totally painless.

Another earlier disadvantage of these syringes was the explosive noise that occurred on injection, but this has been controlled in more recent models.

References

1. Kim, S., Edwall, L., Trowbridge, H., and Chien, S.: Effects of local anesthetics on pulpal blood flow in dogs. J. Dent. Res., *63*:650–652, 1984.
2. Smith, G.N., and Walton, R.E.: Periodontal ligament injection: Distribution of injected solutions. Oral Surg. Oral Med. Oral Pathol., *55*:232–238, 1983.
3. Rawson, R.D., and Orr, D.L.: Vascular penetration following intraligamental injection. J. Oral Maxillofac. Surg., *43*:600–604, 1985.
4. Smith, G.H., and Pashley, D.H.: Periodontal ligament injection: Evaluation of systemic effects. Oral Surg. Oral Med. Oral Pathol., *56*:571–574, 1983.
5. Pashley, D.H.: Systemic effects of intraligamentary injections. J Endod., *12*:501–504, 1986.

Choice of Anesthetic Technique and Causes of Anesthetic Failure

Prior chapters in this text have dealt with various technical considerations of local anesthetic injections and the resulting distribution of anesthesia. However, experienced clinicians normally base both the choice of specific injection technique and the ultimate amount of anesthetic administered on the requirements of the patient and the anticipated procedure. The anesthetic needs for preparing a premolar for an amalgam restoration are quite different from those for oral or periodontal surgery involving tissues with a wider sensory distribution or for the endodontic treatment of inflamed teeth, which are more subject to incomplete anesthesia. Within limits, a simple commonsense rule is that the more extensive a procedure, the more anesthetic will be needed. For example, an occlusal restoration of the mandibular first molar would usually be accompanied by an inferior alveolar nerve block in which 1.0 to 1.5 mL of anesthetic is deposited at the mandibular foramen. However, if lingual and buccal soft tissue trauma is expected to be minimal or absent, the lingual and buccal nerves would not necessarily need any special attention and could remain unanesthetized. As an alternative, a periodontal ligament injection of the specific tooth to be treated could substitute in many circumstances for an inferior alveolar nerve block. In contrast, surgical extraction, periodontal surgery, bone biopsy, and other procedures that include significant manipulation of both the tooth and its adjacent structures require not only an inferior alveolar nerve block but profound anesthesia of the lingual and buccal tissues as well.

Control of hemorrhage is often a factor in the choice of both anesthetic solution and injection technique. Thus, the restorative dentist who desires pulpal anesthesia but expects to perform little or no gingival manipulation can opt for a drug not containing a vasoconstrictor and considerably limit the amount and distributon of anesthetic administered. On the other hand, the clinician performing a quadrant of periodontal flap surgery, intraseptal bone contouring, and root curettage not only needs adequate pulpal and bony anesthesia from the nerve block but will find it most useful to provide extensive soft tissue infiltration with an anesthetic containing a vasoconstrictor. This provides supplementary anesthesia in some cases but, more important, controls the hemorrhage from large areas of exposed soft tissue. The net effect is often better visibility, faster completion of the procedure, and in the end, greater patient comfort.

Anesthesia of the maxillary teeth and soft tissues is an excellent example of technique selection under different operating conditions. Uncomplicated restorative treatment of a minor carious lesion can usually be accomplished with a small amount (0.5 mL) of anesthetic solution administered supraperiosteally adjacent to the specific tooth involved. However, if the tooth has a pulpitis or the adjacent soft tissues are abscessed, supraperiosteal anesthesia may be ineffectual, whether endodontic treatment or surgical removal is planned. In such circumstances, an infraorbital nerve block (anterior teeth) or a maxillary nerve block (posterior teeth) may be required to anesthetize the area to be treated. Likewise, the volume of anesthetic needed will doubtlessly be greater.

The sometimes difficult choice of providing palatal soft tissue anesthesia also depends on treatment needs. Because both the nasopalatine (incisive) and greater palatine nerve block injections are quite uncomfortable for many patients, clinicians tend to avoid their use unless there is an absolute need for palatal soft tissue anesthesia. Thus, uncomplicated restorative treatment of maxillary teeth is often done simply by buccal/labial supraperiosteal anesthesia without the use of these palatal injections. On the other hand, dental extraction or other surgical intervention, gingival retraction or recontouring during crown preparation, and periodontal curettage all require palatal anesthesia. Tables 12–1 and 12–2 list examples of normal recommended anesthetic techniques under different treatment conditions. It should be appreciated from the preceding discussion that several options may be available for any particular set of circumstances.

Failure of Anesthesia

Anesthetic injections in the oral cavity occasionally fail to produce the desired result. If the operator is a novice, the most likely cause of unsatisfactory anesthesia is incorrect placement of the needle, particularly if conventional landmarks are poorly developed or obscured by overlying tissues. Reinjection in such instances will usually solve the problem. However, even the knowledgeable clinician adept in injection technique

Table 12–1. **SELECTED DENTAL PROCEDURES AND ANESTHETIC TECHNIQUE CHOICES IN THE MAXILLA**

Procedure	Supraperiosteal Injection				Nerve Block				
	Single Tooth	Anterior Superior Alveolar	Middle Superior Alveolar	Posterior Superior Alveolar	Infra-orbital	Maxillary	Greater Palatine	Naso-palatine	Partial Palatine
Conservative treatment of incisors/canines	0.5 mL	1.0 mL						0.2 mL*	0.3 mL*
Surgery or extraction of incisors/canines	1.0 mL	1.0 mL						0.2 mL	0.3 mL†
Conservative treatment of premolars			0.5 mL				0.3–0.5 mL*		0.3 mL*
Surgery or extraction of premolars			1.0 mL				0.3–0.5 mL		0.3 mL†
Conservative treatment of molars	1.0 mL‡			1.0–1.5 mL			0.3–0.5 mL*		0.3 mL*
Surgery or extraction of molars				1.5–1.8 mL§			0.3–0.5 mL		0.3 mL†
Surgical or endodontal treatment of abscessed incisors/canines					1.0–1.5 mL	1.5 mL‖		0.2 mL	0.3 mL†
Nonsurgical or surgical (periodontal) treatment of hemimaxilla						1.5 mL¶			

* Optional, if needed for soft tissue anesthesia.
† Alternative, can be used for palatal soft tissue anesthesia adjacent to individual teeth.
‡ May be ineffective in area of zygomatic buttress.
§ Middle superior alveolar injection often needed for full anesthesia of first molar.
‖ If infraorbital nerve block is ineffective or if abscess is large and involves the infraorbital foramen area.
¶ Additional infiltration of soft tissues desirable to reduce hemorrhage.

experiences some anesthetic failures. If the injection is performed with care and the anesthetic agent employed is fully potent, a number of possibilities remain that can explain a lack of anesthesia.

ANATOMIC VARIATION

In humans there is considerable variation in the anatomic location of nerves and contiguous structures. For example, the lingula is generally located less than 1 cm above the occlusal plane, and as a result, injecting 1 cm above the plane (as is often practiced) usually permits the anesthetic to be deposited within the mandibular sulcus. A significant minority of patients, however, have lingulas more than 1 cm above the occlusal plane (Table 12–3).[1] Palpation of the greatest concavity of the coronoid notch is useful in correcting for these variations. In still other people, particularly those with prognathia, the lingula is located even above the coronoid notch and thus above the usual end-point for needle insertion during a standard inferior alveolar nerve block. This anomaly results in deposition

Table 12–2. **SELECTED DENTAL PROCEDURES AND ANESTHETIC TECHNIQUE CHOICES IN THE MANDIBLE**

Procedure	Mental/ Incisive Nerve Block	Standard Inferior Alveolar Nerve Block	Buccal Nerve Block	High Mandibular Nerve Block*	Partial Lingual Nerve Block
Conservative treatment of premolars/anteriors	1.0–1.5 mL	1.0–1.5 mL		1.8 mL	0.5 mL†
Conservative treatment of molars		1.0–1.5 mL	0.3–0.5 mL†	1.8 mL	
Surgery or extraction of anteriors	1.0–1.5 mL	1.5 mL		1.8 mL	0.5 mL
Surgery or extraction of premolars/molars		1.5 mL	0.3–0.5 mL	1.8 mL	
Surgery on lower lip	1.0–1.5 mL				
Surgery on tongue or floor of mouth					1.0 mL

* *Gow-Gates and Vazirani-Akinosi closed-mouth techniques.*
† *Optional, if needed for soft tissue anesthesia.*

of the anesthetic solution below the lingula and medial to the sphenomandibular ligament. Insufficient anesthetic solution then distributes laterally and superiorly to bathe the minimum length of nerve reported to be necessary for a complete sensory block.[2]

Gross anatomic anomalies can often be discovered by palpation, visual inspection, or radiography. Much more difficult (or impossible) to detect are subtle differences in the orientation of fascial planes within an injection site. Although it is true that the closer the needle is to the nerve to be anesthetized the greater is the likelihood for a successful nerve block, this axiom fails to take into account the uneven distribution of anesthetic

Table 12–3. **POSITION OF MANDIBULAR LINGULAR TIP TO THE OCCLUSAL PLANE**

Highest Point (mm)	No. of Cases	Incidence (%)
−3 to +1	63	15.75
+2 to +5	190	47.50
+6 to +9	108	27.00
+10 to +19	39	9.75
Total	400	100.00

Data from Bremer.[1]

Table 12–4. **COMPARATIVE ANESTHETIC SUCCESS OF THE GOW-GATES AND STANDARD ALVEOLAR INFERIOR NERVE BLOCK IN ADULTS**

Study	Technique	Good–Excellent (%)	Poor (Failure) (%)
Watson and Gow-Gates[4]	Std. I.A.	95	5
	Gow-Gates	100	0
Gow-Gates and Watson[5]	Std. I.A.	90	10
	Std. I.A.	92	8
	Gow-Gates	100	0
Robertson[6]	Std. I.A.	71	29
	Gow-Gates	92	8
Levy[7]	Std. I.A.	65	35
	Gow-Gates	96	4

solution that can occur following injection. Indeed, studies of radiopaque dyes mixed with local anesthetics have revealed that, occasionally, an injection can be made within a few millimeters of a nerve without producing any effect, whereas in other instances the solution can be deposited more than 2 cm away and still yield excellent anesthesia.[3] In the former case, the anesthetic spreads over the path of least resistance away from the nerve; in the latter case, it is directed toward the nerve.

A logical solution to these problems is to substitute the use of a high mandibular injection technique such as the Gow-Gates nerve block, as it places anesthetic solution well above the lingula regardless of known variations, and it apparently avoids potential problems associated with variations in soft tissue barriers. Tables 12–4 and 12–5 compare the relative efficacies of the Gow-Gates block and the standard inferior alveolar (lingual) nerve block.[4–8] One should realize that high-block techniques depend on distribution of solution over greater distances than the standard injection technique. Thus, while 1.0 mL of solution can often anesthetize the inferior alveolar nerve in an average-sized adult when injected near the mandibular foramen, a high technique such as the Gow-

Table 12–5. **COMPARISON OF THE STANDARD INFERIOR ALVEOLAR NERVE BLOCK VERSUS THE GOW-GATES MANDIBULAR BLOCK IN CHILDREN AGED 4 TO 16 YEARS**

	Quality of Anesthesia		Injection Pain		
	Good/Excellent (%)	Poor (%)	None (%)	Mild (%)	Moderate (%)
Standard inferior alveolar block	82	18	9	55	36
Gow-Gates block	100	0	64	36	0

Data from Yamada and Jastak.[8]

Gates nerve block requires at least 1.8 mL and occasionally more volume in large adults.

Although probably of less importance than poor technique, aberrant or accessory nerve pathways sometimes contribute to a lack of satisfactory anesthesia. Alternative nervous innervation does have credence, especially in the mandible, but its effect is generally one of incomplete anesthesia of an isolated tooth or group of teeth despite adequate anesthesia of the surrounding soft tissues and adjacent teeth.

The mylohyoid nerve is thought to provide some sensory innervation to the mandibular incisors and possibly posterior teeth in a significant segment of the population. Under normal circumstances, the successful administration of an inferior alveolar nerve block also anesthetizes the mylohyoid nerve. However, in a small percentage of individuals the mylohyoid nerve is believed both to decussate from the inferior alveolar nerve up to 2.5 cm above the mandibular foramen and to enter a separate bony canal in its course along the medial aspect of the ramus.[9,10] The effect of this anatomic variation would be incomplete blockade of this nerve and incomplete analgesia of the mandibular teeth and/or soft tissues of the chin (Figs. 12–1 and 12–2). Again, the simplest solution appears to be the use of a high mandibular block technique, although periodontal ligament or supraperiosteal injections would also provide supplementary pain control.

Another example of alternative sensory innervation occurs in the molar region of the mandible. Several sources of accessory nerve fibers have been described. First, the inferior alveolar nerve may have separate nerve branches supplying the molars, particularly the third molar. In certain instances these nerves apparently branch off from the main trunk of inferior alveolar nerve some distance above its entrance into the mandibular canal and then course inferiorly and anteriorly in separate small canals (Fig. 12–3).[10] Although such variants are clinically unpredictable,

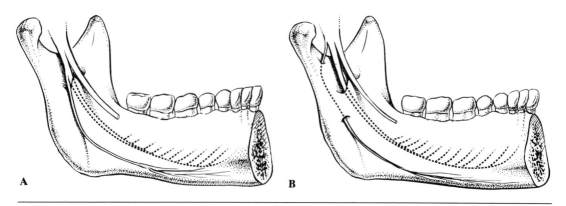

Figure 12–1.   Accessory mylohyoid nerve innervation. **A.** Usual mylohyoid nerve anatomy. **B.** Alternative anatomy (high mylohyoid nerve origin).

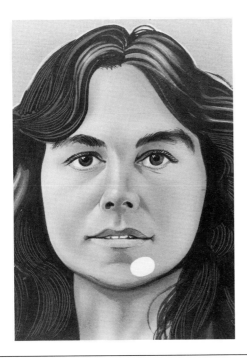

Figure 12–2. Area of soft tissue sensation provided by the mylohyoid nerve (unilateral).

they do occur in up to 2.5% of caucasians[11] and undoubtedly cause difficulty with mandibular molar anesthesia.

Careful dissection has shown that nerve fibers from the temporalis and
other muscles of mastication penetrate the surface of the mandible near
their respective muscle attachments to eventually communicate with the
inferior alveolar nerve or its branches serving the molar teeth. Neurovas-

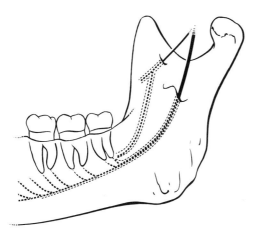

Figure 12–3. Example of an alternative innervation pattern of the mandibular third molar (temporal
crest canal).

cular bundles are especially prominent in the retromolar fossa, near the insertion of the deep tendon of the temporalis. Clinical and histologic investigations have also found that fibers contributed by the buccal and lingual nerves may provide accessory innervation to the posterior mandibular teeth.[12,13] Depending on the exact innervation of the area, supplementary injections are often effective in providing adequate anesthesia. A high mandibular block technique (e.g., the Gow-Gates block) will generally anesthetize accessory fibers supplied by the inferior alveolar, lingual, buccal, and mylohyoid nerves. Injection in or next to the retromolar fossa will catch fibers contributed by the deep temporal nerves, buccal nerve, and perhaps other sources as well. Lingual injection opposite or behind the tooth in question will block the lingual and mylohyoid nerves. In general, buccal and lingual supraperiosteal injections may be useful in securing anesthesia without regard to the actual accessory pathways present.

A few nerve distributions are so highly variable that alternative innervation is to be anticipated. Previously discussed is the tendency for incisor teeth to receive cross-innervation from the contralateral nerve, and the common absence of the middle superior alveolar nerve, resulting in unpredictable innervation of the maxillary first molar. A third such example involves the buccal nerve. Although the buccal nerve normally supplies the buccal gingiva and mucosa up to the first molar or the second premolar, in rare cases its range may extend to the canine.[10] At the opposite extreme, the buccal nerve may not contribute innervation to the mandibular arch at all, its function being taken over by the posterior superior alveolar and mental nerves. Therefore, should a conventional buccal nerve block fail, extensive infiltration of anesthetic solution around the area concerned may very well succeed in anesthetizing the target tissues.

INTRAVASCULAR INJECTION

In addition to the obviously rich vascularity of the human head, there is considerable anatomic variation in the location of arteries and veins. These two factors translate into a relatively high frequency of intravascular placement of needles. Such an occurrence is especially likely when the inferior alveolar, mental, posterior superior alveolar, and maxillary nerves are anesthetized (see Chapter 13). Injection of anesthetic solution into a blood vessel may not produce anesthesia, but often elicits systemic effects. Aspiration before injection should always be practiced.

In the event of an inadvertent intravascular injection, a second attempt to secure anesthesia may be made, provided that the patient is willing and that no serious systemic reaction resulted from the accident.

NEEDLE DEFLECTION

As clinicians use thinner needles in the pursuit of the painless injection, the disadvantages of these needles become more evident. Simply put, the finer the gauge and the greater the flexibility, the larger the deflection of the needle from its intended path on straight insertion and the more difficult it is to accurately redirect the needle once it has been inserted into tissue. Although of little significance with supraperiosteal anesthesia, the use of 27-gauge and especially finer needles for block anesthesia (inferior alveolar, posterior superior alveolar) does result in occasional instances of significant misdirection and failure of anesthesia. Needles will deflect in a direction opposite to the bevel. A fine-gauge needle can deflect 3 to 6 mm when inserted 1 to 2 cm into soft tissue, and this deflection is sufficient in certain instances to cause the deposition of anesthetic solution behind anatomic barriers that limit adequate dispersion toward the target nerve. A prime example of this is the injection of anesthetic solution medial to the sphenomandibular ligament during attempted inferior alveolar nerve block. Here the common recommendation to place the bevel of the needle toward bone actually contributes to medial deflection of the needle. However, the use of a heavier gauge needle (i.e., 25-gauge) will minimize such problems.

INFLAMMATION

Local anesthetics seemingly do not work well in the presence of inflammation. As discussed in Chapter 2, acidic by-products of inflammation can lower the pH of affected tissues and decrease the amount of nonionized anesthetic available for crossing the nerve sheath and membrane. Another aspect of inflammation is that the increased blood flow through the tissue hastens the removal of the drug from the injection site, thereby decreasing the duration and the intensity of anesthesia. A normal strategy in the setting of inflammation is to give a nerve block injection somewhat proximal to the lesion. Unfortunately, this approach is not always successful.

Attention has been focused on the effects of certain mediators of inflammation (e.g., prostaglandins, kinins, adenine nucleotides) on nerve transmission and local anesthetic activity.[14] At least indirectly, these substances can partially reverse a local anesthetic block. Also of significance is the fact that morphologic changes can be found in nerve trunks some distance away from the inflammatory focus and even in the central nervous system. This observation helps to explain, for example, why an inferior alveolar nerve block may not always anesthetize a mandibular canine with a periapical abscess.[15]

A promising experimental approach to anesthetic failure in the setting of inflammation is the use of concentrated local anesthetic solutions. In this regard, the injection of 5% lidocaine with epinephrine has been shown to produce anesthesia of teeth with acute pulpitis when the standard 2% solution with epinephrine failed to do so.[16] It must be emphasized, however, that concentrated anesthetic solutions are significantly more toxic than conventional formulations and are not a substitute for proper injection technique.

MISCELLANEOUS CAUSES

Certain patients appear to be basically difficult to anesthetize. A highly anxious individual may perceive nonnoxious stimuli, such as pressure, noise, vibration, or touch, as being painful. The apparent anesthetic failure in this case is often best managed by reducing anxiety with conscious sedation (e.g., inhalation or intravenous sedation). In other cases the anesthesia appears to be adequate but of very short duration. In some instances using an anesthetic solution with a higher vasoconstrictor concentration (e.g., 1:50,000 epinephrine) or a longer acting local anesthetic (e.g., bupivacaine) may prove beneficial. At times a patient is encountered who seems to be constitutionally resistant to local anesthetics. Although speculation of, and anecdotal evidence for, genetic resistance is occasionally reported,[17] there is no definitive evidence for such a phenomenon. Nevertheless, changing the anesthetic may correct the problem, or, in rare instances, using a higher concentration may succeed where the more usual concentrations do not.

Many chronic drug abusers (e.g., of alcohol, narcotics, tranquilizers, stimulants) are difficult to anesthetize.[18] Although the precise mechanism of the resistance is unknown, drug–receptor interactions,[19] occult metabolic acidosis,[20] and increased sodium channel density[21] have been offered as possible explanations. A most likely explanation is the relative inability of these individuals to tolerate moderate stress.

In a practical sense, the use of behavioral strategies, electronic dental analgesia, and/or conscious sedation again can help many individuals obtain effective pain control. In the most difficult cases, only deep sedation or general anesthesia will be effective.

References

1. Bremer, G.: Measurements of special significance in connection with anesthesia of the inferior alveolar nerve. Oral Surg. Oral Med. Oral Pathol., 5:966–988, 1952.
2. Rood, J.P.: The diameters and internodal lengths of the myelinated fibres in human inferior alveolar nerve. J. Dent., 6:311–315, 1978.
3. Galbreath, J.C., and Eklund, M.K.: Tracing the course of the mandibular block injection. Oral Surg. Oral Med. Oral Pathol., 30:571–582, 1970.
4. Watson, J.E., and Gow-Gates, G.A.E.: A clinical evaluation of the Gow-Gates mandibular block technique. N.Z. Dent. J., 72:220–223, 1976.

5. Gow-Gates, G.A.E., and Watson, J.E.: The Gow-Gates mandibular block: Further understanding. Anesth. Prog., *24*:183–189, 1977.

6. Robertson, W.D.: Clinical evaluation of mandibular conduction anesthesia. Gen. Dent., *27*:49–51, 1979.

7. Levy, T.P.: An assessment of the Gow-Gates mandibular block for third molar surgery. J. Am. Dent. Assoc., *103*:37–41, 1981.

8. Yamada, A., and Jastak, J.T.: Clinical evaluation of the Gow-Gates block in children. Anesth. Prog., *28*:106–109, 1981.

9. Frommer, J., Mele, F.A., and Monroe C.W.: The possible role of the mylohyoid nerve in mandibular posterior tooth sensation. J. Am. Dent. Assoc., *85*:113–117, 1972.

10. DuBrul, E.L.: Sicher and DuBrul's Oral Anatomy, 8th ed. St. Louis, Ishiyaku EuroAmerica, Inc., 1988.

11. Ossenberg, N.S.: Temporal crest canal: Case report and statistics on a rare mandibular variant. Oral Surg. Oral Med. Oral Pathol., *62*:10–12, 1986.

12. Rood, J.P.: Some anatomical and psychologic causes of failure to achieve mandibular anesthesia. Br. J. Oral Surg., *15*:75–82, 1977.

13. Rood, J.P.: The analgesia and innervation of mandibular teeth. Br. Dent. J., *140*:237–239, 1976.

14. Horrobin, D.F., Durand, L.G., and Manku, M.S.: Prostaglandin E1 modifies nerve conduction and interferes with local anesthetic action. Prostaglandins, *14*:103–108, 1977.

15. Najjar, T.A.: Why can't you achieve adequate regional anesthesia in the presence of infection? Oral Surg. Oral Med. Oral Pathol., *44*:7–13, 1977.

16. Eldridge, D.J., and Rood, J.P.: A double-blind trial of 5 per cent lignocaine solution. Br. Dent. J. *142*:129–130, 1977.

17. Geraci, R.P.: Letter. Reg. Anaesth., *6*:123, 1981.

18. Scheutz, F.: Drug addicts and local analgesia effectivity and general side effects. Scand. J. Dent. Res., *90*:299–304, 1982.

19. DiFazio, C.A.: Letter. Reg. Anaesth., *6*:124, 1981.

20. DeJong, R.H.: Letter. Reg. Anaesth., *6*:123, 1981.

21. Scurlock, J.E.: Letter. Reg. Anaesth., *6*:122, 1981.

Chapter 13

Complications and Side Effects

L ocal anesthetics administered carefully and within recommended dosage limits have established an enviable record of safety. Although life-threatening systemic reactions do occur, most adverse effects or complications are largely inconsequential, representing more of a temporary inconvenience than a true hazard.

Incidence of Adverse Reactions

Statistics related to complications and side effects from oral regional anesthesia are meager and subject to error. Because no adequate mechanism exists in the United States to collect the necessary information consistently on a wide scale, available data are subject to regional biases and other distortions.

MORTALITY

Mortality statistics have been obtained in two ways: questionnaires to practitioners and review of local government mortality files. Using the former approach, Seldin found that the mortality for local anesthetics in oral surgery was 1 : 1,450,000 during a period (1950–1956) when procaine was the most widely used anesthetic agent.[1] By sampling the records of the Medical Examiner's office of New York City for the years 1943 to 1952, Seldin and Recant estimated the mortality from local anesthesia in general dental practice to be 1 : 45,000,000.[2] Several more recent investigations conducted after lidocaine replaced procaine as the most popular drug have yielded results similar to those of the two earlier studies (1 : 1,850,000 and 1 : 1,490,000 in oral surgery, 1 : 36,000,000 in general dental practice).[3,4]

Although apparently reproducible, these values are nevertheless open to question. It is likely, for example, that some deaths from local anesthetics go unreported and that others are mistakenly identified as myocardial infarctions, cerebrovascular accidents, or other causation. On the other hand, it is also probable that some deaths imputed to local anesthetics are due to procedural stress or are merely accidents of time and place and not causally related to drug administration at all.

Although some reservations must remain concerning the true lethality of local anesthetics administered intraorally, it is clear that a higher incidence of anesthetic death occurs during oral surgery than in general dentistry. Much of this difference undoubtedly results from the greater stress associated with surgery, the heightened anxiety it generates, and possibly from an increased population of high-risk patients. However, larger amounts of local anesthetics are often injected, and the chances for dose-related toxicity are therefore correspondingly greater. It should be noted that, for similar reasons, regional anesthesia in oral surgery is significantly *less* dangerous than it is in certain other specialities, such as orthopedics and general surgery.

MORBIDITY

Tabulations of nonfatal adverse reactions to regional anesthesia have generally been made at a single clinic, hospital, or school from patients treated by one or several practitioners. When such study designs are coupled with differences in criteria for what constitutes undesired responses, it is not surprising that the reported incidence of untoward reactions varies widely, from 0% to 30%.[5]

In one of the largest and best controlled investigations, Persson recorded adverse effects in 2.5% of 2,960 patients given one to two cartridges of various anesthetic agents.[5] Factors positively correlated with adverse reactions included the number of injections (2% incidence for single administrations, 5% for multiple injections), a lack of anesthesia (2% with complete anesthesia, 4% with partial anesthesia, and 7% with unsuccessful anesthesia), and a previous history of side effects (40%). Because most of the complications observed—pallor, unrest, sweating, fatigue, palpitations, nausea, and fainting—are common manifestations of acute anxiety and may even develop before needle insertion, it is evident that many of the adverse effects ascribed to regional anesthesia are actually generated by the process of administration and not by the drugs themselves.

Systemic Effects

Major untoward responses to injections of local anesthetics are caused by a variety of factors, most of which are not clear at the time of occurrence. Unintentional overdosage, accidental intravascular injection, and allergic responses are all possible. Additionally, procedural stress (particularly in the medically compromised patient), unexpected drug reactions, and pure coincidence also produce emergencies in which the patient's life may be in jeopardy.

OVERDOSAGE

The risk of systemic toxicity from administering too much drug is relatively low in regional anesthesia of the oral cavity. For example, the inferior alveolar or Gow-Gates mandibular nerve blocks normally require 2 mL or less in adults. In contrast, instillation of 20 to 30 mL is commonplace for various general surgical procedures. Even though the concentration of drug is usually less than that used in the mouth (e.g., 0.5% to 1.5% lidocaine instead of 2%), this volume frequently results in patients receiving maximum permissible doses.

Table 13–1 is a compilation (derived from Table 4–3) of maximum doses for local anesthetics. These values are not absolutes and are based on extrapolations from animal studies and statistical analysis of tests involving relatively small numbers of subjects. Because of variations in patient health status, drug absorption, distribution, and elimination, it is still possible that toxic reactions may occur in some patients within the so-called "safe" dosage range. In addition to the above factors and the well-known florid vascularity of the tissues of the mouth, many popular dental anesthetic preparations contain relatively high concentrations of vasoconstrictors. Contrary to prior belief, vasoconstrictors may increase toxicity (when intravascular injection occurs) rather than decrease it. Because of these factors and the relatively modest anesthetic volumes

Table 13–1. **MAXIMUM RECOMMENDED DOSES OF LOCAL ANESTHETICS**

Drug	*Maximum Dosage (mg/kg)*	*Maximum Adult Dose (mg)*
Propoxycaine/procaine	6.6*	
Lidocaine	4.5†	500
	7.0‡	
Mepivacaine	6.6	400
Prilocaine	8.0	600
Bupivacaine	—	90
Etidocaine	8	400
Articaine	7 (adult)	—
	5 (child)	

* Combined anesthetic weight.
† Without vasoconstrictor.
‡ With vasoconstrictor.

Table 13–2. **SAMPLE DOSAGE CALCULATION FOR REGIONAL ANESTHESIA**

Data base: 3 cartridges of 3% mepivacaine (without vasoconstrictor)
Each cartridge = 1.8 mL
3% solution = 30 mg/mL or 54 mg per 1.8 mL cartridge
20-kg child
Maximum recommended dose = 6.6 mg/kg

Dose calculation: 3 cartridges × 1.8 mL × 30 mg/mL = 162 mg drug

Maximum for 20-kg child: 6.6 mg/kg × 20 kg = 132 mg (2.4 cartridges)

needed for most dental procedures, the maximum doses listed in Table 13–1 are rarely approached. On the other hand, they may be exceeded in selected circumstances.

Most true overdoses of local anesthetics in dentistry occur in young children. Table 13–2 illustrates the basis for this assertion. Clearly, three cartridges of 3% mepivacaine are within the permissible range for an adult patient but exceed the maximum recommended dose in the child. Although obvious here, it is very easy to forget that anesthetic quantities suitable for adults may be excessive in children. Mistakes of this kind unfortunately do occur, and the results are often tragic for everyone involved.[6]

Toxic reactions depend on the plasma concentration of drug that is achieved. With lidocaine, these effects normally begin when the plasma titer approaches 5 μg/mL. The two organ systems most affected are the central nervous system (CNS) and the cardiovascular system.

Central Nervous System

Cortical neurons are generally much more responsive to local anesthetics than are the peripheral nerves. Entry of drug into the brain often produces a complex pattern of neurologic excitement followed by depression. This clinical picture is the result of a selective blockade of inhibitory neurons or synapses by concentrations of anesthetic that permit facilitatory pathways to act unopposed. With higher concentrations of drug, depression develops as all neurons become similarly affected.

Systemic responses may be so mild as to go unrecognized as such. At times, a sedative effect in which the patient becomes drowsy and less communicative may even be beneficial. Other initial symptoms of systemic toxicity may include feelings of lightheadedness or dizziness, tinnitus, double or blurred vision, nausea, or a sudden onset of confusion, disorientation, or unexpected anxiety. As drug absorption progresses, preconvulsant manifestations appear: nystagmus, muscle fasciculations, and tremors of the eyelids, jaw, and extremities. At convulsant concentrations (normally over 7 μg/mL for lidocaine), epileptiform brainwave activity originating in the limbic system spreads throughout the cerebral cortex, eliciting generalized tonic–clonic seizures. With excessively high concentrations of drug, a state of profound CNS depression eventually intervenes. Fatal doses of local anesthetics typically cause death by respiratory failure.

Overdose reactions may begin anytime from several minutes to more than 1 hour after drug administration. However, the slower the onset, the milder the reaction will be. The severity of toxicity will tend to parallel the plasma concentration, which normally peaks 15 to 60 minutes after injection.

Cardiovascular System

Cardiovascular effects of most local anesthetics are benign and of little danger, even with concentrations of drug that produce marked CNS derangement. Myocardial depression by lidocaine, for example, normally does not become significant until the plasma concentration is well into the convulsant range. With artificial ventilation, several "lethal" doses of anesthetic may be administered before circulatory collapse occurs.

Although the above characteristics were once thought to apply to all local anesthetics, the high-potency drugs are more cardiotoxic. Thus, cardiovascular depression may coincide with seizure activity in response to an overdose of bupivacaine or etidocaine.[7] Should cardiac arrest ensue, management of the emergency is complicated by the fact that removal of the drug from the bloodstream through redistribution and hepatic clearance is severely impaired.

Management of Overdose

Emergency management of adverse reactions to local anesthetics varies in proportion to the presenting symptoms. If the reaction is mild and transient, little more than observation, reassurance of the patient, and discontinuing the procedure is necessary. However, with increasing severity of response, more aggressive treatment is indicated. Oxygen supplementation and support of respiration are vitally important because inadequate ventilation greatly increases the possibility of seizures and cardiovascular disturbance. Convulsions that do arise are best controlled with a benzodiazepine such as diazepam (Valium) or midazolam (Versed). Short- or ultrashort-acting barbiturates can also be used to terminate seizures, but those drugs tend to produce additional and undesirable CNS depression.

Cardiopulmonary resuscitation is mandatory should respiratory and circulatory collapse occur. Table 13–3 outlines the management of systemic reactions to local anesthetics. Because severe responses are best

Table 13–3.   **MANAGEMENT OF TOXIC REACTIONS TO LOCAL ANESTHETICS**

Severity of Reaction	Symptoms	Treatment
Mild	Sedation, drowsiness	None
Mild	Transient anxiety	Temporarily discontinue procedure; reassure patient
Moderate	Dysphoria, anxiety, nausea, confusion, sensorium disturbances, tremors	Discontinue procedure; reassure patient; monitor vital signs; give diazepam, 5–10 mg IV, or midazolam, 2–5 mg IV, for sedation
Moderate to severe	Disorientation, semiconsciousness or unconsciousness	Discontinue procedure; monitor vital signs; maintain patent airway; provide oxygen supplementation
	Tonic–clonic seizures	Restrain patient from injurious movements; monitor vital signs; maintain patent airway; provide oxygen supplementation; give diazepam IV in 2–5-mg increments until convulsions cease; midazolam in 2-mg increments may also be used
Severe	Respiratory and cardiovascular collapse	Cardiopulmonary resuscitation

treated in a hospital environment, inherent in these recommendations is the need to call for emergency assistance.

INTRAVASCULAR INJECTION

Toxic reactions during regional anesthesia of the oral cavity are much more likely to result from an accidental intravascular injection than from a true overdose. Depositing the anesthetic solution directly into the bloodstream avoids the ordinarily slow process of absorption and markedly increases the systemic toxicity of the drug. Several investigations have documented that intravascular placement of the needle is a common occurrence with certain anesthetic techniques (Table 13–4). Additionally, Table 13–5 represents a composite of data regarding the inferior alveolar nerve block derived from a number of authors.[8–15] The rate of positive aspirations varied among these studies, presumably because of differences in technique or reporting, but positive aspiration is a very common occurrence for most clinicians. Similarly, current experience with the Gow-Gates mandibular nerve block indicates considerable variation in incidence, although early reports suggested a very low aspiration rate (Table 13–6).[16–18] Finally, evidence suggests that during inferior alve-

Table 13–4. **AVERAGE INCIDENCE OF POSITIVE ASPIRATION OF BLOOD BY INJECTION SITE**

Injection Site	Blood Vessels at Risk	Positive Aspirations (%)
Maxilla		
Supraperiosteal	Terminal branches of maxillary artery and vein	1.9
Posterior superior alveolar nerve block	Posterior superior alveolar artery and vein, pterygoid venous plexus	3.9
Palatal injections	Greater palatine and nasopalatine vessels	1.2
Maxillary nerve block	Greater palatine artery and vein (pterygopalatine canal approach); posterior superior alveolar artery and vein, pterygoid venous plexus maxillary artery (high tuberosity approach)	14.3
Mandible		
Inferior alveolar nerve block	Inferior alveolar artery and vein	7.9
Mental nerve block	Mental vessels	7.0

olar nerve block, young patients may be more prone to intravascular needle placement than adults (Table 13–7).[19]

Even with proper aspiration, it is not always possible to avoid intravascular injection. The bevel of the needle, for example, may rest against the vessel wall. Negative force then merely draws the intimal lining of the

Table 13–5. **INCIDENCE OF POSITIVE ASPIRATION DURING INFERIOR ALVEOLAR NERVE BLOCK**

Study, Year	Aspirations Attempted (n)	Positive Aspirations (%)
Harris, 1957[8]	3,085	3.6
Forrest, 1959[9]	577	4.2
Frye, 1963[10]	550	12.2
Shiano and Strambi, 1964[11]	702	11.0
Cohen et al., 1969[12]	1,050	10.6
Bos et al., 1971[13]	2,130	9.4
Bartlett, 1972[14]	994	11.0
Williams and Simm, 1975[15]	1,198	9.3
All studies	10,286	7.9

Table 13–6. **INCIDENCE OF POSITIVE ASPIRATION DURING GOW-GATES MANDIBULAR NERVE BLOCK**

Study, Year	Incidence (%)
Gow-Gates and Watson, 1977[16]	1.6
Robertson, 1979[17]	17.0
Levy, 1981[18]	7.7

vessel over the needle lumen, preventing entry of blood into the cartridge (Fig. 13–1).

Intravenous Administration

Much experience with the intravenous administration of local anesthetics has been gained with the use of lidocaine for treating cardiac arrhythmias. Two to three times the amount of lidocaine in a single anesthetic cartridge can be given intravenously over a 2-minute period without incident in most patients. However, injecting the drug more rapidly than this may elicit convulsions. The incidence of seizures when lidocaine is administered intravenously to control arrhythmias may be as high as 0.6%.[20] Moreover, it should be noted that the epinephrine incorporated into lidocaine solutions may increase the intravenous toxicity of the anesthetic.[21]

In susceptible individuals, an excessively rapid injection of local anesthetic solution into a vein may produce life-threatening cardiac arrhythmias. Without having an opportunity to disperse within the vascular compartment, the agent will reach the heart as a bolus of very high concentration. However, cardiac arrest has even been caused by intravenous "pushes" of physiologic salt solutions that temporarily perturb the osmotic and ionic environment surrounding the pacemaker cells of the heart.

Table 13–7. **POSITIVE ASPIRATIONS DURING INFERIOR ALVEOLAR NERVE BLOCK IN CHILDREN***

Age Range (yr)	Aspiration Attempts (n)	Positive Aspirations (%)
7–12	275	20
13–16	367	12
All	642	15

* Data from Bishop et al.[19]

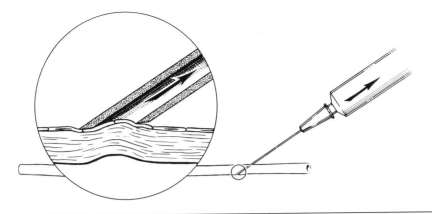

Figure 13–1.   Intimal obstruction of blood aspiration.

Intraarterial Administration

Aldrete and co-workers have suggested that a small quantity of local anesthetic injected intraarterially may cause serious neurotoxic reactions.[22] This hypothesis is contradictory to the usual thinking that normal flow of arterial blood through branches of the external carotid artery and peripheral capillary beds should reduce the risk of systemic responses to less than that posed by intravenous injections. However, rapid infusion with the small-gauge needles used in the mouth may permit the retrograde movement of drug down the external carotid artery and into the internal carotid circulations, thereby exposing cortical neurons to a transient but large concentration of the agent (Fig. 13–2). A similar reaction has been reported involving the backflow of radiographic contrast media from the radial to the subclavian arteries.[23]

The "reverse carotid flow" hypothesis of Aldrete and co-workers, if true, could explain a variety of untoward responses frequently labeled as "allergic" or "idiosyncratic" in origin. In particular, it could theoretically provide an explanation for a local anesthetic fatality reported by Tomlin.[24] The patient, a 22-year-old woman in apparently good health, lost consciousness during the injection of a single cartridge of anesthetic for an inferior alveolar nerve block. Convulsions developed quickly, and death soon followed despite attempts at resuscitation. However, animal studies[25] designed to test Aldrete's hypothesis unexpectedly demonstrated that intravenous toxicity with boluses of lidocaine (with or without epinephrine) were much more lethal than intraarterial injections directly into the common carotid artery. These data suggest that Aldrete's reverse carotid flow hypothesis may possibly account for some aberrant behavioral effects by a direct effect on the CNS, but anesthetic toxicity sufficient to cause death would probably require a different mechanism. Alternative causes of death in the case reported by Tomlin include coincidental myocardial infarction, anxiety-provoked cardiac dysrhythmia, or possibly stroke.

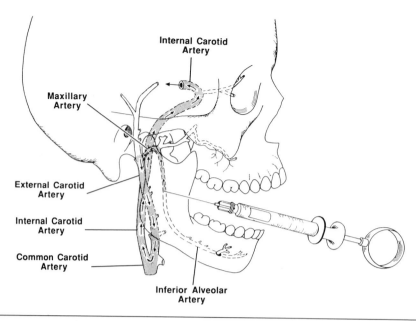

Internal Carotid
Artery

Maxillary
Artery

External Carotid
Artery

Internal Carotid
Artery

Common Carotid
Artery

Inferior Alveolar
Artery

Figure 13–2.   Proposed retrograde flow of anesthetic solution after accidental injection into the inferior alveolar artery.

Management of Intravascular Injection

Adverse reactions to accidental intravascular injections of local anesthetics have a rapid onset. They may occur instantaneously or develop over a period of 1 to 2 minutes. True intravascular reactions also tend to be short-lived, rarely lasting more than 30 minutes, unless the circulation is markedly depressed. The ephemeral nature of intravascular toxicity is based on the distribution pattern of the local anesthetic, as illustrated in Figure 2–18. Local anesthetics gain quick access to the brain (equilibration half-time of 1 minute) because of their lipid solubility and the organ's high vascularity. After several minutes the drug begins to leave the CNS to be redistributed to less well-perfused tissues (with a mean equilibration half-time of 10 minutes). The continued uptake by these tissues (muscle, fat, etc.) permits the plasma concentration to fall to subtoxic levels within a fairly short time.

The management of accidental intravascular injections is similar to that outlined in Table 13–3 for true overdoses. The major difference is that drug intervention to control seizure activity is usually unnecessary, because these convulsions tend to subside spontaneously within several minutes. Should convulsions last longer than that, an anticonvulsant should then be administered.

VASOCONSTRICTOR EFFECTS

Epinephrine or other vasoconstrictors included in local anesthetic solutions rarely produce severe untoward responses, the majority of such reactions being mild and of short duration. Subjective effects mirror those that a person feels after having been strongly startled or frightened: weakness, nausea, nervousness, and so forth. Cardiovascular responses often include tachycardia, mild hypertension with or without bradycardia, and occasionally premature ventricular contractions. The patient, however, can be aware of such palpitations or forceful contractions of the heart and, if anxious about the injection or subsequent dental treatment, may respond in an exaggerated manner. Also, headache can result in the rare occurrence of a severe hypertensive response.

In sensitive patients or under certain clinical conditions, epinephrine-like drugs may cause pronounced tachycardia or hypertension and may elicit dangerous cardiac arrhythmias. The latter outcome is particularly likely when the patient is heavily sedated or under general anesthesia, and insufficient attention is given to respiratory function, permitting arterial carbon dioxide to increase and sensitize the heart to catecholamines.

Management of mild systemic responses to vasoconstrictors is usually simple. Reassurance, temporary discontinuance of the procedure, placing the patient in the supine position, and sometimes mild sedation (diazepam) are of benefit. Because epinephrine is quickly metabolized, responses to intravascular injections rarely last more than 5 minutes, and even true overdoses are of fairly short duration. In the rare event of a life-threatening response—myocardial infarction or cerebral vascular accident—cardiopulmonary resuscitation (if necessary) and hospitalization are required.

ALLERGIC REACTIONS

Historically infrequent, allergic reactions to local anesthetics have been greatly reduced in number since 1948 by the development and marketing of the amide local anesthetics: lidocaine, mepivacaine, and others. The fact that patients continue to claim allergy to one or more "caine" drugs is largely the result of misdiagnosis and patient misinformation, or anxiety reactions that mimic allergic responses but, when adequately evaluated, fail to be confirmed as true allergy.[26,27] In this regard, the majority of patients reporting allergy to local anesthetics also seem to have severe anxiety regarding dental care, and some are even psychologically disabled.

True allergic responses to local anesthetics may be localized or general, immediate in onset or delayed. Their severity can range from a small, inconsequential rash to major emergencies. Most published accounts of allergic reactions to amides (e.g., lidocaine) or to the preservatives added to commercial solutions suggest that the anaphylactic response (type 1 of Coombs and Gell[28]) is the most likely allergic reaction to produce a generalized effect in patients after intraoral injection. In anaphylaxis, combination of the anesthetic antigen with reaginic antibodies bound to mast cells and basophils elicits the release of specific mediators (histamine, leukotrienes, and others) that in turn affect the various target tissues of the body. The most common manifestations of anaphylaxis involve the skin: erythema (redness), pruritis (itching), and urticaria (hives). Swelling at the site of injection or in the form of angioneurotic edema is also possible. Smooth muscle contraction may lead to bronchial constriction (wheezing) and to abdominal cramps and nausea. Death may occur from respiratory embarrassment (bronchial spasm or laryngeal edema) or shock.

Although anaphylactic reactions to local anesthetics may develop almost immediately after drug administration, many skin reactions and even some cases of hypotension do not become pronounced until 1 or more hours afterward.[29,30] This delay suggests that a reactive metabolite of the anesthetic might be the cause; it may reflect the time that is required for the metabolite hapten to successfully form a complete antigen by attaching to an endogenous substrate.

Other types of allergic reactions are also possible. Epidermal rashes of uncertain immunologic origin have been noted, along with isolated case reports of exfoliative dermatitis and thrombocytopenic purpura.[31] The most prevalent allergic response to ester local anesthetics and to topical preparations containing methylparaben is probably the delayed skin reaction. In this regard, most instances of allergy to the ester anesthetic procaine have occurred in practitioners exposed to the anesthetic on a daily basis. The fact that related esters (e.g., benzocaine, tetracaine) are still used for topical anesthesia may be a source for the continued incidence of contact allergic reactions in the mouth.

The management of allergic responses to local anesthetics is outlined in Table 13–8. Although the listing of signs and symptoms in discrete categories is useful for purposes of organization, it is not meant to imply that such divisions are always seen in practice. Thus, it is possible that a patient with a mild skin reaction may also experience some bronchoconstriction and/or hypotension.

ANXIETY REACTIONS

Most systemic reactions during local anesthesia are of psychological origin. A majority of the U.S. population suffers mild anxiety about dentistry, while a sizable minority is highly anxious and, in effect, avoids dental care.[32,33] Needle phobia appears to be high on a list of anxiety-provoking responses in selected populations,[34] and, in a study of fainting during oral surgery, fear of needles was cited by patients as the single most impor-

Table 13–8.   **MANAGEMENT OF LOCAL ANESTHETIC ALLERGY**

Reaction	Signs and Symptoms	Treatment
Localized skin reaction	Local erythema; edema; pruritus	None, or oral antihistamine*
Generalized skin reaction	Pruritus; urticaria; macular rash; angioedema of eyelids, lips	Antihistamine IM*; close observation; consultation with allergist
Respiratory embarrassment	Bronchoconstriction; laryngeal edema; dyspnea	Epinephrine IM or SC†; oxygen; patent airway maintenance; emergency medical assistance and hospitalization if required; supplemental drug therapy‡
Anaphylactic shock	Any of the above, plus marked hypotension and possible cardiovascular collapse	Epinephrine IV†; oxygen; cardiopulmonary resuscitation as indicated; emergency medical assistance and hospitalization; supplemental drug therapy‡

* *Example: diphenhydramine, 25 to 50 mg.*
† *IM or SC: 0.2 to 0.5 mL of 1:1,000 solution. IV: 2 to 5 mL of 1:10,000 solution. May be repeated after 10 minutes if necessary.*
‡ *Antihistamine IM or IV. Example: diphenhydramine, 50 mg. Glucocorticoid IM or IV. Example: hydrocortisone sodium succinate, 100 mg.*

tant cause of their reaction.[35] Anxiety, pain, and other sources of emotional stress elicit physiologic disturbances that, if allowed to progress, may result in loss of consciousness. Terms used to describe the simple faint include vasodepressor syncope, vasovagal syncope, neurogenic syncope, and psychological syncope.

Syncope is best defined as a sudden, transient loss of consciousness. It usually results from cerebral ischemia secondary to inadequate cerebral perfusion. Syncope may also be induced by cerebral hypoglycemia. Although emotional stress is by far the most common inciting factor, a number of other conditions can also precipitate syncopal attacks.[36] These include hyperventilation, excessive coughing, postural hypotension, obstructive vascular disease, severe cardiac disorders, and certain drugs (Table 13–9). Factors contributory to vasodepressor syncope include hunger (low blood glucose), exhaustion, the upright position, and a warm, humid environment. Males between the ages of 15 and 40 seem to have a special proclivity for fainting.[37]

Table 13–9. **CAUSES OF SYNCOPE**

Clinical Syndrome	Provocative Conditions	Prodromal Manifestation
Postural hypotension	Upright position	—
Orthostatic hypotension	Fluid volume depletion	—
Vasodepressor syndrome	Emotional stress	See text
Dysrhythmias*	Exercise (some dysrhythmias)	Palpitation, tachycardia, bradycardia
Carotid sinus hyperreactivity	Manipulation of carotid sinus	—
Cerebrovascular disease	Exercise	Neurologic abnormalities
Aortic stenosis, other anatomic impediments to cardiac outflow	Exercise	—
Hyperventilation, hypoglycemia	Emotional stress, fasting or reactive hypoglycemia	Dyspnea, lightheadedness
Tussive syncope	Paroxysms of coughing	—

* *Various disorders including supraventricular tachycardia (as in Wolff-Parkinson-White syndrome), ventricular tachycardias, premature ventricular contractions, transitory ventricular fibrillation, bradydysrhythmias, and partial or complete heart blocks.*

Overly anxious patients often exhibit prodromal signs of vasodepressor syncope—pallor, sweating, exaggerated yawning, tachycardia—and experience nausea, weakness, and palpitation. Especially in young women, hyperventilation can lead to a syndrome that may require coaching to slow respiration or breathing into a paper bag to reverse.[37] If these manifestations of acute emotional stress are not recognized by the practitioner or reported by the patient, blood (in response to sympathetic-induced vasodilation) may accumulate in skeletal muscle and splanchnic blood vessels to such an extent that venous return to the heart becomes significantly reduced. As the cardiac output begins to fall, the patient often experiences visual and auditory disturbances. Then, in quick succession, the tachycardia abates, the blood pressure drops precipitously, and the patient loses consciousness. Bradycardia is common, and even transient cardiac arrest may occur.

Treatment of vasodepressor syncope is aimed at restoring effective circulation to the brain and oxygenation of the blood. The patient is placed in the supine position with the legs elevated. The patient's neck should be hyperextended to ensure a patent airway. Breathing is further assisted by the administration of oxygen and an ammonia inhalant to stimulate respiration. These procedures normally reverse a simple faint within seconds to a few minutes. Nevertheless, postsyncopal signs of pallor, weakness, and sweating may persist for some time. The more complex causes of syncope outlined in Table 13–9 obviously need further evaluation and management.

Localized Effects

Localized responses to anesthetic injections are fairly common. Most individuals, for instance, have experienced mild soreness at one time or another in the area of injection. However, other side effects are less frequent, and rarely reported complications can be bizarre and difficult to explain.

NEUROPATHY

Because of physiologic differences, rare individuals may experience unusually prolonged anesthesia, even after small doses of drug. This variance is benign and does not require any particular treatment. Of more concern is the finding of prolonged anesthesia, paresthesia (tingling or itching sensation), dysesthesia (painful sensation to nonnoxious stimuli), or hyperesthesia (increased sensitivity to noxious stimuli).

Direct nerve injury from needle insertion is primarily a complication of the inferior alveolar nerve block and, to a lesser extent, the maxillary nerve block via the greater palatine canal. It may also occur with other injections in which the needle is introduced into a foramen containing the nerve.

Although it is impossible to avoid injury in all cases, the incidence of nerve trauma is quite low. However, one must be very careful to identify the true cause of traumatic nerve injury. In this time of frequent litigation, traumatic neuropathy, particularly of the lingual nerve, is one of the most frequent causes of malpractice challenge. Although needle-caused injury is frequently claimed as a cause of lingual nerve injury, the vast majority of such cases involve surgical treatment, especially third molar removal. In this regard, data suggest a substantial incidence of both inferior alveolar and lingual nerve injury, principally due to surgical manipulation. Under very selected circumstances, this incidence can be as high as 22%.[38] In contrast, the true incidence of nerve injury during nonsurgical dental treatment in which needle injury is the only reasonable cause is well under 1%. Moreover, the small-gauge needles employed intraorally almost never totally sever a nerve. Rather, they usually damage a small portion of the fibers. In some instances, pressure or chemically induced injury to the nerve may develop from injecting the solution, or causing hemorrhage, within the nerve sheath. Regardless of the precise mechanism of injury, most needle-induced nerve injuries result in minor sensory deficits that tend to resolve spontaneously over a period of several weeks to a few months and almost never involve the total distribution of the affected nerve.

Impinging on the nerve trunk with the needle often causes an "electric shock" to be felt along the peripheral distribution of the affected nerve. When this occurs, the needle should be retracted slightly before the solution is deposited or insertion along a slightly different pathway is continued. Patients who suffer postanesthetic neuropathy should be told the probable reason for its occurrence and observed periodically for recovery of innervation. Consultation with an oral surgeon trained in this area may be useful. Surgical exploration and repair are rarely indicated unless total anesthesia exists and there is no evidence of regeneration within 3 months.

Accidental nerve damage from contaminated anesthetic solutions is largely a thing of the past. When a single-dose cartridge is used before its expiration date, chemically induced neurotoxicity is most likely the result of the cartridge having been stored in a disinfecting solution. Alcohol and other chemical disinfectants can enter the cartridge through the rubber diaphragm. Injection of alcohol may, in addition to producing prolonged anesthesia, result in local pain and swelling. For this reason manufacturers recommend storing cartridges in a dry container.

TRISMUS

Trismus, or the inability to open the mouth, can result from hemorrhage, muscle trauma (spasm), facial space infection, tumor growth, bony ankylosis, facial bone fracture, foreign bodies, or an enlarged coronoid process. Any of the first three may be caused by regional anesthesia. Of these, the single most common reason for trismus is damage to the medial pterygoid muscle by insertion of the needle too far medially during an inferior alveolar nerve block. Although not widely appreciated, it has been demonstrated that local anesthetics are selectively toxic to skeletal muscle in concentrations employed clinically.[39] Injection of a local anesthetic intramuscularly or even supramuscularly produces a rapidly progressive necrosis of exposed muscle fibers. Similar injections of physiologic salt solutions produce no deleterious effect (Fig. 13–3). Muscle damage is accentuated by vasoconstrictors but is fully reversible. The clinical effects of medial pterygoid muscle damage include pain, myospasm, and difficulty opening the mouth. Additionally, data from experimental animals suggest that masticatory force can be decreased by 30% to 40% for a 2-week postinjection time period.[40]

Hemorrhage and hematoma formation may also restrict jaw opening. Of special interest is the possibility of a fibrous band forming around the medial pterygoid muscle in response to a hematoma in the area.[41,42] Should this occur, maximum opening will begin to narrow 1 to 6 days after injection. Without treatment, this form of trismus will persist indefinitely. Low-grade infection may also generate trismus that lasts until the body's defense mechanisms eliminate the microbial insult.

Treatment of mild postinjection trismus is usually symptomatic (analgesics, warm saline rinses) unless the symptoms are progressive or related to an acute infection, in which case antibiotic therapy and/or drainage may be necessary. If severe trismus occurs, an aggressive regimen of physical therapy, jaw opening exercises, analgesics, and muscle

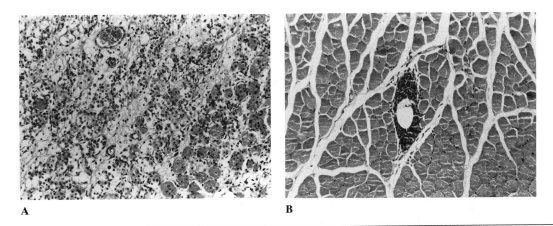

A   B

Figure 13–3.   Skeletal muscle damage after regional anesthesia. **A**. Appearance after intramuscular injection of 3% mepivacaine. The entire field of muscle is necrotic, with edema, fibrin deposits, and numerous macrophages. **B**. Appearance after injection of control vehicle. Damage is limited to an inflammatory response immediately surrounding the needle track.

relaxants is recommended. Mechanical opening of the mouth under general anesthesia may be required in cases unresponsive to more conservative measures. Data from one series suggest that most patients with this affliction are middle-aged, develop trismus in about 3 days, and require an average of 6 weeks to fully recover (Table 13–10).

MUCOSAL IRRITATION

Modern local anesthetic solutions are relatively nonirritating to tissues (skeletal muscle excepted). Nevertheless, local tissue reactions are occasionally observed. Allergic reactions, including Arthus-type phenomena, may account for some circumscribed lesions, while others are from the pharmacologic agents themselves or physical injury. Unusual infections such as impetigo have also been associated with local anesthesia[43] and can be mistaken for allergy or other unrelated problems. On rare occasions, injection of a contaminated anesthetic solution or use of a strong antiseptic before needle penetration is implicated in mucosal damage.

Table 13–10. **ONSET AND TREATMENT COURSE OF POSTINJECTION TRISMUS***

Mean Age (yr)	Nonsurgical Cases (n)	Surgical Cases (n)	Onset of Trismus (days)	Interincisal Opening (mm)	Recovery (wk)
49.5 (range 40–77)	11	5	2.9 (range 1–6)	13.7 (range 5–23)	6.2 (range 4–20)†

* Data adapted from Hinton et al.[41]
† Three cases required manipulation under general anesthesia for resolution.

Topical anesthetic preparations typically contain high concentrations of local anesthetics. Prolonged exposure of the mucous membranes to at least some of these agents may produce irritation. Thus, it is a good practice to wipe off any residual anesthetic just before needle insertion.

Tissue necrosis from injected local anesthetic solutions is usually the result of ischemia. Vasoconstrictors reduce the supply of oxygen to the injected tissue and promote the buildup of acidic by-products of metabolism. The fact that local anesthetic solutions with vasoconstrictors are adjusted to a lower pH than are their plain counterparts (in order to preserve the vasoconstrictor) accentuates tissue acidity. Although local ischemia rarely results in frank mucosal damage, it is germane to note that some patients experience more discomfort during and after injection of drugs with vasoconstrictors than of drugs without.[44]

One of the areas with the highest incidence of ulceration is the palate. A combination of drug effects, blanching of the tissue during injection, and a *relatively* poor blood supply serves to promote tissue ischemia. These lesions normally heal within a period of 2 weeks; a few trophic ulcers, however, may persist for months.[45]

Some blanching of the mucous membrane is to be expected after submucosal administration of solutions containing vasoconstrictors. Infrequently, the skin over the injection site may also lose color (Fig. 13–4). This effect is entirely harmless and disappears as the drug is absorbed into the systemic circulation. Momentary blanching of peripheral tissues supplied by an artery may be elicited by contraction of the blood vessel in reaction to needle impact or by mechanical stimulation of sympathetic vasoconstrictor fibers supplying the area.[46] Blanching distant to an injection of local anesthetic with vasoconstrictor may also occur in response to an accidental intraarterial infusion and reflux flow to nearby branches

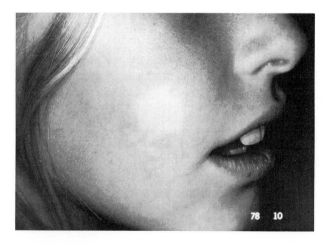

Figure 13–4.   Facial ischemia in response to a maxillary supraperiosteal injection of a local anesthetic with vasoconstrictor. (Courtesy Dr. A.H. Rosenthal, Altanta.)

of the artery. Either mechanism is a possible explanation for the blanching of the maxillary mucosa that has been reported following blockade of the inferior alveolar nerve.[47]

NEEDLE BREAKAGE

Accidental breakage of the disposable stainless steel needle is very uncommon, and the few instances that have been reported involved the thinner (27- and 30-gauge) needles. Typically, breakage is usually the result of a sudden unexpected movement by the patient.[48] Other causes include excessive lateral force applied by the clinician and, rarely, manufacturing defects. When they break, needles usually do so at the hub, which explains why no needle should ordinarily be inserted all the way to the hub. A broken needle is relatively easy to remove so long as the proximal end of the broken portion remains outside of the mucosa. In contrast, a needle fragment that is totally retained within the tissues is very difficult to find and often requires specialized surgical and radiographic techniques to locate and remove. If this complication occurs, and the end of the needle is not visible or easily extracted, the following is advised:

1. Take radiographs of the area from both lateral and frontal planes to help localize the needle.
2. Save the hub for structural evaluation.
3. Record the exact sequence of events in the patient's record.
4. Refer the patient for further evaluation. Unless extensively trained and experienced in surgery of the involved region, practitioners should not try to retrieve the buried needle.
5. Inform your malpractice carrier of the accident.

These recommendations may appear rather extraordinary at first reading, but experience has shown that this type of incidence has a high potential for litigation.

CARTRIDGE BREAKAGE

Excessive force in depositing the anesthetic solution, defects in manufacture, or damage during shipment has resulted in shattering of the anesthetic glass cartridge during injection. In recent years, this has been a particular problem with the repopularization of the intraligamentary (PDL) injection during which high injection pressures are common. In response to this problem, in the mid-1980s manufacturers of dental cartridges began coating the glass with a clear plastic reinforcement to prevent such breakage, and this process appears to have mostly solved the problem.

Because of the design of the aspirating syringe, the cartridge is subject to fracture during the inferior alveolar block injection if the patient, usu-

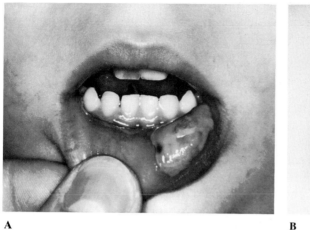
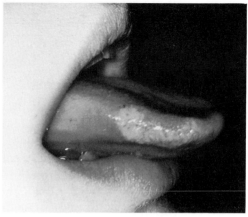

A   B

Figure 13–5.   Self-inflicted injury after inferior alveolar and lingual nerve blocks. **A.** Lower lip.
B. Tongue. (Courtesy Dr. A.H. Rosenthal, Atlanta.)

ally a child, suddenly bites down. To prevent this, the syringe barrel can
be rotated before needle insertion so that the metal sleeve is between the
cartridge and the teeth.

SELF-INFLICTED INJURIES

Patients occasionally injure themselves by biting, chewing, scratching, or
otherwise manipulating anesthetized tissues (Fig. 13–5). The areas of
greatest risk are those supplied by the lingual (tongue), buccal (cheek),
and inferior alveolar (lower lip) nerves. Children are particularly likely to
physically test anesthesia; they and their parents should be warned about
such temptation. Keeping a cotton roll between the teeth until the anesthesia wears off is a good method for minimizing intraoral trauma.

HEMATOMA FORMATION

Hematomas occur with moderate frequency following intraoral injection.
Table 13–4 lists the major blood vessels likely to be punctured or lacerated by a needle.
     The posterior superior alveolar nerve block is particularly likely to
result in hematoma formation. The posterior superior alveolar artery
runs a tortuous course along the posterior aspect of the maxilla. It is
directly in the path of needle insertion and cannot always be avoided.
The signs and symptoms of arterial hemorrhage include rapid swelling, a
sensation of fullness or mild discomfort, facial asymmetry, and perhaps
mild trismus (Fig. 13–6). The pterygoid venous plexus may also be injured during this block injection, especially if the needle is directed too

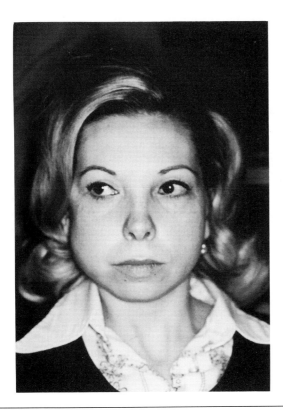

Figure 13–6.   Hematoma after a posterior superior alveolar block injection.

far laterally or deeply. Because the venous system has a low hydrostatic pressure, swelling is slower in onset and often of less severity.

Although sometimes spectacular in appearance, hematoma formation is more of an inconvenience and a cosmetic nuisance than a true danger. Treatment is normally limited to application of ice packs on the day of occurrence in order to restrict swelling. Heat may be applied after 24 hours, but the actual benefit this affords is debatable. Aggressive measures such as drainage or attempted aspiration are unnecessary, since the vast majority of cases resorb spontaneously without lasting morbidity. Indeed, such techniques may be counterproductive, merely succeeding in causing an infection. Because of the potential danger of sepsis, some clinicians recommend prophylactic antibiotics if gross bacterial contamination of a hematoma is suspected.

INFECTION

Bacteria are carried into tissues whenever an intraoral injection is performed. The fact that clinical infection rarely follows is a testimonial to the body's defense mechanisms and to the effectiveness of the unit-dose anesthetic cartridge and disposable needle in eliminating cross-contamination between patients. The few infections that do occur are sometimes the result of poor technique, injection into or through an existing area of infection, or use of a cartridge or needle on more than one patient.

Although a needle can be used for more than one injection in the *same* patient, the incidence of infection does rise when multiple injections are administered in a given area, as may occur in failure to obtain mandibular anesthesia. An increased bacterial challenge coupled with the additional needle trauma probably accounts for this higher incidence.

Insertion of a needle into an area of localized infection may disseminate the disease. Of special concern is the transport of bacteria through fascial planes that normally limit the spread of infection. Fortunately, most cases of infection are low grade, causing pain in the area but few systemic symptoms. These conditions generally resolve without treatment. Acute infections are managed with appropriate antibiotics and, when necessary, surgical drainage.

UNDESIRED NERVE BLOCK

Among the least dangerous but most startling complications of regional anesthesia is the unexpected nerve block. Unpredictable neurologic symptoms may be caused by any of three misadventures: gross misdirection of the needle, accidental intravascular injection, or an unusual pattern of anesthetic distribution (Fig. 13–7). Treatment normally consists of reassuring the patient that the condition is temporary.

Many instances of unanticipated anesthesia occur in response to attempted inferior alveolar nerve blocks. Excessive insertion of the needle may result in deposition of the anesthetic solution within the parotid capsule and anesthesia of the seventh cranial (facial) nerve. The resultant hemifacial paralysis is quite disconcerting to the patient but ultimately regresses without permanent harm. Because the protective lid reflex of the eye is lost, however, it is advisable that the patient be given an eyepatch to wear until motor function is restored.

Inadvertent placement of the needle near the internal carotid artery, or unusual spread of the anesthetic through the lateral pharyngeal space, has been reported to cause blockade of the sympathetic plexus serving the head. The neck and upper arm may also be affected. Manifestations of cervical sympathetic block include ptosis of the upper eyelid, vascular dilation of the conjunctiva and ipsilateral side of the head (and neck and arm), nasal congestion, and pupillary constriction.[49] Concomitant blockade of the recurrent laryngeal nerve will cause hoarseness and a feeling of suffocation.

Ocular effects may arise in response to an accidental intraarterial injection. As shown in Figure 13–8, the middle meningeal artery frequently communicates with the ophthalmic artery or one of its main branches. Infusion of anesthetic solution into the inferior alveolar artery (or perhaps another branch of the maxillary artery) can cause the drug to be

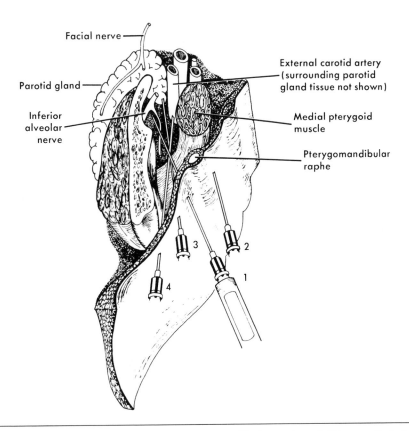

Facial nerve

Parotid gland

Inferior
alveolar
nerve

External carotid artery
(surrounding parotid
gland tissue not shown)

Medial pterygoid
muscle

Pterygomandibular
raphe

Figure 13–7. Needle misadventures in the pterygomandibular region. *1.* The needle is in the correct position for an inferior alveolar block. Any unanticipated neurologic manifestations are the result of an unusual distribution of the injected drug. *2.* Injection within the medial pterygoid muscle leading to possible trismus. *3.* Placement of the needle into the parotid gland. Anesthetic block of the facial nerve and hemiparalysis of the face are likely outcomes. *4.* Intravascular injection. Symptoms will depend on the distribution of anesthetic throughout the vascular tree.

distributed to the orbit through retrograde flow. Dizziness and diplopia from ocular muscle palsies and even temporary blindness from anesthesia of the optic nerve may result.[47] Other injections that have produced transient blindness and/or loss of motor control to the eye are the infraorbital, posterior superior alveolar, and maxillary nerve blocks. While these injection effects on the eye are best explained by retrograde flow through blood vessels, one report described repeated unilateral oculomotor nerve paralysis in a patient who received small amounts of local anesthetic for middle superior alveolar nerve anesthesia.[50] During each supraperiosteal injection, careful aspiration and slow injection ruled out intravascular placement. The only likely explanation in this case was direct extension of the anesthetic solution into the orbital tissues through a bony defect or unusual fascial plane. Another group,[51] describing a similar circumstance, attributed this type of side effect to injury of pe-

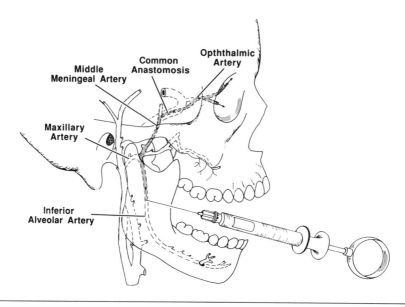

Figure 13–8. Proposed flow of anesthetic solution leading to temporary blindness or paralysis of the motor control of the eye.

ripheral vasculature and its accompanying autonomic nerves. However, the more plausible explanation remains of direct anesthetic diffusion into the periorbital tissues.

Less remarkable but more common examples of unanticipated anesthesia include mandibular numbness after posterior superior alveolar and maxillary blocks and anesthesia of the auriculotemporal nerve by an inferior alveolar injection (other than the Gow-Gates mandibular block).

References

1. Seldin, H.M.: Survey of anesthetic fatalities in oral surgery and a review of the etiological factors in anesthetic deaths. J. Am. Dent. Soc. Anesth., *5*:5–12, 1958.
2. Seldin, H.M., and Recant, B.S.: Safety of anesthesia in the dental office. J. Oral Surg., *13*:199–208, 1955.
3. ASOS Committee on Anesthesia: ASOS anesthesia morbidity and mortality survey. J. Oral Surg., *32*:733–738, 1974.
4. Driscoll, E.J.: Anesthesia morbidity and mortality in oral surgery. *In* Proceedings of the Conference on Anesthesia for the Ambulatory Patient. Chicago, American Society of Oral Surgeons, 1966.
5. Persson, G.: General side-effects of local dental anaesthesia. Acta Odontol. Scand., *27*(suppl 53):1–141, 1969.
6. Berquist, H.C.: The danger of mepivacaine 3% toxicity in children. J. Calif. Dent. Assoc., *3*:13, 1975.
7. Albright, G.A.: Cardiac arrest following regional anesthesia with etidocaine or bupivacaine. Anesthesiology, *51*:285–287, 1979.
8. Harris, S.C.: Aspiration before injection of local anesthetics. J. Oral Surg., *15*:299–303, 1957.

9. Forrest, J.O.: Notes on aspiration before injection of local anæsthetics using dental cartridges. Br. Dent. J., *107*:259–262, 1959.

10. Frye, D.G.: Aspirator syringes—facts and figures. J. Am. Dent. Assoc., *66*:145–146, 1963.

11. Shiano, A.M., and Strambi, R.C.: Frequency of accidental intravascular injection of local anesthetics in dental practice. Oral Surg. Oral Med. Oral Pathol., *17*:178–184, 1964.

12. Cohen, M.B., Gravitz, L.A., and Knappe, T.A.: Twenty five versus twenty seven gauge needles. J. Am. Dent. Assoc., *78*:1312–1314, 1969.

13. Bos, A.L., Coppes, L., Determann, E.J., et al.: Aspiration control in the administration of local anesthesia in dentistry. Ned. Tijdschr. Tandheelkd. Suppl., *6*:24–38, 1971.

14. Bartlett, S.Z.: Clinical observations on the effect of injections of local anesthetics preceded by aspiration. Oral Surg. Oral Med. Oral Pathol., *33*:520–526, 1972.

15. Williams, M., and Simm, W.: Practical aspiration for local anesthesia. Dent. Update, *2*:23–27, 1975.

16. Gow-Gates, G.A.E., and Watson, J.E.: The Gow-Gates mandibular block: Further understanding. Anesth. Prog., *24*:183–189, 1977.

17. Robertson, W.D.: Clinical evaluation of mandibular conduction anesthesia. Gen. Dent., *27*:49–51, 1979.

18. Levy, T.P.: An assessment of the Gow-Gates mandibular block for third molar surgery. J. Am. Dent. Assoc., *103*:37–41, 1981.

19. Bishop, P.T.: Frequency of accidental intravascular injection of local anaesthetics in children. Br. Dent. J., *154*:76–77, 1983.

20. de Jong, R.H.: Toxic effects of local anesthetics. J.A.M.A., *239*:1166–1168, 1978.

21. Åkerman, B.: Effects of felypressin (Octopressin®) on the acute toxicity of local anaesthetics. Acta Pharmacol. Toxicol., *27*:318–330, 1969.

22. Aldrete, J.A., Narang, R., Sada, T., Liem, S.T., and Miller, G.P.: Reverse carotid blood flow—a possible explanation for some reactions to local anesthetics. J. Am. Dent. Assoc., *94*:1142–1145, 1977.

23. Downs, J.B., Reckstein, A.D., Klein, E.F., and Hawkins, I.F.: Hazards of radial artery catheterization. Anesthesiology, *38*:283–286, 1973.

24. Tomlin, P.J.: Death in outpatient dental practice. Anaesthesia, *29*:551–570, 1974.

25. Yagiela, J.A.: Intravascular lidocaine toxicity: Influence of epinephrine and route of administration. Anesth. Prog., *32*:57–61, 1985.

26. Milam, S.B., Giovannitti, J.A., and Bright, D.: Hypersensitivity to amide local anesthetics? Oral Surg. Oral Med. Oral Pathol., *56*:593–596, 1983.

27. Arora, S., and Aldrete, J.A.: Investigation of possible allergy to local anesthetic drugs. Anesth. Rev., *3*:13–17, 1976.

28. Coombs, R.R.A., and Gell, P.G.H.: Classification of allergic reactions responsible for clinical hypersensitivity and disease. *In* Gell, P.G.H., Coombs, R.R.A., and Lachmann, P.J. (eds.): Clinical Aspects of Immunology, 7th ed. Oxford, England, Blackwell Scientific Publications Ltd., 1975.

29. Goransson, K.: Hypersensitivity to prilocaine. Dermatologica, *152*:158–160, 1976.

30. Holti, G., and Hood, F.J.C.: An anaphylactoid reaction to lignocaine. Dent. Pract., *15*:294–296, 1965.

31. Stefanini, M., and Hoffman, M.N.: Studies on platelets: XXVIII. Acute thrombocytopenic purpura due to lidocaine (Xylocaine)-mediated antibodies. Report of a case. Am. J. Med. Sci., *275*:365–371, 1978.

32. Scott, D.S., and Hirschman, R.: Psychologic aspects of dental anxiety in adults. J. Am. Dent. Assoc., *10*:27–31, 1982.

33. Gatchel, R.J., Ingersoll, B.D., Bowman, L., Robertson, M.C., and Walker, C.: The prevalence of dental fear and avoidance: A recent survey study. J. Am. Dent. Assoc., *107*:609–610, 1983.

34. Kleinknecht, R.A., Klepac, R.K., and Alexander, L.D.: Origins and characteristics of fear of dentistry. J. Am. Dent. Assoc., *86*:842–848, 1973.

35. Edmondson, H.G., Gordon, P.H., Lloyd, J.M., and Whitehead, F.I.H.: Vasovagal episodes in the dental surgery. J. Dent., *6*:189–195, 1978.

36. Noble, R.J.: The patient with syncope. J.A.M.A., *237*:1372–1376, 1977.

37. Malamed, S.F.: Handbook of Medical Emergencies in the Dental Office, 3rd ed. St. Louis, C.V. Mosby Co., 1987.

38. Sisk, A.L., Hammer, W.B., Shelton, D.W., and Joy, E.D.: Complications following removal of impacted third molars. J. Oral Maxillofac. Surg., *44*:855–859, 1986.

39. Benoit, P.W., Yagiela, J.A., and Fort, N.F.: Pharmacologic correlation between local anesthetic-induced myotoxicity and disturbances of intracellular calcium distribution. Toxicol. Appl. Pharmacol., *52*:187–198, 1980.

40. Hinton, R.J., Dechow, P.C., and Carlson, D.S.: Recovery of jaw muscle function following injection of a myotoxic agent (lidocaine-epinephrine). Oral Surg. Oral Med. Oral Pathol., *59*:247–251, 1986.

41. Brooke, R.I.: Postinjection trismus due to formation of fibrous band. Oral Surg. Oral Med. Oral Pathol., *47*:424–426, 1979.

42. Stone, J., and Kaban, L.B.: Trismus after injection of local anesthetic. Oral Surg. Oral Med. Oral Pathol., *48*:29–32, 1979.

43. Popowich, L.D., and Brooke, R.I.: Postinjection infection—two unusual cases. *J.* Oral Surg., *37*:494–495, 1979.

44. Petersen, J.K., Luck, H., Kristensen, F., and Mikkelsen, L.: A comparison of four commonly used local analgesics. Int. J. Oral Surg., *6*:51–59, 1977.

45. Hartenian, R.M., and Stenger, I.O.: Postanesthetic palatal ulceration. Oral Surg. Oral Med. Oral Pathol., *42*:447–450, 1976.

46. Kronman, J.H., and Giunta, J.L.: Reflex vasoconstriction following dental injections. Oral Surg. Oral Med. Oral Pathol., *63*:542–544, 1987.

47. Rood, J.P.: Ocular complications of inferior dental nerve block. Br. Dent. J., *132*:23–24, 1972.

48. Fox, L.J., and Belfiglio, E.J.: Report of a broken needle. Gen. Dent., *34*:102–106, 1986.

49. Campbell, R.L., Mercuri, L.G., and Van Sickels, J.: Cervical sympathetic block following intraoral local anesthesia. Oral Surg. Oral Med. Oral Pathol., *47*:223–226, 1979.

50. Petrelli, E.A., and Steller, R.E.: Medial rectus muscle palsy after dental anesthesia. Am. J. Ophthalmol., *90*:422–424, 1980.

51. Kronman, J.T., and Kabani, S.: The neuronal basis for diplopia following local anesthetic injections. Oral Surg. Oral Med. Oral Pathol., *58*:533–534, 1984.

Chapter *14*

Electronic Dental Analgesia

Frederick C. Quarnstrom
Christine L. Quinn

P ain control has traditionally been a major concern of dentistry. By the early 20th century, the development of reliable local anesthesia stimulated the development of modern dental therapy as we know it today. However, even modern local anesthetics possess undesirable side effects, and their administration can be uncomfortable at times. Although the use of electricity for relief of pain has been attempted for centuries, recently electroanalgesia, a specific use of transcutaneous electrical nerve stimulation, has shown promise of reliable, nontraumatic pain control in carefully selected circumstances.

History of Electrical Analgesia

The earliest evidence of the therapeutic use of electricity comes from pharonic Egyptian temples, where drawings depict the use of the Nile River catfish (*Malapterurus electricus*) for medical purposes. In ancient Greece and Rome, the torpedo ray (*Torpedo marmorata*) was specifically used to treat the pain of gout by the direct application of a living ray to the painful extremity.[1,2] The development in the 17th century of electrostatic generators and Leyden jars, which could store electricity, provided a further stimulus for the medical use of electricity.[3] Unfortunately, much of the use of electrical energy for medical therapy was "electroquackery,"[4] with the principal beneficiary being the advocate-practitioner. In this regard, electrical "therapy" was claimed to cure or relieve paralysis, sciatica, headache, renal lithiasis, gout, pleurisy, seizures, and angina pectoris.[3,5-9] With the development of the storage battery, much smaller and more convenient devices became available, permitting the use of electrical current for relief of dental pain. In the mid-19th century, Francis described the use of electrical current for dental extraction.[1] Others recommended electrical therapy for the treatment of neuralgia, tic doloreux, toothache, and other jaw pain. Because of these poorly substantiated claims, as well as prejudice, a conference of the College of Dentists (London) was convened on October 12, 1858. As a result of that group's deliberations, four statements were adopted: (1) electricity is not an anesthetic agent, (2) electricity augments pain, (3) electricity sometimes modifies sensation, and (4) when favorable results are produced, they are due to diversion and not to insensibility. Subsequently, electrical therapy lost popularity and remained obscure until its recent revival with the use of transcutaneous electrical nerve stimulation.

TRANSCUTANEOUS ELECTRICAL NERVE STIMULATION

The reemergence of interest in electrical nerve stimulation roughly coincided with the publication by Melzack and Wall of the gate-control theory of pain in 1965 (Fig. 14–1).[10] This theory provided a possible theoretical basis for the clinical use of electrical nerve stimulation. Transcutaneous electrical nerve stimulation (TENS) specifically refers to the passage of a small electrical current across cutaneous tissues to effect nervous system responses.[11] The use of TENS principally evolved for the treatment of chronic pain. Prior to the routine use of electrical stimulation, partial cordotomy of the ascending spinothalamic tracts was performed in selected patients with intractable pain. The procedure was associated with significant morbidity and a high failure rate. With the publication of the gate-control theory, it was reasoned that direct stimulation of the dorsal column of the spinal cord could possibly inhibit pain signals from ascending to the thalamic and cortical centers. Initially, electrodes were surgically implanted over the dorsal column. In some patients this resulted in broken electrodes, wound irritation, and other complications. Also, it was not always possible to predict which patients would respond favorably. Thus, in an attempt to determine patient acceptance, skin electrodes were used as a preoperative trial. However, it was discovered that

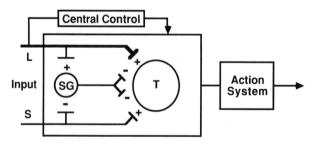

Figure 14–1. The gate-control theory of pain mechanisms as diagramed by Melzack and Wall.[10] S, small-diameter fibers; L, large-diameter fibers; SG, substantia gelatinosa; T, first central transmission cells.

this placement was equally effective and had the benefit of avoiding surgery. Hence, TENS was born.[11]

Because most dental treatment is of relatively short duration (1 hour or less) and most clinically reliable local anesthetics have residual effects beyond that time period, early workers hoped that the use of electrical current could provide a period of anesthesia or analgesia limited to the specific duration of the dental procedure. Also, the promise of pain control without the use of injections was considered a positive attribute from the patient's viewpoint. As a result, several early attempts were made to adapt dental handpieces with electrical current sources.[12–14] The specific techniques and the amount of voltage or current used differed, and these devices were often cumbersome and unreliable. However, when successful, patients liked the use of electrical pain control and tended to prefer it to local anesthesia. More recently, handpiece-delivered current has been replaced by various intraoral or extraoral electrodes, both of which are more reliable and less cumbersome to use.

Several mechanisms of action have been hypothesized for electrically induced pain control. The most prominent remains a form of gating action in which the electrical current selectively stimulates large sensory fibers (Aα, Aβ), "closing the gate" and preventing pain stimuli that travel via the small Aδ and C fibers from reaching the brain.[10] However, alternative explanations include electrical stimulation of endogenous opioid release (endorphins, enkephalins),[15] release of 5-hydroxytryptamine (serotonin),[15] and frequency-dependent conduction block.[16] In fact, a combination of some or all of these hypotheses may be necessary in selected circumstances to produce electrical analgesia.

Electronic Dental Analgesia

The basic machine used for dental pain control is a variant of the medical TENS unit. However, a variety of waveforms are currently in use, although little research data exists documenting particular advantages to any one format. Early handpiece-mounted units used direct current, but all modern TENS units use alternating current so that no net positive or negative charge will build up that could drive bacteria or toxic ions into the tissue. Contemporary devices deliver single impulses or pulse bursts (multiple impulses at lower amplitude).

WAVEFORMS

A balanced, symmetric, biphasic, and exponentially decaying waveform has been marketed as the H wave® (Fig. 14–2). Superficially, this waveform has some similarity to the H-reflex, a biphasic postsynaptic waveform reflex primarily found in infants. Although claims have been made that its analgesic effect is related to its similarity to the human H-reflex,

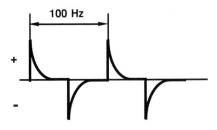

Figure 14–2.   H-wave®.

in fact this reflex has nothing to do with pain transmission, perception, or control, and the similarity of shape is unrelated to its effectiveness. Many devices, especially in the medical TENS market, utilize a balanced asymmetric square wave (Fig. 14–3). While useful for dental electronic analgesia (EA), patients perceive it as an intense, sharp vibration that is somewhat less comfortable than other waveforms. Other formats in use include a 16-kHz wave grouped into 16-Hz pulse trains and balanced by a 16-Hz square wave of opposite polarity (Fig. 14–4); balanced positive and negative pulses of a 3.2-kHz sine wave (Fig. 14–5); and, most recently, the use of two 16-kHz sine waves applied to the dorsum of each hand with a third electrode placed over the tooth to be treated. This latter device depends on an interference signal of 130 Hz generated between the two 16-kHz waves to produce the analgesic current (Fig. 14–6).

Although insufficient information is available to select a specific waveform as preferable or more reliable than others, some data exists on patient comfort. In most instances, patients will not notice differences or express a preference unless direct comparisons are made during the same treatment. In trials where patients switched back and forth among three different types of waveforms, patients did occasionally express preference for the H-wave® in terms of initial comfort but otherwise had difficulty perceiving any preference in terms of analgesic success (Quarnstrom, F. Unpublished data.)

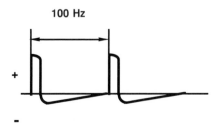

Figure 14–3.   Square wave.

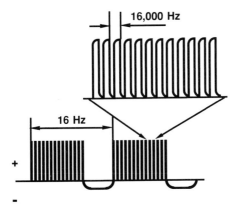

Figure 14–4. Composite wave.

FREQUENCY

Some EA devices are designed to change the frequency of the electrical signal produced. Clinical experience has allocated the use of higher frequencies (e.g., 55 Hz or greater) for control of acute procedural pain, while lower frequencies (e.g., 2 Hz) are usually used for deep muscle soreness. A 2-Hz frequency produces a noticeable pulsing sensation to the patient, with muscle contraction thought to be beneficial to circulation and removal of metabolic by-products.

POLARITY

Most EA devices permit reversal of signal polarity. Patients occasionally report the sensation of electrical stimulation only at one electrode. Al-

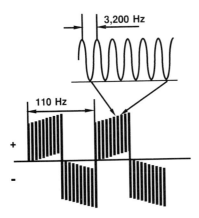

Figure 14–5. Composite square wave.

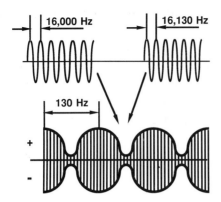

Figure 14–6.   Composite sine wave with 130-Hz interference signal.

though this may be caused by variations in tissue conductance or electrode contact, polarity reversal can sometimes correct this effect, especially in devices that have asymmetric signals in which the positive waveform is configured differently from the negative form.

POWER SOURCE

All contemporary devices use either nickel-cadmium (Ni-Cad) or lead acid batteries as a power source. This permits greater portability and enhances electrical safety. Ni-Cad batteries maintain a constant voltage until they are nearly discharged, and if recharged before complete discharge they tend to develop a charge-limiting "memory." Lead acid batteries, on the other hand, do not develop a memory, hold more charge, and are less expensive than Ni-Cads, but they are much more bulky and thus may limit the degree of unit miniaturization possible. The voltage output of the lead acid battery decreases proportionately to its degree of discharge and thus provides the clinician with several hours' warning before a recharge is necessary.[17–19] Several devices use disposable 9-V or 1.5-V D cells. The advantage to this is lowered cost and the convenience of quick replacement without a lengthy recharge.

CONTROLS

Most contemporary EA devices come with two complete circuits (channels), each with amplitude and frequency controls. The small medical TENS devices usually have just one frequency control that is designed to adjust both channels. These devices also have a wave-width control and a mode control. The wave-width control is set for the widest signal (maximum), as this is the most comfortable setting for the patient. The mode control is generally used by physical therapists; for dental analgesia purposes, it should simply be set on N (normal). Most units have a battery condition indicator, and those with internal batteries have a charging circuit.

The intensity of the signal is altered by the amplitude control. These units generate an "adequate stimulus," meaning that they can create stimuli that will equal or exceed the threshold for a nerve action potential. The amplitude (voltage) is proportional to the intensity of the sensation felt by the patient. The amplitude control is turned up until the patient starts to feel a sensation, referred to as the "threshold." The patient then is given the "patient control" or, in the case of miniature units, the complete device. Patients should be encouraged to increase the signal strength to the maximum tolerable point. After approximately 1 minute of stimulation, it is usually possible for the patient to further increase the signal strength. It is at this level that patients will have maximum analgesia. Also, patients in whom EA is most successful tend to adjust the intensity signal in relation to the perceived pain.

ELECTRODES

Electrodes, which are critical to both patient comfort and ease of use, have been the greatest problem in the delivery of electronic dental analgesia. The ease of placement of electrodes and particularly the ease of working around them are important factors in determining whether the clinician will continue to use this technique long enough to develop the necessary skills for success. Although most systems use some form of intraoral electrode, recent studies increasingly include extraoral electrode placement. Intraoral electrodes come in three types: sponges, a conductive fabric, and adhesive materials.

Initially, all electrodes were attached to 8 × 120 mm cotton rolls that enclose a plastic rod for increased stiffness. Sponge electrodes are attached to one end of the cotton roll by elastic bands. A third band is used to keep the wire in place along the cotton roll. This band is positioned about 2 cm from the end of the roll opposite from the electrode. (With children, it is often necessary to reduce the length of the cotton roll.) The cotton roll is bent into a U shape and saturated with water before insertion into the mouth. They are quick and easy to place, can be removed and reversed to use in the opposite arch, but are rather bulky and often a nuisance to work around (Fig. 14–7). Several attempts have been made to use clamps to grasp teeth and hold sponges in contact with the tissue. One design was shaped much like a rubber dam clamp. Unfortunately, the plastic material did not have sufficient strength to hold the clamp in place. Other electrode types utilized wire clasps much like orthodontic retainers. This is more successful but requires adjusting for each tooth placement. It is, however, particularly useful in patients with exaggerated gag reflexes who have difficulty tolerating cotton rolls (Fig. 14–8).

Adhesive electrodes are a more recent development and have the advantage of directly adhering to the mucosa. They are quite thin (6 mm ×

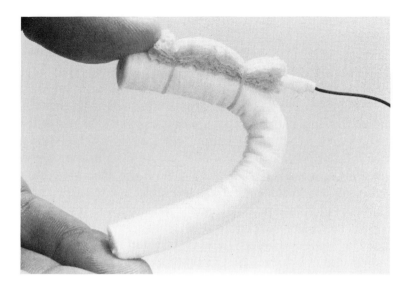

Figure 14–7. Cotton roll with attached sponge electrode bent into a U-shape configuration for placement into the patient's buccal vestibule.

25 mm). Use of these electrodes requires that the mucosa be dry and free of the mucopolysaccharide coat usually found in the mouth. Unfortunately, this coating reforms very rapidly, making it necessary to place the electrodes within a few seconds of drying the mucosa. This task is complicated by the electrodes' tendency to stick to everything they touch, including latex gloves. A gauze square can be placed over the electrode

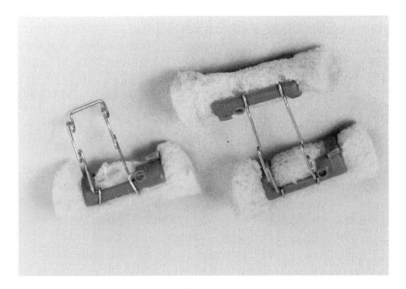

Figure 14–8. Wire-clasp electrode holders. This style requires individual adjustment to fit different arch sizes.

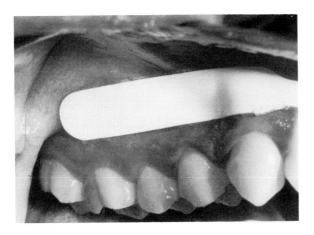

Figure 14-9. Adhesive electrode placed over the maxillary vestibular mucosa.

once it is in place to help keep it dry. Also, it is important to clip the leads onto the patient's bib to minimize any tension that might be placed on these devices (Fig. 14-9). In an attempt to alleviate the problems of intraoral electrodes, extraoral electrodes are also being used (Fig. 14-10). There have been no controlled studies reporting which technique is superior, but clinical experience suggests that they are equally reliable. Before the skin electrodes are placed, the site should be cleaned with alcohol to remove skin oils and makeup. To place skin electrodes, the patient's mouth should be opened widely. When treating mandibular teeth, electrodes are best placed over the roots of the first premolar to the

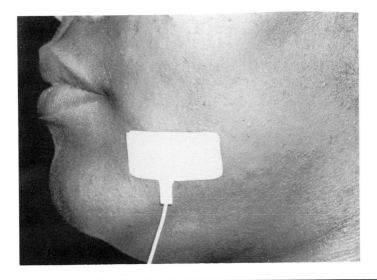

Figure 14-10. Extraoral electrode placement for treatment in the left mandibular region.

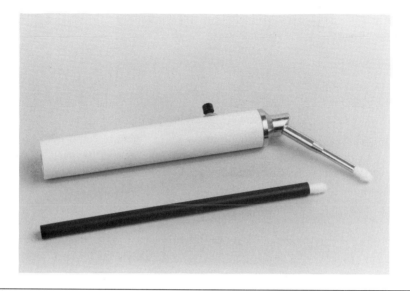

Figure 14–11.   Two types of hand-held wand electrodes for use prior to local anesthetic injections.

first molar. For maxillary teeth, the upper edge of the electrode should be at the base of the zygoma from the cuspid area extending distally to the first molar. Finally, hand-held probes can be used in place of topical anesthesia prior to local anesthetic injections (Fig. 14–11). With this device, all types of injections can be done virtually pain-free if a careful, slow injection technique is used. Two wands are held like chopsticks with the tips about 1.5 cm apart over the area where the needle will be inserted.

Patient Selection

There are few reports of adverse effects with TENS.[20] The only complication personally seen (in over 4,000 uses over a period of 5 years) has been a traumatic ulcer from dry cotton roll electrodes sticking to the mucosa. There are, however, some relative contraindications that should be considered before using EA devices.

CARDIAC PACEMAKERS

It is possible that the EA current could interfere with demand pacemakers (patients may not know which type of pacemaker they have). Depending on the type of demand pacemaker, TENS devices could stimulate either a very fast or very slow cardiac rate. However, theoretically this should occur only if the electrodes are placed on the thorax. Asynchronous pacemakers provide a signal that results in heart depolarization at a fixed rate. Unlike demand pacemakers, these pacemakers are not affected by TENS signals.[21]

CARDIAC PLEXUS AND CAROTID BODY

It is currently thought that electrical stimulation of the cardiac plexus or the carotid body could provoke severe hypotension. It is also possible to stimulate the recurrent laryngeal nerve, resulting in upper airway obstruction from laryngospasm. For this reason, EA electrodes should not normally be placed on the neck.

PREGNANCY

While TENS has been used in labor and delivery, its effects in pregnancy are unknown. The release of endogenous opioids (a possible mechanism of EA) is a natural process. Electrical current, if it accidentally came in contact with the gravid uterus, would be conducted harmlessly through the surface amniotic fluid and probably would never affect the fetus. Nevertheless, until EA in pregnant women is fully approved, caution must be exercised in its use with this group of patients.

CEREBROVASCULAR PROBLEMS

TENS devices have been shown to increase blood flow in the extremities and theoretically could do so elsewhere in the body. Thus, their use should be avoided in patients with known aneurysms and those with a history of cerebrovascular accident. Some manufacturers also warn against their use in patients who suffer from transient ischemic attacks.

EPILEPSY

Seizure disorders are known to be triggered by pulsing lights, sounds, or electrical current. Thus, EA devices should not be used in patients with a history of a seizure disorder.

Indications for Use

EA is best suited for procedures in which there is a high probability of success. Both clinical experience and controlled clinical research have suggested that simple restorative procedures, particularly on anterior teeth, and nonsurgical periodontal procedures, such as root planing, scaling, and comprehensive probing in sensitive patients are very comfortably performed with EA. Also of value is the use of EA for seating crowns or bridges, and, when local anesthesia is required, preinjection usage, especially in the palate, to significantly reduce the pain of injec-

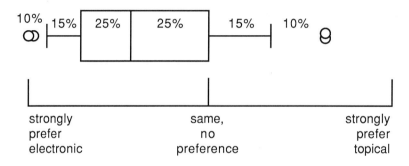

Figure 14–12. Visual analog scale of patient preference for electroanalgesia versus topical anesthesia in relieving pain of local anesthetic injection. Numbers represent percentage of patients with preference.

tion. In a recent study comparing the use of topical anesthesia versus EA prior to injection of a local anesthetic, (Quarnstom, F., and Libed, E. Unpublished data), 75% patients preferred EA (Fig. 14–12). Finally, symptomatic control in patients with myofascial pain is possible with EA. However, cure of intraarticular pathology causing clicks, pops, or crepitus is unlikely.

Recent evidence suggests that the more complicated and extensive a restorative procedure becomes, the higher will be the failure rate of EA.[22] Figures 14–13 through 14–15 illustrate data obtained from patients subjected to one- through five-surface alloy or composite restorations, crown and bridge preparations, and seating of crowns and bridges. Although EA was successful in more than 90% of single-surface procedures, its use in multisurface preparations (three or more surfaces) was much less reliable. Similarly, EA was successful in only 60% of crown preparations but highly effective and convenient for seating and cementing crowns and bridges.

TENS can be combined with other analgesic modalities, such as nitrous oxide, to enhance its usefulness. A large-scale clinical study of

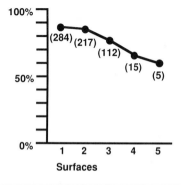

Figure 14–13. Success rates for electronic analgesia during preparation and placement of alloy restorations. Bracketed numbers indicate teeth treated.

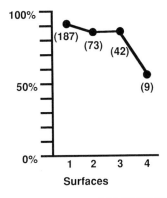

Figure 14–14. Success rates for electronic analgesia during preparation and placement of composite restorations. Bracketed numbers indicate teeth treated.

patients who underwent various restorative or periodontal procedures compared EA alone, nitrous oxide sedation/analgesia alone, and a combination of the two techniques.[22–24] The dental procedures evaluated were not specifically selected for increased success with either analgesic method and included both complex and simple procedures in all groups. The combination of nitrous oxide with EA resulted in a very satisfactory success ranking that neither EA nor nitrous oxide alone was able to match. Other authors have reported high patient acceptance percentages without the use of coagents such as nitrous oxide.[24–28] However, EA is much more likely to be unsatisfactory in patients with high indices of apprehension or skepticism or very low pain tolerance.[24] Thus, patients' expectations appear to be very important in determining the applicability of this technique.

Children aged 5 through 12 years are much more successfully treated with EA than adults. The practitioner must adjust the amplitude control (in young children) until the orbicularis oris muscle begins to contract, then back the stimulus off just enough to relax this muscle. At this inten-

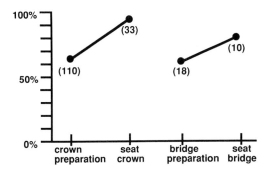

Figure 14–15. Comparative success of electronic analgesia in tooth preparations versus prosthesis placements. Bracketed numbers represent teeth treated.

sity, analgesic failures are rare, even for the placement of stainless steel crowns and pulpotomies. Additionally, when two "injection probes" are used, one on the buccal and the other on the lingual, primary teeth with 50% or greater root resorption can be extracted without pain.

Conclusions

In time, the clinician can develop sufficient experience with the use of EA to predict fairly accurately in which patients this modality can be used successfully. EA is almost always successful in patients who dislike the effects of local anesthesia but are otherwise cooperative, and it is often successful in patients with a needle phobia. Simpler and less invasive procedures are far more successfully performed with EA than are complex procedures or highly invasive ones such as endodontic or surgical therapy. In general, the patient's attitude toward dentistry is an important determinant. In this regard, dental phobics are the least predictable group of patients because their overwhelming fear results in little trust in any dental procedure.

It is doubtful that EA will replace local anesthesia as a mainstay of pain control for dental procedures. It will, however, reduce the need for local anesthesia, especially in patients who have less complex treatment needs or who prefer not to receive local anesthesia. Even if EA as the sole analgesic technique fails, its use will enhance the pain-free administration of an injected local anesthetic.

References

1. Kane, K., and Taub, A.: A history of local electrical analgesia. Pain, *1*:125–138, 1975.
2. Stillings, D.: The piscean origin of medical electricity. Med. Instrum., *7*:163–164, 1973.
3. Rowbottom, M., and Suskind, C.: Electricity and Medicine: History of Their Interaction. San Francisco, San Francisco Press, Inc., 1984.
4. Malamed, S., and Joseph, C.: Electricity in dentistry. J. Can. Dent. Assoc., *15*:12–14, 1987.
5. Taylor, E.: The electrified hand: Psychotherapeutic implications. Med. Instrum., *17*:281–282, 1983.
6. Ersek, R.A.: Pain Control with Transcutaneous Electrical Neuro Stimulation (T.E.N.S.). St. Louis, Warren H. Green, Inc., 1981.
7. Stillings, D.: John Wesley: Philosopher of electricity. Med. Instrum., *7*:307, 1973.
8. Stillings, D.: John Wesley: Electrotherapist. Med. Instrum., *8*:66, 1974.
9. Stillings, D.: A medical cure by Benjamin Franklin. Med. Instrum., *10*:27, 1976.
10. Melzack, R., and Wall, P.D.: Pain mechanisms: A new theory. Science, *150*:971–979, 1965.
11. Cady, R., and Shealy, C.N.: Electrotherapy in medicine. J. Calif. Dent. Assoc., *15*:22–26, 1987.

12. Suzuki, K.: New dentin-desensitizing technic by means of electro anesthesia. J. Jpn. Stomatol. Soc., *19*:56–69, 1952.
13. Brooks, B., Reiss, R., and Umans, R.: Local electroanesthesia in dentistry. J. Dent. Res., *49*:298–300, 1970.
14. Ehrlich, R.D.: Electricity in local anaesthesia: Test of "sin dolar." S.A.A.D. Dig., *2*:50–51, 1973.
15. Mayer, D.J., and Price, D.D.: Central nervous system mechanisms of analgesia. Pain, *2*:379–404, 1976.
16. Phero, J.C., Raj, P.P., and MacDonald, J.S.: Transcutaneous electrical nerve stimulation and myoneural injection for management of chronic myofascial pain. Dent. Clin. North Am., *31*:703–723, 1987.
17. Utz, P.: The black art of batteries: Part 1. Gel cells and Ni-Cads. AV Video, *9*:51–53, 1987.
18. Utz, P.: The black art of batteries: Part 2. Gel cells and Ni-Cads. AV Video, *9*:67–70, 1987.
19. Utz, P.: Ni-Cad batteries in depth: Part 1. AV Video, *10*:30–36, 1988.
20. Katch, E.M.: Applications of trancutaneous electrical nerve stimulation in dentistry. Anesth. Prog., *33*:156–160, 1986.
21. Eriksson, M.S., Schuller, H., and Sjolund, B.: Hazard from transcutaneous nerve stimulation in patients with pacemakers. Lancet, *1*:1319, 1978.
22. Quarnstrom, F.: Electrical anesthesia. J. Calif. Dent. Assoc., *12*:35–40, 1988.
23. Donaldson, D., Quarnstrom, F., and Jastak, T.: The combined effect of nitrous oxide and oxygen and electrical stimulation during restorative dental treatment. J. Am. Dent. Assoc., *118*:733–736, 1989.
24. Quarnstrom, F., and Milgrom, P.: Clinical experience with TENS and TENS combined with nitrous oxide-oxygen. Anesth. Prog., *36*:66–69, 1989.
25. Clark, M.S., Silverstone, L.M., Lindemuth, J., et al.: An evaluation of the clinical analgesia/anesthesia efficacy on acute pain using the high frequency neural modulator in various dental settings. Oral Surg. Oral Med. Oral Pathol., *63*:501–505, 1987.
26. Hochman, R.: Neurotransmitter modulator (TENS) for control of dental operative pain. J. Am. Dent. Assoc., *116*:208–212, 1988.
27. Jensen, M.: A clinical evaluation of electro-dental anesthesia: Patient selection, wave form, and frequency. Presented at the First Annual Symposium on Electrical Anesthesia, University of Southern California, February 26, 1988.
28. Malamed, S., Quinn, C., Torgersen, R., and Thompson, W.: Electronic dental anesthesia for restorative dentistry. Anesth. Prog., *36*:195–198, 1989.

Index

Note: Page numbers in *italics* refer to figures; entries followed by a 't' refer to tables.

Diacylglycerol, 67
Diazepam, 188
Digitalis glycosides, 78
Disinfectants, cartridge contamination by, 162
Disinfection, of equipment, 162–163
    vs. sterilization, 154
Disposable needle collector, *167*
Dissociation constant, 27–28
Distribution, of anesthetics. See also under specific
        drugs.
    during nerve block, *28*
    neurophysiology of, 8–11, *10*
    pH strategies for, 116
Distilled water, pyrogen-free, 87
Diuretics, 78
Dosage, calculation of, 290t
Drug addiction/abuse, 140, 284
Drug allergy, 133–135
Drug identification label, for anesthetic cartridges, 155,
        156
Drug interactions, 129–133, 131t, 132t
Duranest. See *Etidocaine.*
Dyclonine, 27, 115
Dysrhythmias, diuretics and, 78
    use-dependent blocks and, 37
    vasoconstrictor-induced, 75, 137
        periodontal ligament injection and, 265, *266*

ECG (electrocardiography), vasoconstrictor-induced
        changes in, 74
Electrical analgesia, 326
    controls for, 318–319
    during pregnancy, 323
    electrodes for, 319–322, *320–322*
    for children, 325–326
    frequency for, 317
    history of, 313–314
    indications for, 323–326, *324*
    machine for, 315
    patient selection for, 322–323
    polarity for, 317–318
    power source for, 318
    success rates for, *324,* 324–326, *325*
    transcutaneous electrical nerve stimulation and, *314,*
        314–315
    waveforms for, 315–316, *316–318*
Electrocardiography (ECG), vasoconstrictor-induced
        changes in, 74
Electrochemical gradients, across neuronal membrane,
        9–10, *10*
Electrotonic currents, 12–14
EMLA (eutectic mixture of local anesthetics), 118
Endocarditis, 136
Endocrine disorders, 137–138
Endoneurium, 7, *8*
Epilepsy. See *Seizures.*
Epinephrine, absorption of, 79
    adrenergic receptor activation and, 65
    as chemical tourniquet for cocaine, 24
    bronchial smooth muscle relaxation and, 76
    cardiovascular disorders and, 136–137
    cardiovascular effects of, 71, *72–75,* 74–76
    differential binding of, 68–69, 68t
    distribution of, *79,* 79–81
    dosages of, for inhalational general anesthesia, 130–
        131, 131t

Epinephrine (*continued*)
    gluconeogenesis and, 77
    glycogenolysis and, 77
    lidocaine peak blood concentrations and, 62–63,
        63
    metabolism of, *79, 80,* 79–81
    monoamine oxidase inhibitors and, 133
    neuromuscular transmission and, 77
    pulpal blood flow and, 264, 264t
    rationale for, 61
    side effects of, 297
    skeletal muscle and, 77
    systemic metabolic effects of, 77–78
    tricyclic antidepressants and, 132–133
    uterine contraction and, 77
    with articaine, 106
    with prilocaine, 98–99
Epineurium, 7, *8*
Equipment, disinfection of, 162–163
    jet injector, 150–152, *150–152*
    needles. See *Needle(s).*
    periodontal ligament syringe, 152–153, *153*
    sterilization of. See *Sterilization.*
    syringes. See *Syringes.*
Erythroxylon coca, 23
Ester anesthetics. See also specific ester anesthetics.
    metabolism of, 52–53, *53*
    structure-activity relationships of, 26t, 27
Ethyl aminobenzoate. See *Benzocaine.*
Ethylene oxide, 154
Etidocaine, advantages of, 103
    chemical name for, 103
    disadvantages of, 103
    distribution of, 104
    dosages of, 90t, 104, 289t
    duration of action of, 89t, 103
    excretion of, 104, *105*
    formulations of, 103
    injection volumes for, 91t
    median lethal dosage of, 89t
    metabolism of, 54, 104, *105*
    peak blood concentrations for, 104
    pharmacokinetic parameters of, 54t
    physicochemical/clinical properties of, 27
    potency of, 104
    pregnancy and, 104
    pregnancy risk category for, 92t
    structure of, 26, 103
    toxicity of, 44t, 104
    trade name for, 103
Eutectic mixture of local anesthetics (EMLA), 118
Excretion, of anesthetics, 53–54, 54t. See also under
        specific anesthetic.
Experimental drugs. See *New/experimental drugs.*

Factor VIII, 139
Fainting, 298–300, 300t
Famotidine, 130
Fat metabolism, 77
Felypressin, 81–82, *82*
Field block anesthesia, 185–186
Fifth cranial nerve. See *Trigeminal nerve.*
Foramen rotundum, 173
Free nerve endings, *2*
Frequency-dependent block (phasic block; use-depen-
        dent block), 31, 35, *36,* 36–37, *37*

AMSA ~ between premolars. Applied w/ cotton swab pressure.

ASA ~ above infraorbital nerve below eye. Pressure with free fingers = apply pressure for 1 min. after injection

PSA ~ inwards, backwards, upwards. @ 2nd molars.

infiltrate ~ at apical of target tooth.